Scholarship in the Discipline of Nursing

HMWAA (Gra)

Scholarship in the Discipline of Nursing

Edited by

Genevieve Gray

RN CM MSc(Nsg)(Manch) DipNEd(NSWCN) DipAdvNsgSt(Manch) FCN(UNSW) FRCNA
Professor of Nursing and Dean, Faculty of Nursing and Health Studies, University of Western Sydney, Nepean

Rosalie Pratt

RN CM DNE(Cumb) BA(Macq) MHPEd(NSW) FCN(NSW) FRCNA
Associate Professor, Faculty of Nursing, University of Sydney

Foreword by

Jocalyn Lawler RN BSocSc MEd PhD FCN(NSW) FRCNA
Professor of Nursing, Faculty of Nursing, University of Sydney

CHURCHILL LIVINGSTONE

MELBOURNE EDINBURGH LONDON MADRID NEW YORK TOKYO 1995

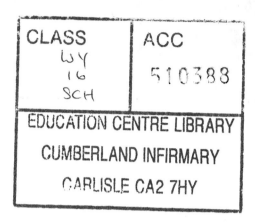
CHURCHILL LIVINGSTONE
An imprint of Pearson Professional

Pearson Professional (Australia) Pty Ltd
Kings Gardens, 95 Coventry Street, South Melbourne 3205 Australia

National Library of Australia Cataloguing-in-Publication Data

Scholarship in the discipline of nursing

    Bibliography.
    Includes index.
    ISBN 0 443 05109 7.

    1. Nursing - Practice - Australia. 2. Nursing - Study and
    teaching - Australia. 3. Nursing - Australia.
    4. Learning and scholarship. I. Gray, Genevieve, 1943-. II. Pratt, Rosalie.

610.730690994

For Churchill Livingstone in Melbourne
Publisher: Judy Waters
Editorial: Pam Jonas
Copy Editing: Mignon Turpin
Desktop Preparation: Sandra Tolra
Typesetting: Sandra Tolra
Production Control: Anke Liebnitz
Design: Churchill Livingstone
Indexing: Max McMaster
Produced by Churchill Livingstone in Melbourne
Printed in Australia

The
publisher's
policy is to use
**paper manufactured
from sustainable forests**

Foreword

It is a pleasure and an honour to write a foreword to a collection of works edited by Rosalie Pratt and Genevieve Gray. Not only are they our country's pre-eminent editors of collected nursing works, they are also our most prolific. Again, they have gathered together a collection of works and authors to further commit nursing to the written record.

This particular collection is a celebration of our willingness to rise above those things that will hold us to the past; it is a collection which, by daring to put the words 'scholarship' and 'nursing' together, lays claim to a place for good thinking in and about nursing and amongst nurses. It is a collection which brings together some of our best scholars and their thoughts about nursing. It is a bold and creative collection of works from some of our most courageous and insightful writers.

Scholarship in the Discipline of Nursing takes a different direction from previous edited volumes by Gray and Pratt and it comes at a very good time for nursing; it is a decade after the decision to transfer nursing education out of the hospitals and into mainstream academe. The 1980s were heady years for nursing in Australia and we were aware that the international nursing community was watching, and waiting, to see what would happen. Not only were we thrust—without much warning when the decision finally came—to move education into the higher education system, we were also thrust into an environment in which we felt a need to articulate what it was about nursing that gave it a (legitimate) place in these important institutions. Matters of a 'higher' scholarly nature were not things that nurses individually or collectively had enjoyed; nor were they universally accepted as the rightful business of nurses.

With the benefit of hindsight, it is not surprising that during the 1980s nurses in Australia, like nurses elsewhere, were engaged in what sometimes felt like (and which I later came to see as) a futile, meaningless, and laborious project to define what nursing was. We laboured under the belief that if we did not know what nursing was, we could not possibly research it, articulate it or teach it in an informed and scholarly way. Our collective and universal history, as nurses, has been characterised by a struggle to be recognised as good thinkers and scholars. Indeed we are still distracted, from time to time, by the remnants of anti-intellectualism and suspicion about those of us who seem too bright (to be nurses) or who enjoy the intellectual challenges of nursing.

I wonder now if we were more concerned about these things than were the generalised 'other' whom we have felt a need to convince. That is not to say, however, that our place in the scholarly havens of the country was not challenged, questioned, debated, undermined and contested. Nor is to say that our ability to be scholarly as nurses, and about nursing, was not also regarded with some degree of scepticism. This collection of works puts that scepticism to one side.

If the 1980s represented the period when we contemplated the meanings and definitions of nursing, the 1990s are possibly going to be remembered as the decade when we contemplated our philosophical points of anchorage and their relationships to ways of researching nursing—it has been our philosophical period. In the heat and pressure to find a space/place in which to research nursing we have, at times, paid less attention to good scholarship in and of itself. We have not had a lot of time, in Australia at least, to simply think about nursing; rather, we have been preoccupied, necessarily, with consolidating our place in the academy and establishing our research program. Scholarship, which I think is akin to good thinking, is inherent in and fundamental to teaching and research but it can be overlooked and taken for granted.

Now it is time to reflect on and think about nursing, and allow ourselves to let go of old ideas and practices. It is the time to consider how we might anchor nursing in relation to our historical and epistemological roots and to find new ways to make nursing knowledge transparent and transferable to others. The writers whose scholarly works appear here are making major contributions to these ways forward.

There are several distinguishable trends emerging in the scholarly works of Australian nursing. The first and most obvious trend is an exploration of postmodernism and how it offers us a way to address the dynamic of our invisibility. This is most clearly evident in the works of Judy Lumby, Judy Parker and Colin Holmes, but it is also apparent throughout the collection.

The second trend is the willingness to challenge taken-for-granted or received wisdom about how we 'should' (and I use the term advisedly) articulate nursing—in this, Margaret Dunlop's work is prominent and, often, profound. In *Scholarship in the Discipline of Nursing*, we see a body of work that takes us beyond the more accepted and safer patterns of knowing and thinking; we are invited, by this book, into critical and political debates which traditionally have not been mainstream concerns of nursing. We are invited to challenge, explore and be discerning about what is offered to us as knowledge and wisdom in nursing.

The third trend that runs through this collection—a trend that reflects nursing scholarship in Australia more widely—is a willingness to explore troubling and troublesome questions about our philosophical roots, ways of experiencing the world, and the places from which we derive meaning(s) as nurses. We have been engaged in a systematic and ordered process of coming to a sense of who we are and how we (can) identify ourselves as nurses and how we can better understand the knowledges that inform nursing practice.

This book, *Scholarship in the Discipline of Nursing*, adds substantially to our capacity to have mature debates and to enjoy the intellectual life of nursing.

Jocalyn Lawler

Preface

Continuing the journey

In the Epilogue to *Towards a Discipline of Nursing*, which we described as a 'journey-within-a-journey', we left readers on a rise in the Australian nursing landscape, contemplating a 360 degree 'view-in-the-round'. This enabled a wide variety of perspectives which included the foreground, middle distance and far horizons in whichever direction one faced. Moreover, there was a tantalising sense of possible nursing worlds opening up as the journey continued.

This promise has been realised in *Scholarship*. In exploring the notion of scholarship in nursing (quintessentially a **practice** discipline) the authors have adopted a richness of perspectives which encompass not only many points on the circle from 0 to 360 degrees, but also many focal lengths stretching towards infinity. Excitingly, in so doing they have journeyed 'beyond' in a number of senses. For some the perspective has become much more 'close-up'—the view intensely personal and infinitely detailed. For others the perspective has incorporated a new dimension: plumbing the **depths** of the discipline's resources. Still others have urged readers to contemplate the foreground of our landscape through the lens of the **background**, i.e. nursing's past. From all of these many perspectives, it becomes clear that the essence of scholarship itself as a concept is being explored, opened up and potentially re-defined.

Similarly, a re-conceptualisation and re-construction of nursing is invited. Readers themselves will come to this volume with a variety of personal and professional perspectives. These will be variously challenged, confirmed, modified or even radically changed as they journey through the chapters. Whichever, the conjunction of the ideas and the thinking of both writers and readers can scarcely fail to ensure that perspectives on nursing itself are transformed. Certainly, readers will find within the pages of this book the depiction of the milieu which we foreshadowed in *Discipline's* Epilogue as being crucial to transformation, i.e. one characterized by a 'connected' profession where uncertainty, tentative thought and conflict will be expected, ambiguity tolerated and a diversity of viewpoints accepted as a part of the pattern of progress and a basis for growth.

The development of the discipline through scholarship is critical not only to the profession itself but to the achievement of improved health outcomes for our consumers. As has been suggested previously, we need to be able to demonstrate the difference that nursing care makes to health outcomes for our patients and the contribution that nurses make to the health care agenda. The development of our knowledge base through scholarship, and the consequent empowering of our practitioners and consumers through access to this knowledge, is crucial to achieving health gain.

But how will we view scholarship? The authors in this book provide a diverse range of views and approaches to scholarship. The traditional view of scholarship in universities has been the construction or invention of new knowledge through basic research. This view has been challenged by nurse academics who consider that this conception of scholarship, which is equated with the conduct of research on the cutting edge of a discipline and its publication in a refereed journal, often fails to take account of an essential element, that of its relevance to society. Authors in this volume explore, and set into context, a new conception of scholarship which gives it a broader meaning and encompasses the four complementary elements of scholarship of discovery, integration, application and teaching. If the nursing profession, both within Australia and at the global level, were to endorse this view of scholarship and see it to be relevant for all nurses whatever their role and practice situation, there would be an emergence of a whole new range of scholarly activities.

So we invite you, whether practitioner, teacher, manager or researcher, to critically examine the ideas presented by the authors in this book. Consider both the rigour of the authors' ideas and their application to practice because, however exciting the ideas are, they have to be applied to practice. Expect to be challenged by these multiple perspectives, to be charmed by some, and to feel uneasy about others, but do not expect to find certain answers. Our main hope is that you will be stimulated to examine the perspectives and issues raised on nursing scholarship. Our wish is to develop scholars who will influence the global world of the future, creating a better tomorrow for its inhabitants. The essence of scholarship is, we believe, in the development and exercising of intellectual powers in a way which will produce independent thought while enabling others to travel with you and learn from the experience; in fostering effective modes of inquiry which promote critical thought and analysis; in the creation of a healthy respect for differing views and theoretical positions; and in the exercising of scholarly humility and intellectual honesty. Our hope is that nurse scholars, in exercising scholarship, will push out the boundaries and open up new worlds for the discipline of nursing.

Genevieve Gray and Rosalie Pratt

Contributors

Elizabeth Cameron-Traub RN BA(Hons) PhD(Flinders) GradDipNursSt(Ed)(Armidale) FRCNA FCN(NSW) MAPsS
Professor and Dean, Faculty of Nursing, University of Technology, Sydney

Julianne Cheek PhD
Senior Lecturer/Research Fellow, Faculty of Nursing, University of South Australia

Lyn Coulon MHPEd(UNSW) BA(NSWIT) DipNursEd(CCHS) RN FCN(NSW) FRCNA
Head, Department of Professional Nursing Development, Australian Catholic University, New South Wales

Graeme Curry BA(Hons)(Syd) BD(Qld) RPN DipEd(SCAE) MA(Syd) MCN(NSW) FRCNA FANZCMHN
Senior Lecturer, School of Nursing Health Studies, Faculty of Nursing, University of Technology, Sydney

Elizabeth Davies RN BSc(Griffith) DipAppScNsgEd(QIT) MEd(UQ)
Head, School of Nursing, Australian Catholic University, McAuley Campus

Margaret Dunlop BA MEd(Hons) DrNurSci RN CM
Professor, Faculty of Nursing, Griffith University, Queensland

Carolyn Emden RN BEd GradDipEdCounselling MEd FRCNA
Senior Lecturer, University of South Australia

Judith Godden BA(Hons) PhD DipEd
Senior Lecturer, Department of Behavioural and Social Sciences in Nursing, University of Sydney

Jennifer Greenwood RN RM DipN RNT DipEd MEd PhD FRCNA
Professor of Nursing and Head, Division of Nursing, Faculty of Health, University of Western Sydney, Macarthur

Barbara A. Hayes DipNEd BA(Hons) MSc DNSc RN RMN RPN FRCNA FANZCMHN FACTM
Professor of Nursing and Head, Department of Nursing Sciences, James Cook University, Queensland

Liza Heslop RN DipNsg(Coll.Nur.Aust) BAppSc(AdvNsg)(Lincoln) BA(Gipps) IAE
Lecturer, Caroline Chisholm School of Nursing, Monash University,
Peninsula Campus

Colin Adrian Holmes RPN BA(Hons) TCert(Manc) RNT MPhil PhD
Senior Lecturer, School of Nursing, Deakin University, Geelong

Jane Jacobs RN CM DipAppSciNurEd(QIT) BAppSciNur(QUT) MEnvCH(Griffith)
Lecturer, Faculty of Nursing, Griffith University, Queensland

Kaye Lont BA(Ed) RN MNurS
Lecturer, School of Nursing, Deakin University, Geelong

Judy Lumby RN ADNE(Armidale) BA(UNE) MHPEd(UNSW) PhD(Deakin) FCN(NSW) FRCNA
E M Lane Chair of Surgical Nursing, Faculty of Nursing, University of Sydney and
Concord Repatriation General Hospital, Sydney

Sandra Lynch RN DipNsgEd(NSWCN) BA(Hons)(UNE)
Head, Department of Professional Nursing Development, Australian Catholic
University, McAuley Campus

Helen Millican RN BA(Melb) BAppSc(AdNsg) FRCNA
Lecturer, Faculty of Health Sciences, La Trobe University, Bundoora

Jennifer Oates RN DipAppSc(CommHlthNsg)(Preston) GradDipAdvNsg(LaTrobe) MNsg(RMIT)
Lecturer, Caroline Chisholm School of Nursing, Monash University,
Peninsula Campus

Janice Jocelyn Owens DipTeach BEd MEd RN RM FRCNA FCN(NSW)
Senior Lecturer, Department of Nursing Sciences, James Cook University
of North Queensland

Judith Parker RN PhD
Professor, School of Nursing, Faculty of Health Sciences, La Trobe University,
Abbotsford

Kathryn L Roberts RN BNSc MA PhD FRCNA FCN(NSW)
Professor, School of Nursing, Northern Territory University

Trudy Rudge RN RPN BA(Hons)
Faculty of Nursing, University of South Australia

Colleen Smith RN DipT(NEd) BEd MEd
Lecturer, Faculty of Nursing, University of South Australia

Fran Sutton RN RPN DipT(NEd) MEdAdmin FRCNA
Associate Professor, Faculty of Nursing, University of South Australia

Lesley M Wilkes PhD(UNSW) MHPEd(UNSW) GradDipEd(Nurs)(SCAE) BSc(Hons)(Syd) RN
RenalCert MCN(NSW) FRCNA
Head, School of Nursing and Human Movement, Australian Catholic University,
New South Wales

John Wiltshire PhD
Reader, Department of English, La Trobe University, Bundoora

Linda Worrall-Carter RN(UK) CoronCareCert(UK) BEd(La Trobe)
PhD student, La Trobe University

Contents

1

Clinical, conceptual and empirical aspects of nursing practice

ELIZABETH CAMERON–TRAUB

Scholarly activities have long been associated with the belief that the pursuit of knowledge and wisdom is an activity related to leisure, and that 'leisure is an essential condition' for contemplation, reasoning and argument (Speake 1979). Thus, learning and learnedness were the privilege of those who had the time, interest and disposition to deploy themselves in intellectual endeavours such as scholarly enquiry, critique and discourse. Pressures and demands associated with working and doing had to be reduced or eliminated if scholars were to give their attention and skills to thinking, to activities of the intellect.

This dualist position that thinking is antithetical to doing, as learning is to working, is perpetuated by our differentiation today between academics and practitioners in practice disciplines such as nursing. In Chinese philosophy it is argued that there are indeed necessary conditions for thinking and human achievement, and these go beyond a dualism of thought and action. According to The Great Learning (de Bary et al in Kessler 1992) one must have a 'fixed purpose' in order to achieve 'calmness of mind'; then with 'serene repose' one can carefully deliberate on matters. This argument focuses on an intellectual and spiritual calmness, given by having a sense of purposiveness and direction. If leisure, repose and purpose are basic ingredients for scholarly activities in nursing, perhaps it is less a question of thinking and doing in nursing than explicating a purpose which would enable learning and learnedness to be grounded in the domain of nursing. Indeed, distinctions between scholars and practitioners, thinkers and doers, theory and practice, academics and clinicians must be broken down if we are to maximise achievements through scholarship in nursing.

This chapter explores some aspects of nursing knowledge, practice and scholarliness. In particular, discussion will focus on issues pertaining to scholarship in nursing as a practice discipline, some considerations drawn from theoretical positions and arguments in the discipline of philosophy, and possible frameworks and methods for nursing enquiry and the development and substantiation of nursing knowledge.

Schultz and Meleis (1988) propose that there are three types of knowledge in nursing, namely, conceptual, empirical and clinical knowledge. In some respects a suggestion to categorise knowledge along conceptual–empirical lines is to perpetuate the long standing debate about the nature of knowledge obtained through thought and that obtained through interaction with 'the world out there'. Thus, this proposal has overtones of the idealism-materialism, and rationalism-empiricism debates which, although still evident in philo–sophical literature, seem to have been diminished in significance by the advent of alternative or competing approaches (e.g. pragmatism, phenomenology) in ontology (i.e. theories of existence) and epistemology (i.e. theories of knowledge). Nevertheless, the framework proposed by Schultz and Meleis may well be a useful guide for scholarly endeavours in the development of nursing knowledge, research and practice. Therefore this discussion also explores some attributes of and possible relationships between clinical, conceptual and empirical modes of enquiry as pertaining to nursing, and scholarship in nursing.

Philosophical perspectives

On human enquiry

In a dialogue about the nature of knowledge Meno asked Socrates how he would enquire into what he did not know, and how he would know that what he found was that which he did not know (Plato in Pojman 1993). These questions suggest that the process of enquiry involves identifying the subject matter, determining the method by which to pursue the search for truth or knowledge, and finally substantiating (to oneself and others) how what is eventually known is indeed known. Nurses today are faced with such challenges implicit in human enquiry as they endeavour to identify, define, examine and critique phenomena or information of concern to nurses, nursing and those to whom nurses are accountable for their practice. Fortunately nurse scholars today may benefit from some of the outcomes of philosophical thinking and discourse over the centuries. However, they may have to be wary of translating unresolved concerns in the discipline of philosophy to the process of enquiry in the discipline of nursing. Discourse and theory in philosophy do not necessarily present answers to many questions that nurses may ask. Consequently, if we seek guidance from philosophical theory or principles we may find that confusion or disenchantment is the result, rather than clear and useful direction. Nor is it always clear where philosophy ends and science begins as we attempt to make sense of our world.

Kessler (1992) defines philosophy as 'the rational attempt to formulate, understand, and answer fundamental questions'. He suggests that Western philosophical discourse has effectively reduced the concept of 'rational' to that which is logical, generally rooted in Aristotelian logic and reliant on logical tools or procedures to clarify thinking, appraise the validity of argument and examine the veracity of claims to knowledge.

The development of most branches of linguistic, logical and philosophical enquiry are attributed to scholastics who, using a method of question and answer through oral debate, structured a teaching/learning experience for the student with the learned scholar (Speake 1979). Methods for enquiry have been explored extensively over the centuries, culminating in the divergence of philosophy and science as competing approaches to the development and verification of knowledge. Scientific enquiry is expected to proceed in accordance with prescribed method and procedures involving formulation of the question, gathering of evidence, interpretation and evaluation of the process and outcomes. Indeed, logical thought and systematic appraisal of empirical information are key features of scientific procedures. However, science as an activity to discover, test and extend knowledge has moved well beyond the realms of philosophical enquiry, and the pursuit of knowledge through reasoning as the primary method. Science itself has become the topic of philosophical enquiry (e.g. Harre 1985, Althusser 1990, Laudan 1990, Boyd, Gasper & Trout 1991).

Nursing has become entwined with developments in medical science and practice, increasing technological advances and changing awareness of the nature of humankind, human concerns and human needs. Since only scientific information based on sound and repeated empirical evidence is accorded recognition and value as knowledge, or truth (Chinn & Jacobs 1987), nurses may feel constrained by the supposed legitimacy of different forms of knowledge, and in the methods of enquiry which they could adopt.

On knowing in nursing

A number of authors have identified types (or categories) of nursing knowledge, or ways of knowing, One of the earliest and often cited classifications was proposed by Carper (1978) who suggests that nursing entails personal, aesthetic, ethical and empirical knowledge. As outlined earlier Schultz and Meleis (1988) identify three types of knowledge or theory in nursing, namely, conceptual, empirical and clinical. Belenky et al (1986) suggest that women have four ways of knowing; these are classified as silence, received knowing, subjective knowing and constructed knowing. These authors also differentiate separate and connected forms of knowing, and describe women's behaviours which are consistent with these categories. Bishop and Scudder (1990) propose ways in which nurses may understand or know, according to the practical, personal or moral sense of nursing. Undoubtedly there will be more suggestions coming forth in nursing literature which may help to elucidate the nature of knowledge (product or outcome) and knowing (process) in nursing. Indeed, given an extensive literature in the discipline of philosophy on epistemology and metaphysics which has bearing on what may be known, and how knowledge may be substantiated, nurse scholars have considerable choice in philosophical perspectives and possible frameworks for the study or classification of nursing knowledge, the ways nurses may know in their practice, and how they may evaluate the truth or usefulness of their knowledge. I will look more closely at these matters in later discussion.

On nursing practice

Nursing is a multifaceted discipline. Nurses are involved in various activities which contribute to the realisation of nursing as a professional practice, and which are engendered by the health related caring needs of society and legitimised by the service provided by nurses to members of the community. Thus, nurses fulfil nursing roles and functions in a variety of ways in the context of clinical practice and the delivery of care as well as in academic and administrative contexts. Meleis (1991) identifies aspects of the domain of nursing according to primary activities which may be undertaken by nurses. She suggests that these areas comprise consultation, administration, teaching, practice, research and theory. All of these areas of activity would be related to and constituted by whatever we believe to be the domain of nursing.

Cameron–Traub (1993) suggests that nursing could be likened to a crystal form (e.g. an iolite gem, Mercer 1990) which gives an observer the impression of many colours or hues in its interior. As different facets are turned to face the observer the colours or predominant shades seen by the observer may vary. Yet those effects are due to prismatic effects on rays of light which, through refraction and dispersion, yield a spectrum of colour as a function of the characteristics and qualities of the form. In the case of a diamond 'white light is therefore broken up into the whole "rainbow" of colours, "violet, indigo, blue, green, yellow, orange and red"' (Wood 1977).

If each of the areas of activity in nursing were like a facet of a crystal then these activities might well be recognised by the hues seen on observation from different perspectives. Perhaps those nurses involved in clinical practice, looking at the crystal through the facet for practice as delivery of care, would see predominantly one portion of the colour spectrum, whereas those looking from the perspective of nursing administration would see mainly another part of the spectrum. Similarly, the perspective for nurses involved in educational activities preparing nurses for practice may differ from that of nurses primarily involved in research activities.

Each perspective on nursing, and its corresponding practice area, is needed if the potential of nursing as a profession, a discipline and a community service is to be realised through the activities and achievements of its various members. Moreover, one portion of the spectrum of nursing activity as one of many facets need not be treated as more important than any other since the appearance of difference would be due to the attributes or properties of the facets working interactively to give rise to the sensory impressions of different colours from different perspectives. Thus, interaction of areas in nursing may be likened to the interaction of light rays of different wavelengths, which may merge and blend into one another to give an appearance of blended or diffused colours. In this analogy it is important to remember that this effect is a function of the medium through which white light is transmitted; the light itself is essentially the same were it not for the crystal. Thus, scholarship may be likened to the white light which, when beaming on the crystal, may give rise to colours due to the properties of the medium through which it passes. So too with nursing, its properties (or indeed essence) may be exemplified through scholarship.

The science of crystallography entails a theoretical description and prescription specifying the criterion of symmetry by which objects may be classified as crystals (Polanyi 1962, Mercer 1990). Only those which fit into one of the 32 classes are classified as crystals, yet there are many variations in the size and shape of objects which are so designated. Perhaps it is not desirable to decide that one form is superior to or more pleasing than others. Nevertheless, it would be possible, with theoretical precision, to determine criteria and to select the form which we considered to be the one most analogous to our idea of what nursing is (or what we may like it to be). In addition, we could develop a theoretical conceptualisation of nursing as entailing certain attributes, and excluding others, in a similar vein to crystallography.

To some extent I believe we have been examining the form of nursing as our practice has been shaped through the centuries, but the efforts and circumstances of nurses and nursing may not have led directly to how we believe nursing should be today. Were we to formulate a theoretical position which would define and explicate the nature of nursing then, as a profession, we would be in a position to test any object, event or situation from many perspectives for its consistency with our ideal form, and so decide whether it does, or does not constitute an aspect of nursing.

On scholarship in nursing

Nursing scholarship is a challenge for nurses as they seek to analyse, differentiate, integrate and synthesise the aspects of nursing which may be identified through the professional activities of nurses. Meleis (1991) argues that 'scholarliness combines theory, research, philosophy, and, in disciplines such as nursing, practice, and it is reflected in the synthesis between a discipline's different components'. Thus, one would expect that dissociation, incongruence or discord between theory, research, practice, or philosophy in nursing would detract from the excellence of disciplinary activities, thereby limiting the integrity and scholarliness of nursing as a discipline.

In order to encapsulate in scholarly work the diversity and complexity of nursing practice today it would be desirable to encourage exploration of nursing phenomena specific to each area of practice but, at the same time, seek to identify commonalities and shared concerns, beliefs and values in and about nursing. If indeed all areas of practice (or activities of nurses) reflect aspects of the domain of nursing, then there should be core beliefs and knowledge which would integrate, even unify the areas so as to constitute a world view congruent with or epitomising the essence of nursing (Cameron–Traub 1991). Furthermore, by identifying similarities and acknowledging and explaining any differences in perspectives between components such as theory, research, philosophy and practice, nurses should be in a position to offer a synthesis between them, thus delineating and explicating the domain of nursing.

Through nursing scholarship directed toward achieving a synthesis, as discussed by Meleis (1991), it should be possible to differentiate the discipline and practice of nursing in varied societal, multidisciplinary and multi-professional contexts. It is not enough for us individually to believe that we know what nursing is and what it is not, what constitutes our practice, and what does not. Nursing practice has to be explicated, and our supposed knowledge tested and confirmed, rejected or modified, so that the integrity of nursing can be recognised unequivocally, not only by nurses themselves, but also by members of the wider community.

Nurses as critical thinkers

By intensive and extensive critique of information from internal or external sources nurses may contribute to the validation and refinement of nursing knowledge. Through sensory and perceptual processes, conceptual activities and reflection on their experiences in nursing practice, nurses will be exposed to a wide range of information. Thus, the status regarding truth or falsity, validity, reliability and credibility of the information has to be determined. In doing so nurses have to examine the evidence conceptually and empirically, and refer to other sources (e.g. people, literature or their own experience) which may be expected to provide support for, or refute, the information. However, there may be many times when nurses accept information as true or valid statements about the world, and thus incorporate new ideas into their practice only to find, sooner or later, that the ideas are incorrect, inappropriate or need further critical examination before being adopted in nursing thought and action.

The Mexican philosopher Vasconcelos (1882-1959) identified at least four types of knowledge, namely inductive (empirical or experiential), ethical (related to human ends or outcomes), aesthetic (synthesising experience involving emotion) and intellectual (involving formal, logical or mathematical processes) (Kessler 1992). These categories differ from Carper's (1978) nursing categories only in one area; she did not identify intellectual (or conceptual) knowledge, but rather personal knowledge. Vasconcelos was indeed concerned that personal knowledge be recognised as legitimate knowledge, in particular aesthetic knowledge. However, personal knowledge may be obtained or developed from a number of sources and by a variety of processes, and comprise a harmony or integration of various types of knowing within and by the individual. In contrast, intellectual knowledge would be specifically the outcome of thought processes, and in particular the processes of reasoning. One would expect that this type of knowledge would be specific, even idiosyncratic to the individual person, unless formal modes of reasoning, following specific rules (e.g. logic), were used. Nevertheless, knowledge may be shared with others, for example, through the use of language. Thus, intellectual or conceptual knowledge may be unique in the sense that it arose from, or was created through, the mental activity of an individual. Yet, some intellectual knowledge may be similar or shared between people if indeed intellectual processes are similar, or yield similar outcomes (e.g. words, sentences, arguments, conclusions).

One of the challenges to nurses in scholarship, research and practice is to be able to share their ideas with others. Since ideas originate within the person, and are sustained or modified by his/her intellectual processes, there needs to be some way (or ways) of determining the veracity or credibility of ideas as generated by an individual, and conveyed to and received by another. This discussion would go well beyond the scope of this chapter and it may suffice to say that critical thinking in nursing may involve various techniques of logical, rational and empirical analysis and verification in order to help nurses to make judgments about information or possible knowledge. Bandman and Bandman (1988), for example, outline some of these approaches and techniques.

In addition to variation between individuals, nurses from different areas of clinical practice may differ in what they believe constitutes nursing knowledge. Nurses in one field of specialised and specific knowledge may share general knowledge about nursing and health care with nurses from other areas, but there would also be aspects of nursing knowledge which would differ from one field or area to the next. Moreover, the concerns of nurses may well differ between different practice areas, perhaps not in their overall goals (e.g. concern for improving the health or comfort of individuals) but in the specifics of who, what, how, when and where. In other words, using Polanyi's (1962) framework, nurses in different areas of practice may be focally aware of different aspects of their nursing situations, and perhaps only aware in a subsidiary manner of phenomena (objects, events or ideas) which would be of prime importance to nurses in other fields.

This situation may be exacerbated by the focus of medical specialties, which perpetuate, through nomenclature and discourse, a dualism of mind and body in Descartes' view, or soul and body according to Plato's dualist notions. Medicine is concerned with medical phenomena such as disease entities, symptomatology and aetiology, and technological, materialistic innovations and modes of bodily intervention. Since nurses usually work closely with medical doctors, assisting, supporting or following on from medical procedures, it would not be surprising if such a dualism were an influence on how nurses conceptualise clinical phenomena, or the way they make judgments about the efficacy, clinical appropriateness or moral 'rightness' of medical or related nursing actions.

Philosophical discourse offers some suggestions which may help nurses understand the assumptions they make or the positions they adopt when receiving or reviewing information they presume to be knowledge. Perhaps being aware of some of the major positions espoused and debated in philosophy would help nurses to participate critically in discussions about nursing and health care when different perspectives are (or could be) used.

Philosophical positions

Here I have selected some philosophical positions which have been extensively debated in philosophy; references for the material outlined (but not as applied to nursing) include Ayer (1956), Sprigge (1985), Dancy (1988), Hospers (1988), Lehrer (1990), Boyd et al (1991), and Carruthers (1992).

The concept of foundationalism relates to the philosophical position that what we know (or may know) is built on basic ideas which are truths about the world. A strong form of foundationalism would be that we cannot know anything which is not built on basic true ideas, which are indeed self–evident, (i.e. needing no proof), and may be innate and so form the basis by which we come to know the world through interpretations of our experiences. The expression that 'nurses are born not made' reflects an assertion that to be a nurse we must have certain inborn predispositions (inborn knowledge), and ideas not given in or through experience, which would form the foundations for nursing knowledge and practice. A weaker form of foundationalism would be reflected in an argument that nurses must undergo a course of training or education in order to gain the knowledge base necessary and sufficient for practice. In other words, this idea would mean that sufficient nursing knowledge is not inborn; necessary knowledge must be acquired through appropriate teaching/learning experiences; practice would only be at an acceptable standard and constitute nursing if such a knowledge base is present; and future learning would build on a foundational knowledge base gained through education and experience in nursing.

Three theories of truth are often discussed in philosophy. Correspondence theory asserts that we can confirm the truth of our beliefs by reference to objects or events which we take to be phenomena in the world. We can only obtain knowledge about worldly phenomena through evidence given in our experience with them, i.e. through the sensations which occur during these experiences. If, when we refer to the world around us to test our beliefs, we find that they are supported by sensory or perceptual evidence, then the truth of these beliefs would be substantiated. Scientific procedures are designed to test such beliefs or hunches, and are based on the idea that the delineation of scientific phenomena through observation and measurement will correspond to whatever is reality.

An alternative theory adopts a coherentist standpoint from which we can argue that as long as our ideas form a coherent (albeit theoretically consistent) system, usually based on logical argument, then we may assume that our beliefs are true. For example, we may claim that nursing is about caring for people, nurses provide care for people, and a nursing act is a caring act. Hence, when a nursing procedure seems to be inflicting discomfort or pain, a nurse could argue that if this is an unintentional or unavoidable aspect of her nursing action, and the nature of the action is consistent with assertions about nursing, then her action was a caring action.

A third theory of truth is based on pragmatism, a philosophical theory arguing that what is true is what is useful to know, i.e. information that would lead to valued or desirable outcomes as a consequence of being known. Perhaps nurses would like to deliberate on this notion, since it may resemble the position adopted when we decide what information to accept or reject depending on its apparent relevance to practice at a given time.

Realism is a philosophical position claiming that objects or entities may have an existence beyond what we perceive (or do not perceive) through our sensory experience. However, the best we can know about objects is through information given through our perceptions, and our interpretation of our experiences as sensory, perceiving and thinking beings. Thus, the only reality we can know about or understand is through our perceptions or experience of the world.

Phenomenalism stands in contrast to realism by representing the view that, because we can only know things through our experiences, these objects or entities are reality, that reality is indeed constituted by these experiences. There is nothing necessarily beyond them and, indeed, objects are only given to us through our perceptions of sets of phenomena or attributes. Only what we experience is meaningful and thus constitutes our truth, our reality. In nursing there is a growing interest in phenomenology and perhaps there is a need to explore more fully the implications of realist or phenomenalist standpoints on what is real (i.e. existing) or not, and what can be known, especially when it comes to understanding and practising holistic nursing care. Moreover, how do these positions concur or conflict with philosophical viewpoints about reality or truth from the perspective of medical science?

Although scepticism is sometimes regarded as impractical (e.g. Schultz & Meleis 1988) arguments from a sceptic's viewpoint may well be employed to oppose the position of dogmatism. Dogmatists claim that argument (or reason) can and does establish knowledge (Musgrave 1993). Scepticism is the position that, although objects or events may be knowable, we can never be sure that what we experience reveals the true nature of these phenomena, or that we really know them. Therefore we must reserve judgement on whether or not we know something; moreover, we must doubt the truth of our supposed knowledge since we can never be sure that we do know what we think we know, nor can we necessarily demonstrate the truth of these beliefs. The sceptic's position may be reflected in situations in which nurses (or others) argue that experiences in clinical practice, administration or education do not really yield knowledge, or that practices are based on beliefs rather than truths. If the sceptic's viewpoint is taken seriously why have scholarly pursuits at all?

From the above summary of philosophical viewpoints it should be evident that philosophy is concerned with critical and varied argument, rather than with providing definitive perspectives, theories or indeed answers to questions about knowledge, knowing, life or reality. The diversity of theoretical positions and conceptualisations about the world and people offers nurses a rich array of possible viewpoints. However, answers to questions which may seem to be vital and determinant in nursing may only be marginally or contentiously addressed through diverse scholastic views in philosophy. It may be more useful in nursing to limit ourselves to a more simple, differentiated view of the world of thinking and discourse about knowledge and knowing. Issues linked with differentiating clinical, conceptual and empirical processes will now be considered, and a framework discussed, as it may contribute to our understanding of nursing knowledge and practice.

Substantiating nursing knowledge

Nurse scholars or teachers, practitioners or researchers, clinicians or administrators will seek to substantiate the information they gain on a daily basis, and in the longer term, to verify information as it becomes knowledge impacting on or influencing their practice. Nurses may choose to substantiate their knowledge by examining various assumptions, as well as critically evaluating evidence for correspondence to or coherence with their beliefs about reality. They may choose to explore knowledge claims through a conceptual approach, or an empirical one. Although Meleis (1991) suggests that there may be overlap or interaction between these modes when it comes to theory development, this may not be the case when considering them as approaches to the substantiation of knowledge held by individuals or groups.

As I have argued elsewhere (Cameron–Traub 1991) conceptual and empirical approaches to theory development may well be considered as discrete, independent in form and method. Indeed they are based on two competing views about how knowledge is obtained and what constitutes knowledge, and are associated with opposing views about how information may be substantiated as knowledge or true information about the world. The conceptual approach is linked with rationalism and idealism, the latter position maintaining that ideas may constitute knowledge, and the former that the truth value of statements or beliefs about the world can be, and should be, deduced by logical argument and appraisal. In contrast, an empirical mode or approach is based on the position that we can only know objects, events or phenomena through our experience. Indeed according to an empiricist standpoint we cannot know the world unless we obtain information about it through our senses and perceptions of worldly objects and events. The accumulation of such information gives us the knowledge upon which we base our interpretations of future experiences as we interact with and in the world. It may be evident to the reader that these approaches are linked with opposing philosophical positions or arguments, as outlined in earlier discussion.

A conceptual approach entails material which is essentially intellectual, created within and through the mind, envisioned through creative or analytical thinking, imagination and thought construction. In contrast, the method by which empirical information is gathered and tested is essentially materialist, observational, and associated with measurement of sensory or perceptual phenomena yielded by objects or events. The scientific method is based on an empiricist approach, as opposed to a rationalist approach, since it requires that we think about phenomena only in so far as we can describe and examine them through measurement, observation and sensory/perceptual information. Scientific knowledge is not built on our thought processes or ideas and beliefs alone. The empirical truth of concepts or relationships between phenomena is determined by testing empirically how they appear to be in the world. Thus, the scientist aims to establish that the information obtained or constructed resembles a reality according to prespecified rules, and thus, constitutes true statements about the world as judged normatively against scientific criteria.

A clinical approach to theorising as proposed by Schultz and Meleis (1988) at first glance appears to stand apart from conceptual and empirical approaches to the discovery of knowledge. However, clinical knowledge or theory developed from clinical experience may well be consistent with a number of philosophical positions. Clinical experience may give the nurse ideas about phenomena in practice and may be appraised conceptually for validity or truth by reference to the coherence of information. (e.g. consistency of ideas, concepts, relationships). Then such a clinical theory would have been developed primarily by a conceptual approach. Alternatively, the nurse's ideas arising from clinical experience may have been based on observations pertaining to phenomena, possibly involving objective or subjective evaluation. If the nurse sought to verify the truth or relevance of these ideas through further experience or outcomes (e.g. tests of correspondence), then the clinical theory would have strong empirical overtones. Finally, clinical theory based on clinical experience may well involve both conceptual and empirical substantiation, and thus would be a prototypical amalgam of these approaches. In other words, how the nurse thinks about phenomena and what the nurse experiences may come together to build clinical knowledge, and thus various forms of clinical theory based on various combinations of conceptual and empirical activities.

Foucault (1973) argues that when it comes to clinical practice in medicine the process is one of objectification, whereby the person undergoing a medical examination becomes 'the object' of the clinician's gaze, and the clinician seeks to objectify any thoughts or ideas about the person, and to read the signs or indications without making subjective inferences. Hence, the notion of objectivity means to stand back, stand outside of one's immediate experience, and attempt to read and interpret clinical information as another person would. In doing so personal characteristics, beliefs or values would not influence the interpretation of information being given to the practitioner through sensory processes. According to this view any medical practitioner should be able to observe the same phenomenon and reach the same conclusions as another. In contrast, subjective interpretation would be specific to the individual practitioner, and thus may not be interpreted in the same way by another.

When nurses describe or explain a clinical situation to others, when they seek endorsement or clarification of their clinical judgment by others, or when they convey information to others about their observations, they may be assuming that their knowledge about phenomena is objective in the sense that others too may share or similarly experience such phenomena if they had the opportunity. In other words, if others were to have had the same experience, their interpretations or meanings would be congruent with (even identical to) those of the nurse who initially experienced that clinical situation. When we hear nurses say 'I know exactly what you mean. I have just had that experience recently in my practice…', we are listening to a claim of congruence between two nurses, and taken a step further, a claim to objectivity in the meanings ascribed to separate experiences.

Husserl (in Gadamer 1976) sought to develop a phenomenological method which would allow a person to 'bracket' phenomena, that is to stand back and consider the 'real' or 'true' nature of an object or event, without distorting it through description or interpretation influenced by subjective factors such as beliefs, values, expectations or prejudices of the beholder. This method is similar to other approaches designed to attain objectivity, rather than allowing the object of one's study to be clouded or distorted by subjective influences (e.g. unique attributes and prejudices of an individual). However, the focus and purpose of the action of 'bracketing' in phenomenology is less on removing the subject, (as is sometimes argued to be the case in science) and more on clarifying the nature of the object or phenomenon under study. Cameron-Traub (1994a) suggests that nurses and persons cared for by nurses may perceive (or think about) phenomena in nursing situations very differently.

According to Husserl's theory this discrepancy may be due to a difficulty in 'bracketing' or phenomenologically reducing information so that the meaning of an object or event is understood similarly by each individual.

Information which may arise from clinical practice and is taken to be nursing knowledge or theory would be more acceptable to others if they too could find it credible, if it were consistent with their knowledge base and their view of or understanding about the world. Nursing knowledge, including clinical knowledge, developed through a strategy incorporating both conceptual and empirical approaches, should lead to acceptance and recognition by others (including people receiving nursing care) as a foundation for nursing practice.

A framework for knowledge and knowing in nursing

Given the above discussion it may be useful to consider how conceptual and empirical processes could (and do) contribute to the development or establishment of nursing knowledge. However, I would argue that such approaches should also be linked with aspects of nurses' knowing in their practice environments. Differentiating between conceptual and empirical approaches for characterising theory development or research, respectively, would invite separation rather than interaction of these components of nursing. Furthermore, nurses in their day–to–day clinical practice would be engaged in forms of conceptual and empirical enquiry, and thus to envisage that a clinical approach is somehow separate or distinct from the other two approaches may not be conducive to the discovery or substantiation of nursing knowledge. Conceptual and empirical processes would both be involved in clinical nursing encounters, in assessing client needs, selecting possible nursing actions, and evaluating client outcomes. Therefore, the following framework may be useful to nurses in the development, extension and refinement of both theory and practice, and in the conduct and critique of research activities within various paradigms.

It could be argued that there are three processes mainly related to an internal conceptual approach:

1 Creating information through formulating ideas, notions and new conceptualisations of phenomena
2 Constructing information as a result of rational thought
3 Commenting critically on information and new conceptualisations (see Fig. 1.1).

In contrast three processes may be primarily associated with an external empirical approach to knowledge development:

1 Consuming information in order to expand or refine one's knowledge base, similar to the received knowledge as described by Belenky et al (1986), or the empirical knowledge described by Carper (1978) and Schultz and Meleis (1988)
2 Confirming information (i.e. testing it)
3 Consolidating information following demonstration that information is empirically supported (i.e. empirically reliable and valid information).

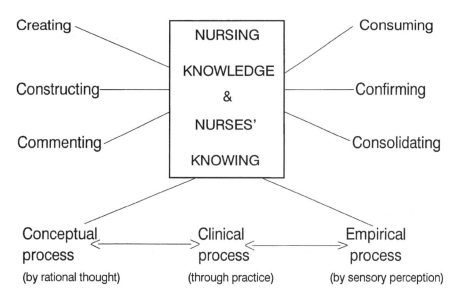

Fig. 1.1 Scholarly activities towards developing and substantiating nursing knowledge and nurses' knowing in theory and practice

These processes are not necessarily in an hierarchical order of importance, nor would they necessarily occur sequentially. To some extent the processes may be ongoing simultaneously depending on the focus and process of enquiry. However, creating information would be an internal productive process whereas consuming information would rely on input from an external source. Constructing information would be an internal activity whereby knowledge and meaning would derive from generative conceptual processes, whereas confirming information would be categorically evaluative of information received from sources external to the individual. Finally, commenting on information would be an ongoing internal process of critical examination and evaluation of conceptual phenomena (e.g. evaluating the coherence of ideas or correspondence to worldly phenomena), whereas consolidating information would be in the form of documentation and personal or public storage as empirical evidence for future reference.

Finally, this model suggests that all six processes may be involved in and contribute to the development of clinical knowledge. Accordingly, the formation of clinical knowledge and the process of clinical knowing may be envisaged as a summative outcome of all six processes. Schultz and Meleis (1988) suggest that criteria should be developed to evaluate conceptual, empirical and clinical knowledge. Nursing theorists have outlined criteria for theory evaluation (e.g. Chinn & Jacobs 1987). Moreover empirical knowledge, as it is uncovered through scientific procedures, has long been subjected to evaluation according to scientifically acceptable criteria. If clinical knowledge is a special form of, and combination of, conceptual and empirical knowing and knowledge, then perhaps the criteria for evaluating clinical information should be a composite of those aforementioned criteria.

13

Towards scholarliness in nursing

If scholarship is to link, integrate or merge together components of nursing as a discipline it may best be guided by a sense of purposiveness as well as appropriate methodology in scholarly pursuits. Just as philosophers through the centuries have endeavoured to determine ways to develop, refine and substantiate knowledge, so too nurses today could continue to develop the philosophical and empirical aspects of nursing through continued and purposive scholarly activities. Through nursing scholarship the components or aspects of practice should be integrated or synthesised so as to facilitate the creation and evolution of nursing's identity. If nurse scholars (academics and practitioners alike) share goals which are addressed through scholarly activities the uniqueness of nursing as a discipline should be demonstrated. Following is a discussion on some approaches which may be helpful toward achieving such goals.

Dialectical method in nursing enquiry

The idea of a dialectical process involving thesis and antithesis may be useful in the pursuit of nursing enquiry. The philosopher Hegel argued that an entity is constituted not only by the positive or confirming aspect but also by the nature of qualities or features of its opposite. Dialectical thinking involves recognition that 'every concept contains within itself its own negation' (Kessler 1992) and we can only understand a concept or thesis by understanding its negation or antithesis. However, dialectical thinking entails more than consideration of both aspects, or opposites, and it is more than an oscillation back and forth between two aspects or phenomena. According to Hegel, a further step is required in dialectical thinking, specifically, that we must endeavour to synthesise the thesis and the antithesis. Hegel believed that in doing so we would 'arrive at a higher more complex understanding of the concept' (Kessler 1992), that we would transcend any understanding we would have of the concept through consideration of the thesis or antithesis alone.

Following Hegel's argument, if we are to think only about what we believe (or would like) nursing to be we will not have a complete or adequate understanding of the concept 'nursing'. When we attempt to conceptualise the negation of the concept of nursing, (i.e. define what nursing is not) we may be in a stronger position to understand what nurses know and do, and what nursing is. However, only by the further step of synthesising nursing and not–nursing into our understanding, so that we come to know the concept in its entirety as a conjunction of thesis and antithesis, will we really have a full conceptualisation of nursing.

Finally, expositions of nursing following a dialectical method, as with any other exposition, would have to be meaningful to nurses regardless of their practice orientation. It is likely that nurses involved in clinical practice, education, research or administration would share some common beliefs about nursing, especially given that they undertake education programs to prepare themselves for nursing, and they are socialised into their professional role through similar education programs and practical experience. Indeed, if nurse scholars focus on differentiation rather than synthesis we may find that delineation of the concept or essence of nursing may elude us regardless of our literary or scholastic efforts. Perhaps we need to use a dialectical approach to delineate nursing from not–nursing, and then to synthesise our concept of nursing from our understanding of both components. This process should enable us to define and explore nursing as it relates to ourselves and others.

Reductionism and holism

One of the problems in attempting to define or describe nursing as a group of elements (or components such as areas of practice or activity) is that there is, in effect, a reduction of the concept of nursing to a number of more simple, differentiated elements. While this approach may seem to make dealing with a complex concept more manageable (or palatable), if the levels of description or exploration differ then identification of various parts need not accurately or completely reflect the whole. Nor can we be assured that such atomistic reduction will fully differentiate nursing from other disciplines contributing to or involved in health care.

In his novel *Siddartha* Herman Hesse (1954) wrote about how a ferry–man's awareness was raised by 'listening' to the multiple voices of a river. Despite the many voices, with differing passions and expressions, the river continued to flow toward its goal, its next turn, and future inevitable goals. Yet as Siddartha listened intently the voices seemed to become interwoven, entwined, and all of them constituted 'the stream of events, the music of life'. A river is the same river both downstream and upstream, and although individual droplets that pass over one's hand at any point on the river's course are different to droplets elsewhere at that time, nevertheless, as the river flows these droplets all merge to constitute the river as an entity. So, too, we can envisage elements or voices of nursing and the 'river' of nursing as it follows its course through historical and social contexts, and merges over time and space to constitute nursing as an entity today.

Commonalities and differences between the thoughts and actions of nurses in different places and at different times need to be synthesised in order to encapsulate the essence of nursing regardless of daily orientations or preferences in past or current working environments. In addition nurses in a given context, e.g. hospital nursing practice, may experience conflict or frustration leading to a compromise in providing care for people (e.g. technical biomedical care versus psychosocial care) rather than experiencing opportunities to provide holistic care in their practice (Cameron–Traub 1994b). We need to work toward an understanding of how aspects of nursing merge, how they may blend to become a unity within any practice context, and over time. And above all, we need to create an awareness or understanding of nursing as an holistic practice discipline, following its course towards some end, some outcome for members of our community who are the actual or potential recipients of nursing care.

Purposiveness in nursing scholarship

As members of the nursing profession, nurses communicate with each other by oral or written discourse, and through such interchanges nurses can share ideas, beliefs, and information which may influence their practice. Nurses interact as learners and teachers interchangeably as they explore forms and modes of communication and traverse various pathways to knowledge and understanding. In addition, nurses exchange information with others from different disciplines or professions as well as with members of the public. Thus, purposiveness and future directions in nursing should take into account social needs, expectations and beliefs about nursing and nurses, as well as how nursing may best contribute to community needs through various local, regional and international strategies in various contexts (Cameron–Traub 1994c).

A number of nursing theorists have developed the idea of purpose or purposiveness in nursing. For example, Orlando argued that nursing practice is deliberative, and King's theory suggests that nursing practice should be goal–directed (Marriner–Tomey 1989). Husserl argued that actions are only meaningful because of the intentions which give rise to them (Gadamer 1976). Cameron–Traub (1989) found that nurses were often in favour of teleological or purposive reasons in accounting for nursing actions in practice. They often preferred to explain actions such as dressing a wound or talking with a patient as purposive from the nurse's point of view. The ideas of intending or trying to improve the patient's comfort, keep the wound clean or provide information to the patients were purposive explanations of these nursing actions. Thus, if nursing scholarship is to facilitate or assist nurses to find meaning in their practice it will need to help delineate purpose or intentionality as being intrinsic to practice.

Gadamer (1979) writes 'that practice has to do with others and co–determines the communal concerns in doing'. Further, he argues that while practice may be motivated and prejudiced, as determined by the individual, the nature of practice entails a challenge to a 'critique of prejudices'. Thus, human actions such as nursing may well be self–conscious, self–critical and mediated by personal, professional and social expectations. Moreover, practice in nursing would be influenced by the past, present and future expectations, values and beliefs not only of the nurse but also of others involved in or affecting the nature of one's practice. Professional, personal and community intentions and motivations in conjunction with nursing practice would all contribute to defining the purpose and direction for nurses and nursing in the future.

Perhaps one of the greatest challenges for nurses today is to undertake and adapt nursing practice so that it reflects the nurse's and nursing's goals, and at the same time concurs with society's needs and expectations. Understanding critically and wholeheartedly where we have come from, and how, is probably a precursor to focusing future practice goals and accountabilities in nursing on sound epistemological and ontological foundations, regardless of our philosophical predilections. We should not be determined (or hindered) by the strengths or weaknesses of our past, nor should we appear captive of forces beyond our control in the future. When we can frame our purpose in recognition of our heritage and in anticipation of our future as significant practitioners in health care and community service, we may find the 'serene repose' and 'calm deliberation' attributed to scholars in Confucian writings (e.g. Kessler 1992). Then, and only then perhaps, may we work towards fulfilment of our visions for nursing in the future.

Dimensions for nursing scholarship

Building on the proposal by Schultz and Meleis (1988) and Meleis (1991) regarding conceptual, empirical and clinical modes for the development of nursing theory and knowledge, the following discussion explores possible relationships between them. The aim here is to provide a framework for scholarly activities in nursing which would acknowledge the contributions of different forms of knowledge, different realities, and different intentions, actions and outcomes.

The following framework focuses on the conceptual and empirical modes, and how they may contribute to nursing scholarship if each is characterised as a dimension along which scholarship may vary at any time, or with individual scholars. I have treated each dimension independently: the philosophical dimension is similar to Meleis' conceptual mode and the pragmatic dimension contains elements of the empirical mode, including phenomenological perspectives. While one mode is represented as a thinking, reasoning or intuitive approach, the other is concerned with, and characterised by, the state of the world and identifiable outcomes. However, when expanding the notion of two modes or approaches to theory development so as to apply to nursing scholarship, I suggest that a third dimension would be useful, namely, a purposive dimension (see Fig. 1.2). This third dimension may be considered an integrative construct which should enable scholars to envisage a synthesis, an intentional unification of phenomena pertaining to the conceptual and empirical dimensions. In addition, the notion of purpose or intentionality in nursing scholarship would be a driving force toward the integration of professional and personal purposiveness. Thus, through attention to these three dimensions (i.e. philosophical, purposive and pragmatic) nursing scholarship may bridge and integrate various activities in nursing. Regardless of where the scholar's main focus may be (i.e. theoretical, educational, research, administrative or clinical practice) through scholarly investigations and discourse, nurse scholars may evoke a synthesis of areas in nursing by addressing the philosophical, purposive and pragmatic dimensions of nursing thought and action.

The philosophical dimension would comprise ideas, assumptions and propositions based on conceptualisations of nursing. Nurse scholars may assume that they are building on pre–existing knowledge which forms a foundation for their analyses and conclusions. In addition they may, through reasoned argument, formulate proposals which are essentially created through deliberation on and about nursing, their interpretations of experiences in nursing, and their suggestions for new approaches, or modifications to existing theory and practice, as derived by processes founded in rationalism, idealism and foundationalism.

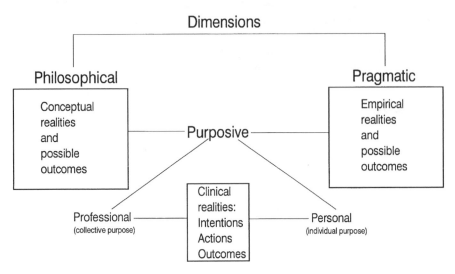

Fig. 1.2 Philosophical, pragmatic and purposive dimensions for nursing scholarship toward an integration of conceptual, empirical and clinical approaches to nursing theory and practice

In contrast, the pragmatic dimension would involve consideration of empirical realities, such as the potential or actual aspects of nursing contexts, the people involved and possible or desirable outcomes. The focus in pragmatic analyses would be on how practice could be effected (i.e. instrumented) in order to produce desirable outcomes and prevent or reduce the likelihood of undesirable outcomes. Alternatively, the focus may be on the phenomenological experiences of the people involved (i.e. the nurse, the person cared for or others) and any perceived implications for them from a pragmatic (i.e. outcome or experiential) point of view.

Finally, the dimension of purposiveness would have professional and personal components, the former being reflected in collective goals, practices and standards of the profession, and the latter in the intentions, actions and outcomes as these may relate to individual nurses. These phenomena would be characterised as and constitute clinical realities, the meanings associated with clinical experience, given the beliefs, values, expectations and interpretations of clinical nursing phenomena. Through a systematic and comprehensive exploration of nursing phenomena, nurse scholars may achieve a synthesis of generic attributes and also achieve delineation of specific attributes of nursing by addressing all these dimensions.

Usefulness and outcomes in nursing

The information and views exchanged through scholarly activities in nursing may assist nurses to explore and critically examine aspects of their practice in professional working environments. Therefore, through scholarly discourse nurses may enhance their practice and be increasingly informed. Outcomes of nursing scholarship may well be a measure of success in terms of stimulating enquiry and guiding practitioners as they make nursing what it is, and could be, in the context of continuing social, cultural and technological change. Thus, scholarly activities must not only build on past efforts (e.g. cumulatively as suggested by Meleis 1991) but also be responsive to the present and proactively directed towards the future (i.e. purposiveness).

Ideas and critical analyses offered by nurse scholars, whose work seeks to provide possible direction for nurses, would probably be welcomed by those who are seeking alternatives and choices in nursing theory, research, administration and clinical practice. By outlining the way in which scholarly proposals or arguments may have bearing on various nursing issues, readers may find new directions following critical appraisal of the information in scholarly texts. Nursing scholarliness would then be more likely to be useful if it offers new insights, amends or replaces outmoded beliefs, and suggests new pathways for practice. However, as outlined in this paper, there are a number of approaches nurses may take to test information, conceptually or empirically, in their practice environments. Many ideas may appear interesting to nurses, but unless they are able to appraise and implement them, these ideas would be rather futile, at best misguided, and at worst erroneous for certain nurses or nursing situations. Furthermore, nurses need to be aware that their arguments for substantiating nursing knowledge or nurses' knowing may depend on the philosophical positions they hold in critical thinking and discourse, and the assumptions they make in evaluating oral or written information. These positions may not be held by others with whom nurses communicate during their practice or scholarly discourse. Therefore, where nurse scholars indicate critically the scope or limitations of their ideas or arguments in conceptual, empirical or clinical terms the contributions of nurses' scholarly efforts should be of greater utility.

Conclusion

Nursing practice is multifaceted and each area (e.g. clinical practice, education, administration, research) may contribute to explication of the discipline and enhancement of nursing as a socially sanctioned professional activity. Learning, learnedness and the development of nursing knowledge and practice in nursing may proceed most effectively through the collective efforts of nurses working together and interactively to enhance nursing. Moreover, through seeking a balance between conceptual (or intellectual) and empirical (or experiential) approaches in scholarly pursuits and enquiry in practice, nurses may achieve epistemological and methodological integration, even synthesis, which would generate and strengthen nursing knowledge and nurses' knowing in various practice contexts. Through scholarly endeavours which address philosophical, pragmatic and purposive dimensions, nurses should contribute to clinical practice, education, research and administration through a systematic and comprehensive pursuit of wisdom and truth in and for nursing. Thus, a hallmark of nursing in the future may be nurses' achievements in the delineation and explication of nursing as a practice discipline, through conceptual, empirical and clinical approaches to scholarly endeavours arising from, and impacting on, nursing thought and action in all areas of nursing practice.

REFERENCES

Althusser L 1990 Philosophy and the spontaneous philosophy of the scientists (trans). Verso, London

Ayer A J 1956 The problem of knowledge. Penguin, Harmondsworth

Bandman E L, Bandman B 1988 Critical thinking in nursing. Appleton & Lange, Norwalk, Connecticut

Belenky M F, Clinchy B McV, Goldberger N R, Tarule J M 1986 Women's ways of knowing. Basic Books, US

Bishop A J, Scudder J R 1990 The practical, moral, and personal sense of nursing. State University of New York, New York

Boyd R, Gasper P, Trout J D (eds) 1991 The philosophy of science. Massachusetts Institute of Technology, Cambridge, Massachusetts

Cameron-Traub E 1989 Nurses' reasons for their practice: an empirical evaluation. Full report to The Victorian Nursing Council (Unpublished)

Cameron-Traub E 1991 An evolving discipline. In: Gray G, Pratt R (eds) Towards a discipline of nursing. Churchill Livingstone, Melbourne

Cameron-Traub E 1993 Effective collaboration in nursing: processes, problems and pathways. In: Proceedings of the First National Nursing Conference, Effective collaboration: effective practice in nursing. Charles Sturt University-Riverina, Wagga Wagga

Cameron-Traub E 1994a Phenomenology and shared lifeworlds in nursing practice. In: Proceedings of the International Nursing Research Conference, Vancouver

Cameron-Traub E 1994b Nursing in hospital practice: conflict, compromise and care. In: Proceedings of the International Nursing Research Conference, Vancouver

Cameron-Traub E 1994c Challenges in nursing: an analysis from four perspectives. In: Proceedings of the Third International Middle East Nursing Conference, Irbid, Jordan

Carper B A 1978 Fundamental patterns of knowing in nursing. Advances in Nursing Science 1(1):13–23

Carruthers P 1992 Human knowledge and human nature. Oxford University Press, Oxford

Chinn P L, Jacobs M K 1987 Theory and nursing, 2nd edn. C V Mosby, St Louis

Dancy J (ed) 1988 Perceptual knowledge. Oxford University Press, Oxford

Foucault M 1973 The birth of the clinic. Sheridan A M (trans) Tavistock, London

Gadamer H–G 1976 Philosophical hermeneutics. Linge D E (trans, ed) University of California Press, Berkeley

Gadamer H–G 1979 Reason in the age of science. Laurence F G (trans) Massachusetts Institute of Technology, Boston, pp 82

Harre R 1985 The philosophies of science, 2nd edn. Oxford University Press, Oxford

Hesse H 1954 Siddhartha. Rosner H (trans) Picador Classics, London

Hospers J 1988 An introduction to philosophical analysis, 3rd edn. Routledge, London

Kessler G E 1992 Voices of wisdom. Wadsworth, Belmont, California, p 7

Laudan L 1990 Science and relativism. University of Chicago Press, Chicago

Lehrer K 1990 Theory of knowledge. Routledge, London

Marriner–Tomey A (ed) 1989 Nursing theorists and their work, 2nd edn. C V Mosby, St Louis

Meleis A I 1991 Theoretical nursing development and progress, 2nd edn. J B Lippincott, Philadelphia, pp 116

Mercer I F 1990 Crystals. British Museum (Natural History), London

Musgrave A 1993 Common sense, science and scepticism. Cambridge University Press, Cambridge

Pojman L P 1993 The theory of knowledge. Wadsworth, Belmont, California

Polanyi M 1962 Personal knowledge. University of Chicago Press, Chicago

Schultz P R, Meleis A I 1988 Nursing epistemology: traditions, insights, questions. Image, Journal of Nursing Scholarship 20(4):217–221

Speake J 1979 A dictionary of philosophy. Pan Books, London, pp 315

Sprigge T L S 1985 Theories of existence. Penguin, London

Wood E A 1977 Crystals and light, 2nd edn. Dover Publications, New York, pp 132

On being a scholar

CAROLYN EMDEN

Introduction

'Being a scholar' conjures up different images. For one, perhaps library stacks, manuscripts and Tibetan monasteries come to mind; for another, images of tattered note pads, warm beer and noisy corner pubs might surface. For most of us, it's an intuitive matter: modestly, we tend not to class ourselves as scholars and kindly, we are not inclined to prod our scholarly friends about their lives. Be this as it may, the terms 'nursing scholar' and 'nursing scholarship' are to be found with increasing frequency within nursing literatures, their presence providing an air of seriousness and maturity—or perhaps, a 'coming of age' of a nursing discipline. But what of the lived-worlds of scholars? What do we know of their ways of thinking and how they came to be scholars? And what can be learned from their experiences—nursing and non-nursing?

These and other questions prompted a phenomenological inquiry into the lives of four scholars (whose real names have not been used): Helen and Mark are both professors of Nursing; Alison is a senior lecturer within a Department of Women's Studies; and Craig is an associate professor within a School of Education where he teaches religion studies. Each scholar works in a different Australian university; all hold doctoral degrees.

Through a process of phenomenological interviews, narrative analysis of data and creation of core stories, followed by further thematic analysis and contrasting of core stories, a set of 'hallmarks' characterising the four scholars was eventually derived. *Hallmarks of a scholar* had not been a specific topic of conversation with the scholars, but the following common characteristics and experiences were found to make up their lived-worlds:

- intense curiosity
- disenchantment with, and effort to improve, prevailing systems

- tenacity for progress within one's scholarly life
- ability to move between disciplines and their respective schools of thought
- holding a viewpoint, and (linked to this)
- an openness to scrutiny from peers.

The scholars' stories as told and interpreted through these hallmarks provide an indication of the kind of people (scholars) with whom we mix in our professional lives, their backgrounds, aspirations, and working habits. They indicate the diverse historical, social, and political contexts in which scholars develop and produce scholarly work. They provide insight into the transdisciplinary nature of scholarship and they reveal the scholars' viewpoints on several relevant topics. The chapter includes an 'exchange' between the scholars based on their reactions to one another's stories and the derived hallmarks. As well, a further viewpoint on scholarship from Afaf Meleis is discussed, together with its implications for nursing education. This 'backstage' insight into the lives of scholars begins, then, with Helen talking about her early childhood curiosity.

Intense intellectual curiosity

Helen remembers curiosity beginning at an early age with her father encouraging her 'to work out why things are the way they are'. In fact, she cannot remember when she hasn't been interested in the world of ideas and recalls how, in her nursing training, which was taught as facts to be memorised, she 'unpicked the knowledge and put it together in a way that conceptualised it'.

Mark also was not impressed with his nursing training ('a lot of it was routinised knowledge, a list of things to be learned and rules of various things'), and it was only when he later went to university that he found his curiosity satisfied and learning stimulating: 'I was good at it; I enjoyed academic debate, and particularly writing assignments'. Now he is concerned with promoting curiosity in others: 'we should be setting people free to pursue their scholarship. I have little time for building constraints around people, or directing people; the fire for scholarship comes through personal experience, personal motivation, and intense interest in particular problems'.

Craig ponders as to whether he could be like a chap he met when he was on study leave from Oxford. 'He's the world expert on Samaritans and he's got this huge set of microfiches, with text and writings and commentaries and everything he'd ever want on Samaritans; and as he says, if someone asks for a paper, he pulls this and that out and puts something between and he's got a paper'. Craig admits although it is an attractive proposal: 'maybe I'm too curious and wouldn't be satisfied'.

Alison's curiosity is exemplified in many anecdotes: her first sense of being an intellectual and going to political meetings and films; remembering the excitement of finding in the letterbox the journal put out by the History Workshop Movement ('it was a wonderful thing to read'); recalling 'some wonderful seminars' in London with the Women's Feminist History Group at 'some dark spooky place' after which she would have to catch the late train back to Colchester; her passion for bringing to light early Australian female writers and constant hope of 'finding a secret cache of letters somewhere'.

Disenchantment with prevailing systems

Of the four scholars, Craig probably experienced the greatest upheaval in his scholastic career. Having established himself as a respected theologian with extensive education and five years of teaching experience at theological colleges, he faced a major crisis:

> I had reached a point where I'd fallen out with the church authorities; academically I had come to conclusions which were no longer acceptable within the Roman Catholic church. I'd had a whole series of confrontations between myself and the Catholic authorities; I realized all I was doing was waiting for some final confrontation at which I would walk out and that wasn't really honest, so I announced I would be leaving. Psychologically, it was putting tremendous pressure on me—the pressure of thinking one thing and being forced to say another—I've never felt such suffocation as I felt then.

Craig eventually went on to explore, within his PhD, 'where religious ideas come from, and how it is that they are able to control human beings and human activity'. Now he is aiming to establish a centre for the study of early Christianity in the university, where masters and PhD students can study particular areas.

An example of Helen's resolve to improve the prevailing system lies in this curriculum anecdote:

> At one stage we got this strange request from interstate to put something on nursing theory in our Diploma of Nursing Education curriculum or they wouldn't recognize the course...Because of my background in feminism and the philosophy of science, when I looked at this [nursing theory] literature I really did think, 'Good heavens, this is dreadful stuff'; I became a critic and the course I put together on it largely criticized what had happened to nursing theory. I got the sense that nurses were operating on a very primitive notion of what science was all about; in trying to produce these theories on the model of physical science, they weren't producing anything much scientific at all. I also started to think about the fact that it was women who were trying to develop a body of knowledge and I came to see the problems at the intersection between philosophy of science and feminism.

Mark's experiences from holding senior posts in several countries have led him to be particularly critical of the bureaucratic constraints upon nursing and to envisage alternative ways of functioning:

> I moved to a health authority where I began to understand the bureaucratic constraints upon nursing and the insularity of nursing; and to see nursing from the outside, and see the lack of flexibility in very senior nurses, in terms of collaborating with other people...I would recommend to any nurse leader, to spend some time outside of nursing, working with nurses, to get a different perspective of how nursing is perceived from the outside...Nursing has been burdened for too long by hierarchic structures...The restructuring of nursing has to start with the way schools are managed, and the way students learn;

only when we've got those right, can we expect practice to become looser and nurses to have more autonomy. The nursing structures in practice areas need to become a lot looser; I'm particularly interested in nurses transferring from an employee status to a self-employed status; setting themselves up as independent practitioners and contracting with health agencies to provide the nursing required.

Alison has been an active campaigner for women's rights since becoming involved in the women's movement when she was 21 years old: 'Your feminism evolves, you get deeper understanding; it was very much part of my identity since the early seventies'. At this time there was only a tentative network among feminist scholars as her experience shows:

> I was teaching in a history department where I was the only woman; I was the one who was a tutor for two years, the other guy was a tutor for just one year before getting promoted. I feel in a sense I've served my apprenticeship for far too long already; I don't want to see other women missing the opportunities and encouragement that I should have had when younger, and not being taken seriously. I want to see them have support and encouragement to work in areas they see as important.

Alison attributes her lack of confidence about her work partly to her own character and family background, but also to a lack of role modelling in society, and the position of the woman scholar in Australia within a masculinist university. She has numerous anecdotes about efforts to change complacent attitudes towards women, for example:

> Then some of us formed a group and started campaigning about the lack of material around women's history particularly to do with our State; we harassed [personnel from] a TV channel who were doing a show on local history, saying 'but there are no women in it' and they got terribly nervous and ran around and plugged bits in; as a result of that the ABC did a three part program for schools on women and history.

Tenacity for progress within one's scholarly life

Any perception that scholars have an easy time in reaching their scholastic goals is dispelled by listening to these four individuals. All reveal dogged determination, with Alison having possibly the toughest experience:

> After history honours I asked the professor how I'd performed and said I was thinking of starting a part time masters, and he said 'People like you who only get a 2A shouldn't really bother' ...I've never forgotten that. I started a research masters part time but it was very unsatisfactory; my supervisor was having a nervous breakdown at the time and was unable to give any support and I felt very ambivalent about doing it. Somehow I finished after about four years and actually got quite good reports.

A second masters degree in social history at a British university was to follow:

> I did my thesis on 'British women at home in World War Two' which meant I had to go down to Kew to the Public Records Office; I would catch the train after nine when it was cheaper, then travel to the western side of London on the underground until it was actually overground; I used to get there about half past ten and go hammer and tongs all day on the records, and then come back. Other days I would cycle to Uni with the baby on the back; I got a tremendous amount out of that course; it was the first time I had been taught by a woman at tertiary level in the subject I really cared about...my supervisor, an esteemed feminist historian, became very important in my work.

Alison finished her thesis after she returned to Australia from her year's study leave, by which time she was expecting her second child. Within two years she was embarking on a PhD which took ten years to complete:

> ...it sounds like a long time but there were years when I didn't do terribly much; my thesis was on South Australian women writers in the nineteenth century; I could buy their books in second hand stores and work on them at home...when you've got two young kids and you work out of town, and the archives are only open from ten to four, that means a lot. When I was getting on in the thesis I remember feeling I was scrabbling around in the bushes in the wrong direction; I felt diffident talking about what I was doing and I'd think 'why am I doing it for god's sake?'. Then suddenly, instead of scrabbling among the bushes I found myself on the main highway. Writing that PhD and getting really good reports, and realizing my judgement had been very good about picking and developing that topic, with little support, has given me a great deal of confidence; now people are urging me to publish it.

Mark recalls (with disarming honesty) his entry to higher education:

> I was invited to be a tutor, and therefore began to teach. I hadn't been teaching long, when I realized I didn't actually know anything to teach anybody; I could read the book the same as anyone else could; I could give my lectures and practical sessions and do clinical education, but it wasn't really predicated on any indepth knowledge about anything...on that basis I decided to go to university and develop some strengths in academic disciplines...I actually did two degrees at the same time; one mainly in sociology and economics, and one mainly in psychology and education. When I finished these degrees, I was about 27, I was awarded a research scholarship and embarked on my PhD over a five year period, during which I also worked part-time as an administrator and an educator. The ideas in my thesis were mainly a Marxist interpretation of what was happening in nursing.

Mark is frank about his struggle to come to terms with what knowledge has meant to him over time:

I experienced knowledge as a student nurse as if it was outside of myself; as if there was knowledge which existed and needed to be assimilated in some way; and that knowledge was about facts, such as the bones of the skull, those sorts of things. Then at university I experienced knowledge as more related to social processes and social structures; I began to experience knowledge as the expression of power relationships; and more recently I've experienced knowledge on a much more personal basis, in terms of knowledge being the outcome of personal creativity; therefore knowledge has become more of a reflection upon myself than a response to what's going on outside. It's very hard to put into words because it's absolutely core to who I am and what I do.

After matriculation Craig studied theology for eight years ('all oriented towards a church career') and then was told he was to teach in a seminary and would have to study overseas. He undertook masters studies in theology and biblical studies at two universities in Rome, and then a postgraduate course in biblical studies and archeology in Jerusalem. It was in Jerusalem that he had his first inkling of being in the world of scholarship ('I was mixing with real scholars who were publishing and sharing ideas') and on his return to Australia he almost immediately began giving public lectures and serious writing.

When his major rift with the church authorities came five years later, Craig was without a job: 'It looked as though any academic career was coming to an end because all my qualifications were geared towards theology and the Roman Catholic church'. Eventually, on advice from friends, he decided to move into history and was able to enter a masters degree in this area:

I was assigned as supervisor a famous archeologist and even though as a supervisor he gave me virtually no help whatsoever, I enjoyed his company; he was an eccentric and we got on quite well together. The history department also offered me a tutorship to try and keep ends together, so I was tutoring in ancient history and writing a thesis in ancient history. My thesis was on the social structures of ancient Israelite society...the problem is still with me today...I worked on it solidly for two years and eventually ended up with a very good thesis which has stayed as a sound foundation for other work since.

After getting a job teaching religion studies in another State, Craig decided he needed a PhD, partly because he wanted to consolidate his position within his new institution and partly because he had become security conscious with the arrival of his first child; also, 'There was specific research that I wanted to do and I thought I had a good backdrop against which to do it'. He accomplished this in four years part-time while also running a department of religion studies. Craig's views on the value of PhDs are interesting:

I never saw my PhD as the requisite for being a scholar; in fact at my university there were people who actually despised PhDs, and saw them as something that people who needed to prove something went and did. My MA supervisor for example, who was world renowned as an archeologist and who had written many books, had a MA from Oxford full stop, and as far as he was concerned that was sufficient for anybody...he didn't ever dirty his hands with a PhD. When I did biblical studies, it was never expected that you would do a doctorate until you had been working for quite a long time. To get masters degrees in biblical studies presupposed that you already had a masters degree in theology, and the idea was that if you had those degrees, then you taught; you did research; you wrote; and only after ten, fifteen, or twenty years would you go back and do a doctorate; the doctorate came after quite a period of mature research and thinking.

Helen's father was the first person who always thought she could do better: 'If you came second in class, "why didn't you do better?"; and when you did come top, "It must be a pretty weak lot this year"'. After her general and midwifery training she left nursing to have a family and thinks it took her up to five years to recover from the hardening effects of her nursing experience:

> When I had children, all of a sudden it was brought home to me that you could lose someone you loved; I realized that I'd built a shell around myself to protect myself from death and suffering. I can remember howling my eyes out one morning about the thought that one of my children could die, or my husband could die; and suddenly realizing the shell that was warding my feelings off had gone from around me, and I made a resolution never to allow it to build up again.

Adult education classes were attended and work eventually resumed; and then Helen managed to win two scholarships in the same year: to attend nursing college for a diploma of education and university for an arts degree. Part-time work was continued together with the degree studies and then a further scholarship was won to complete the degree full-time:

> I chose subjects that I wanted to do, English and philosophy; I also picked up a minor in medieval history by accident. In third year I started doing an honours in philosophy and then transferred to education honours, and because of the English as well, I was doing double honours. In the midst of all this I took a good look at myself and realized that what I was trying to do would stretch a twenty year old—so I ended up with education honours. I wrote my thesis on the problems of nursing education in my State; I was able to take material from one area and apply it to another; that got me into the habit of looking at bodies of knowledge outside of nursing and seeing how they apply to nursing.

Helen went on to complete a masters degree in education; she could have undertaken a doctorate but: 'There really was no supervision; basically in what I did, you had to educate your supervisor before you started and I didn't want to do a doctorate in that situation'. Her thesis was on why there is always a shortage of qualified nurse educators: 'it was more or less in sociology; some people never go outside the nursing journals and nursing text books...I tend to read the nursing literature only to the extent that I need to see how it fits with other knowledge, particularly from women's studies. Helen later undertook a doctorate in nursing science overseas that had its shortcomings:

'Most people were striking for the first time the sort of stuff that I had actually been living with for a long time in my teaching, about problems in nursing knowledge development. Basically I discussed the problems of developing nursing knowledge, using philosophy of science and feminist literature'.

Ability to move between disciplines and their respective schools of thought

All scholars spoke of personal mobility between and among different disciplines, but Craig's experience is probably the most striking. After his theological training, advanced study in this area, and eventual study of history, Craig recalls:

> At that stage I realized I was now an historian: I was tutoring in ancient history; I was rubbing shoulders more or less as a peer with people teaching ancient history at university; and so, suddenly I found myself as an academic but in a different secular university and in a different discipline to that in which I began...I became as it were, ensconced in a different circle.

Over time, Craig realised there was a strand running through his academic work: 'The biblical studies I'd done overseas moved off into the history thesis, and the history thesis then moved off into the PhD thesis; there's been a direction to what I was doing. As a result I'd become a great generalist'.

People view him according to the context in which they know him, for example some still see him as the biblical studies scholar because he's written in certain circles, and has kept this up: 'I was at an international conference in Melbourne a couple of months ago where I gave a paper on the literary structure of the Letter of James'; some see him as the ancient historian: 'A week ago I was asked to talk to teachers of classical studies at one of their inservice days'; while others think of him as an Egyptologist: 'At Christmas I'm leading a study tour to Egypt'. Because people have known him only in one or other context 'They get absolutely freaked out when they find that I also teach biblical studies courses or that I'm supposed to be an Egyptologist'. Craig admits to at times not really knowing what he is, but:

> The areas are meshed together; there's an overarching set of values and thinking that keeps them in place and to me it's fairly unified...I don't think the disciplines are as discrete as we think them to be; secular religion studies, biblical studies, and history particularly have a certain commonality and I feel quite comfortable in moving from one to the other.

Helen is a firm advocate of using bodies of knowledge from different disciplines to enhance nursing knowledge. She has studied several areas outside the field of nursing to satisfy her learning interests, including English, philosophy, history, sociology, education and feminism. She believes scholarship is having a broad background with which to look at a particular area, or, as she says:

> ...developing ideas so they are a new synthesis, or a new way of putting together, sometimes old ideas and sometimes new ideas...scholars need

imagination and in a sense, it's seeing how you can follow an idea through and apply it to a different set of circumstances. So you might be reading in a particular area and think 'yes, if you follow that line of reasoning then such and such and so and so will bring consequences for nursing'.

Helen particularly is interested in new ways of looking at knowledge and the limits of knowledge. She sees nursing as lying outside 'the dominant model of what knowledge is about in our society' because it is largely women's work, but is heartened by feminist critiques of the structure of knowledge: 'the excitement is being part of a whole movement of rethinking the common assumptions that we've had about the world...nursing is an important part of rethinking the ordering of knowledge, and is a very good example of what's involved in female work and what happens as a result of under recognition'.

Alison talks about moving disciplines: 'I started being an historian and did honours history...[later] I became very interested in women's feminist history and that is the discipline I'd locate myself in, although more broadly in women's studies'. She refers to 'a whole critique of the divisions of the disciplines' and is not critical of her movement over the years. There were anxious moments nevertheless, for example when publishing some research: 'I sent the paper off interstate to the people who put out a literary journal; here I was, an historian, straying into literature and I was terrified I would make a fool of myself—but they said they'd publish it'.

Mark pursued his interest in different disciplines when he went to university after his nursing training. He studied sociology, psychology, philosophy, economics, and education; all of which he then put to use in his work as an administrator and later, as an educationalist and academic. He openly recommends nurses to seek out experiences and knowledge beyond their immediate realm in order to better understand their work within nursing. Mark has found this ability to move beyond the boundaries of his field invaluable to his career: 'I got a good handle on how decisions are made at the highest level...and a thorough grounding in the politics of health; then I went...[overseas] where I became sensitized especially to the importance of multicultural perspectives and feminist scholarship; then I came to Australia, where I'm putting together all those various elements'. For him, 'immersion in text, reading widely and deeply, and writing' are essential activities of nursing scholarship and he is critical of some higher degree students in nursing who 'would prefer not to have to think widely and critically about issues'.

Holding a viewpoint

With little prompting, all scholars proffered viewpoints on a range of topics, in lucid and convincing tones. Because these viewpoints were instructive in terms of the broader concerns of the study, one viewpoint from each scholar is (in part) retold here.

Mark is very interested in leadership issues, including his own leadership philosophy and style:

I spend a lot of time in reflection; I keep a journal and read a lot. I'm interested in how I actually put things together and the way I try to influence the school; all the time facing this issue of my lived experience as the Head of a school of nursing and the lived experience of others in the school; and the extent to which it is possible to take their experiences into account, and the kinds of management processes I can use to ensure I do that to the extent I want to; which is something I work at constantly. I have no problem thinking about what direction we should go in, my problem is to be sure there is sufficient support for the ideas of others; and that their ideas are given equal prominence in the way I think about things.

It was not hard to draw Alison's views on postmodernism:

Yes, in a way I'm a postmodern feminist but I find some of the theory extraordinarily difficult; it can become an elitist reactionary tool whereby some use it like a blunderbuss, to hit others and show how clever they are. I don't think it should be the only ideology; I still find a socialist analysis very important; and a liberal analysis which is about some of the changes you can achieve in the sort of society we live in, an analysis about progress and rights is very important. I've come to an understanding and accommodation where I can take the bits that please me. I like a very grounded understanding; people who can tell you about Lyotard and Derrida do not necessarily have an understanding of how it works in relation to something else in a grounded sense.

With much current discussion about a discipline of nursing, Helen's views in this area were timely:

A discipline is simply any area in which people wish to study. There have been traditional ways of delineating disciplines and some disciplines are seen as more prestigious than others; but basically any area of human thought or human activity is worthy of study, and the sort of thinking and experience that accumulates around that is what we call a discipline. I don't have any problem in seeing nursing as a discipline; the problem is that some disciplines have been privileged over others. The disciplines that have been privileged are the ones attached to the occupations that have been privileged; nursing is an underprivileged occupation carried out by an underprivileged group of people, and therefore people raise their eyebrows if you talk about the discipline of nursing, whereas they don't if you talk about the discipline of medicine or the discipline of theology, or the discipline of whatever else, dentistry or law perhaps; because basically these are occupations that have been built up in a male dominated world and have been privileged over those that have been formulated and developed in the female world. There is no reason to continue using these standards for judging disciplines.

Finally, Craig offered a viewpoint for aspiring scholars:

As far as advice to aspiring scholars goes, once they've decided what area they are going to work in, I stress that it is necessary to get all the skills required to be a self sufficient person. You must work out whether you are going to need ancient languages: if you are going to be an Egyptologist, you must go away and do hieroglyphics; if you're going to work in the biblical field, you must have Hebrew and Greek, and have them well. Then secondly, they also need to have control of secondary literature, so that means that they must have the main languages such as French, German and to a lesser extent, Italian, those at least, so again, you're not at the beck and call of someone else who says 'Oh look, the very latest trend over in France is such and such'; you can go yourself and find out what it is and understand it. Then, depending upon the sort of work that you're going to do, you must formulate a methodology; it might be that you want to move into a historical methodology, or phenomenology, or you might be interested in feminist hermeneutics, but you must find what you regard as the attractive methodology, where it differs from other methodologies, and what its capabilities are. It's only when that ground work has been done that you can go ahead and start doing something worth while.

An openness to scrutiny from peers

Linked to the scholars' obvious possession of views on various matters, was their clear willingness to 'go public' with their professional viewpoints—as indicated by fragments of stories to do with publication and presentations. Although willing, and indeed wishing, for public scrutiny from peers in this regard, the actual production of ideas for public presentation appeared to be a challenging process for the scholars. As Helen says:

> At the moment I'm writing a book...people say I write well and I think that's probably true, but I put a lot of work into it. The end product seems almost effortless and because it just flows off the page, people think it just flows onto the page. I agonize over a particular idea until it comes in the right words to make it clear; once I get the right words, it looks effortless— but actually a lot of effort goes into it.

Mark talks not so much about his writing but about what it means to be a professor in his field, that is, to publicly profess: 'Our core values are what's really important. I think anybody who is a professor of nursing has to hold core values about nursing, and if they don't then I don't think that they have the inner resource to actually lead in nursing. This is no place for the faint hearted'.

Alison recalls her first publications coming out of talks she gave early in her career, and of many papers since: 'I find one has this expectation of conference papers, that they are going to be brilliantly well received or that you're going to be damned, and really neither ever happens; there are a few desultory questions and occasionally you find someone who really is interested'. She remembers being prodded by her thesis supervisor as to what was happening about publication of her master's thesis, and the excitement of the eventual publication of part of it in an international journal. Anecdotes of involvement in several books reveal some agonising experiences, for example:

We hired a freelance writer for three months but the manuscript was huge and in very poor shape, no publisher would have taken it; then the writer had to leave and so a couple of us worked on it and became co-authors...it hasn't sold a million but it's being used as a text book here at university and it's quite a good book really.

Despite an extensive publishing record, Craig admits to some reluctance with his writing:

It wasn't that I deliberately set out and said 'I will write as part of my scholarly life'; it's almost as if I've been pushed into it, particularly books...people would come to me and say 'Look, you've got a flair for writing text books' and I would feel pressured. It's happening right at the moment; yesterday I met with a publisher in the morning and a publisher in the afternoon, both of them saying 'These are the projects we've got, will you be interested?' and so on. Writing books is particularly time consuming; I'm getting used to using a computer and that makes things much easier, but it still takes time; for weeks now I've been at my desk at five o'clock in the morning.

His writing style has been a mixture of 'a popular mode and much more serious stuff and includes something like sixteen books'. Nevertheless when reflecting on his writing, Craig concludes: 'the serious articles I've published are much more at the cutting edge of my own research and, if I was going to be judged, I'd prefer to be judged on the articles rather than the books'. He also provides a valuable clue to his writing success:

It's been a great advantage belonging to a circle of scholars; they are very friendly, honest people whose opinion I respect. If I'm writing something I'll send a draft to two or three of them and they'll kindly read it and send it back with suggestions and questions and on the basis of that, I'll redraft it and begin to see it from their point of view and in the end it will be a much better piece than it was before.

On being a scholar

On being gently pressed as to how they viewed themselves as scholars, all became similarly reticent. It was as if, despite stunning accomplishments, 'being a scholar' is not something one flaunts, but rather continually aspires to. Mark comments:

I don't think of myself as a scholar primarily...I believe I made appointment to professor on the grounds of my academic qualifications and performance; research track record, particularly for external funding; and the leadership I can bring enriched by experiences that might not be available to many nurses. So I'm perfectly comfortable with the title of professor, but less comfortable with identification as scholar. In my career, various things have detracted me from scholarship; what was missing was mentoring or steering and I now feel a responsibility to mentor and support, and not leave nurses in the situation I was in.

Alison recalls that at an early stage in her career: 'I had then more a sense, not so much of being a scholar, but an intellectual, where your work and interests are tied together'. She refers to there being only 'a tentative network among feminist scholars through the early seventies' (of which she was a part), but then later, her exhilaration at the attendance of two thousand women at the Women and Labour conference held in Adelaide (at which she presented a scholarly paper). Helen says:

> I haven't ever really thought of myself as a scholar, except fairly recently when people have started to refer to me in that way; its just doing what seemed at hand, and getting qualifications that you need for the job. People now seem to think that maybe there's something in what I'm saying if only because I'm now a professor; but yes, I suppose I do have a little bit of scholarly nous.

Craig admits to a sense of scholarship only when he arrived back from overseas 'able to read ancient Greek, Hebrew, and Aramaic' and also having a 'good reading knowledge' of German, French, and Italian, as well as having learnt textual criticism. As he says with convincing simplicity (and significance for young scholars): 'I think it was a feeling of self sufficiency that meant to me I was a scholar'.

Reactions and reflections

The four scholars may well have enjoyed an opportunity to meet one another after perusing the above analysis of their stories (and indeed but for their far flung geographic locations this would have been a possibility within the design of the study). Instead, they reacted in writing to one another's stories, as presented around the concept of 'hallmarks of a scholar'. General comments included 'extremely interesting'; 'really interesting'; and 'self-revealing and accurate'. Alison thought there may be further hallmarks; Helen was relieved that 'consistency is not required among scholars' (or 'even within scholars' as she humorously commented); Craig thought that I may have 'chanced on individuals who had found self sufficiency in the "academic world"'—knowing that others have felt 'tied down by its restraints, which were ultimately tied up in its administration'.

More specifically: in relation to 'intense intellectual curiosity', Craig ponders that there is 'little evidence of self-satisfaction' in the stories, for example there is 'no mention of seeking money or position etc.; lectureships, professorships etc. seem to have come unawares'. Helen 'strongly agrees' with Mark's ideas about the 'fire for scholarship' coming from within and finds that it ties in with her 'experience of research supervision'. She also admits to having felt she 'should be more like' Craig's chap from Oxford with the huge set of microfiches, but like Craig, thinks that it 'just would not satisfy' her. Mark is reminded of hours spent in the medical library as a student nurse, reading about psychiatry: 'special permission was required and it was quite a ritual to get the key'.

On 'disenchantment with, and effort to improve prevailing systems', and in response to Mark's point about the need for nurses in independent practice, Helen is 'ambivalent' because she believes this approach tends to 'commodify nursing'. Helen also states a shared interest with Alison in feminism, arising about the same time or a little earlier. Craig's experience with the Catholic authorities prompts Mark to recall his times of being thoroughly disillusioned with nursing but then, 'when I have worked in non-nursing positions, I have always felt immediately drawn back to nursing'. He also finds Helen's anecdote about not wishing to teach some nursing theory reflects part of his own experience when he felt drawn back to study sociology, 'because it seemed to offer the stimulation of radical perspectives' needed in nursing.

On 'tenacity for progress within one's scholarly life', Mark's comments about what knowledge has come to mean to him 'strikes a chord' with Alison:

> It was only when I did my DipEd and was becoming involved with social and feminist ideas that I really had the sense of integrating my learning within me and related it to a sense of values...I think that is why women's studies is so exciting to many students because they are learning something about which they care; it relates to the fabric of their lives and identities and values.

Helen comments that Mark's experiences about knowledge were 'reversed' for her in that 'knowledge as creativity came before knowledge as power'. Helen also shares something of Craig's 'religious struggle' having had one of her own ('fundamentalist rather than Catholic') arising at a similar life-stage; but as she says, 'Craig had more at stake occupationally'. She also shares Alison's 'very female struggle to combine family, work and study'. Helen comments that she had something of Craig's experience of mixing with scholars when she was overseas, but thinks 'it is an area where nursing is relatively weak yet'. She also acknowledges that in response to Craig's comments about not pursuing a doctorate until late in one's career, part of her 'protests that this should still be the case'. Craig observes it is apparent that all the scholars experienced 'satisfaction in progressive research'. Mark agrees that the road to scholarship 'winds uphill all the way', but that eventually the path narrows to where 'one must dare to stand alone'. Helen's mention of her father's encouragement also prompts Mark to comment on his wife's encouragement for him 'to achieve something of his potential'.

On 'ability to move between disciplines and their respective schools of thought', Craig observes that all the scholars have used skills from one area in another or others. He sees this almost like a 'personal revolution', like Kuhn's 'scientific revolution', and muses whether this could be the basis for 'a model of scholarship'. In terms of 'holding a viewpoint', Alison finds Mark's views about leadership 'interesting and relevant to her own situation as head of department'. Helen strongly agrees with Alison's views about some postmodern theory becoming 'an elitist reactionary tool' and that a 'grounded understanding' is necessary. In an equally enthusiastic vein, Alison strongly agrees with Helen's comments about disciplines, especially the notion that a discipline is 'simply any area in which people wish to study' and that some disciplines have become privileged over others because they have been built up in a male dominated world. Alison also agrees with Craig's ideas about scholars needing to become self-sufficient through a sound study of relevant areas; as she says: 'When you read a great book and look at the footnotes you can see the broad and deep base which is being drawn upon; my regrets are that I haven't done this more'. Concerning 'an openness to scrutiny from peers': Alison expresses doubt as to whether all scholars are open to scrutiny. She suggests many fear it and admits she usually feels 'quite anxious about giving and publishing papers'. In response to Craig's anecdote about passing draft work among a friendly circle of scholars, Helen suggests this is another area that 'nursing has not yet developed well'.

Another viewpoint

By the nature of their 'discussion' the scholars validated the proposed hallmarks—at least as being valid among themselves. It is interesting therefore to consider a further view:

> A scholar is a thinker, one who conceptualizes the questions as well as pursues the answers. A scholar is able to see the questions as parts of the whole of the discipline. A scholar has a sense of history, a vision of the whole, a commitment to a discipline, and an understanding of how scientific work is related to the discipline's mission and to humanity as a whole. A scholar has a lifelong commitment to the development of knowledge in the discipline and therefore is always engaged in a systematic program for knowledge development. A scholar is flexible, has a well-developed theoretical orientation, and seeks and engages in pertinent philosophical debates (Meleis 1992).

Although advocating flexibility, Meleis is very concerned with 'the discipline' (nursing discipline), suggesting that all efforts must be directed towards this end. The participants in 'On being a scholar', in contrast, appeared to be more open minded as to how or where knowledge may be useful.

Meleis (1992) goes on to outline a curriculum for students enrolled in a doctoral program in nursing that has three components: coursework, socialisation and independent work. While acknowledging not all programs at this level have a coursework component, Meleis believes with an 'increasing volume of scholarly research and theoretical debate in nursing' seminars are the most efficient and effective way to develop knowledge in these areas. A doctoral program should also offer students the opportunity to develop 'a scholarly identity' that includes a sense of belonging to a scholarly group and research experiences such as research grant writing and presentation of research findings—in conjunction with mentors. Independent work involves the expectation that students will be able to develop and defend a proposal; complete an independent piece of research that makes a substantial contribution to the field; and communicate and defend the findings. Issues raised by Meleis as requiring ongoing attention include: the difference between

PhD and Doctor of Nursing Science programs; relationships between mentors, sponsors, and doctoral students; finding a balance (for graduates) between being well versed in a wide range of methodologies and possessing indepth expertise in any one (Meleis is concerned that some faculty 'who religiously defend one world view and one philosophy may limit students' options too early'); and ownership of research areas and data, especially with long term research residencies and research teams becoming a way of life.

These thoughts on formal preparation of scholars are relevant to the hallmarks of the experiences scholars discussed earlier: if there is an appreciation of hallmarks, then it follows that education can reasonably be directed towards exhibiting these. For example, by what means are nursing students (at all levels) encouraged to: develop their curiosity; challenge prevailing systems; overcome obstacles to their progress; read beyond their discipline; defend a viewpoint; and invite critique of their work? Meleis (1992) suggests that preparation for a scholarly career happens in a 'puzzle-fitting fashion' whereby the puzzle pieces fit together over time. This is in keeping with the dialogue of the participants in 'On being a scholar': over time (indeed from young ages), and as a result of various events in their lives, they came to recognise in themselves a sense of 'being a scholar'.

Conclusion

Being a scholar, it appears, is a highly personal experience. There seems no single route or preferred pathway to being a scholar; indeed, diversity and multiplicity may be the best clues to a scholarly life. The scholars in this study reported a diversity and multiplicity of study pursuits, work experiences, professional interests, reading habits, writing modes and viewpoints. Within the wide ranging nature of the scholars' lives, however, some elements of conversion are suggested. The scholars who participated in this study possess an intense curiosity about matters of interest to them, often from an early age; they find they are often disenchanted with the systems within which they work and live, and are willing to expend considerable energy on improving these systems; they have a tenacity for progress within their scholarly lives, even in the face of significant opposition; they have a remarkable ability to move with ease between different disciplines and schools of thought; they hold clear viewpoints on various topics that fall within their areas of expertise; and they are willing to expose themselves to scrutiny from their peers on these viewpoints.

The scholars also are prone to the human frailties of uncertainty of purpose, fear of failure, mistrust in personal ability, laziness, disappointment in standards achieved, insularity, procrastination, and the host of other feelings and habits that beset most of us a lot of the time. The scholars told different stories as to how they manage to pass through their dark periods into productivity, such as: having mentors at different career stages; being deeply committed to their field; having supportive family and friends; experiencing success; and belonging to a circle of like minded scholars. Clearly, scholars' lives do not fall into place without effort and intention—a common misconception of younger discipline members. On this basis, education for scholarship is a realistic prospect.

Somewhere along the educational pathway the fire for scholarship is lost, as evidenced by the small proportion of students who proceed to higher degree study. Teachers' attitudes towards scholarship may be critical to how students view scholarship: Do we seek to inspire students towards scholarship? Do we provide an example to nursing students through our own scholarship? Are we prepared to mentor nursing students? Do we include the skills of scholarship such as critical thinking, reading and writing within all topics taught as a matter of course? Do we introduce these aspects of scholarship from the very beginning of a nurse's education? The answers to these questions are of course mixed; some of us consistently seek to educate for scholarship, some of us sometimes do, some of us would like to but don't, and so on. One small study has demonstrated that individuals can reach high levels of scholarship from very different, and unexpected, beginnings; while generalisations are difficult, it can nevertheless be said with confidence that with an increased understanding of scholars' lives, of their lived-worlds, nurses are better placed to fulfil their own scholastic goals.

ACKNOWLEDGEMENTS

The four scholars who participated in this study are sincerely thanked for their generous interviews and sustained interest. Advice from Professor Judith Parker also is gratefully acknowledged.

REFERENCE

Meleis A I 1992 On the way to scholarship: from master's to doctorate. Journal of Professional Nursing 8:328-334

3

Critical theory scholarship and nursing

KAYE LONT

During the last 40 years there has been an exploration occurring to determine a suitable philosophy on which to base nurse education and research. The days of empiricist philosophy as the only theoretical grounding on which to base nursing knowledge are fast receding. Nurse scholars have sought to legitimise nursing knowledge as being more extensive than just knowledge of physiological changes in disease processes. A search has been underway for philosophies which allow the exploration of nursing as an ethical, aesthetic art as well as a science. These need to be comprehensive enough to enable understanding of how nurses know what they know, a grounding for research and the search for new knowledge.

One aspect of scholarship is about learning, and initially nursing is learned through the implementation of curricula in undergraduate programs. This chapter will discuss curricula from Schools of Nursing, from around Australia. In addition, the ideologies underlying curricula will be examined, because critical scholarship challenges assumptions that underpin nursing and can contribute to research by bringing alternative perspectives for exploration. Critical nursing scholarship can lead to a redefinition of the processes which currently ensure the reproduction of existing social relations of nursing with medicine and the institutions in which nurses practise.

Historical background to critical theory

During the 1930s there was a group of philosophers known as the logical positivists (the Vienna Circle). They espoused knowledge as being formulated through the testing of scientific hypotheses and emphasised objectivity, measurement, instrumentality, reliability and validity of the scientific method. Their aim was to theorise about phenomena in nature through description, explanation and prediction. This methodology has relevance today as it did

60 years ago, although it is limited when considering human phenomena and many aspects of nursing.

Around the same time there was another school of philosophers known as the Frankfurt School, and their aim was to show that there were other forms of knowledge than that provided by the positivists. Early critical theorists (Lukács, Horkheimer, Adorno and Marcuse) were part of a group of philosophers in the Frankfurt School. This group's aim was to generate theories which would show that different experiences provide differing realities, for instance, positivist or empirical knowledge provides an objective reality, whereas historical-hermeneutic knowledge provides understanding of subjective experience. Held (1980) explains the Frankfurt School's motivation as laying 'the foundation for an exploration, in an interdisciplinary research context, of questions concerning the conditions which make possible the reproduction and transformation of society, the meaning of culture, and the relation between the individual, society and nature'. In order to lay these foundations, these critical theorists believed that through the examination of social and political issues, they could critique prevailing ideology and aid in constructing a more rational and just world. In many ways these authors' ideas and writing were very distinctive and Habermas in particular, reworked the notion of critical theory.

An overview of Habermasian critical theory

Habermas is one of the most significant proponents of critical theory in the 20th century. In developing a theory of critical social science, he aimed to show that knowledge is made up of a priori ideas and concepts that an individual brings to every thought and perception. Knowledge does not occur in a vacuum but is gained through the compilation of human 'interests' in satisfying needs which have been developed and shaped by social and historical conditions. Therefore, according to Carr & Kemmis (1986) '...knowledge is the outcome of human activity that is motivated by natural needs and interests'.

Habermas' (1972) theory follows in a direct line from the philosophies of Descartes [1637] 1986, Hume [1739] 1969 and Kant [1781] (1929). These philosophers attempted to give accounts of how we know and what we can know. Kant appeared to tread the middle ground between Descartes' rationalism and Hume's empiricism. Kant's theoretical position did not wholly agree with Descartes' notion that reason alone gives us knowledge. In addition Kant's ideas differed from those of Hume, who believed that authentic knowledge only came through sense experience. Kant showed that reason and experience must work together in order for us to have understanding. However, Kant's philosophy did not explicate the role of social interaction in understanding and knowledge. He tended to philosophise on the level of the lone individual contemplating the complexities of the universe in solitude, whereas Habermas was to write that knowing subjects are also social and that social experience mediates the knowing. Therefore, the processes of knowing are inextricably interwoven in the usage of everyday language in every human interaction (Pusey 1987).

40

Habermas contended that '...we apprehend reality ground [in] three categories of possible knowledge: information that expands our power of technical control [technical knowledge constitutive interest]; interpretations that make possible the orientation of action within common traditions [practical knowledge constitutive interest]; and analyses that free consciousness from its dependence on hypostatized powers [emancipatory knowledge constitutive interest]'. Knowledge is not detached from individual concerns, it is constituted through everyday needs and interests that are shaped by social and historical conditions. Further, he said that these knowledge constitutive interests take form in the social organisation of the species, through work (modern society exists through labour), language (through tradition bound social interaction and language), and power (through social control and sanctions of individuals who do not conform to group norms).

Critical pedagogy

The Frankfurt school has provided theories for radical pedagogy to ed–ucationalists, particularly those educational theorists who are critical of Tylerian or systems approaches to education, which are based in the positivist paradigm (Giroux 1983). This is an aspect on which Freire based his work.

Freire's (1972, 1973) writings are an enticement to struggle against oppression which is historically built into consciousness. He strives to make overt the ways in which oppression is continued through cultural oppression. He raises the possibility of liberation through the formation of a critical consciousness. His method is to problematise taken for granted reality. He believed that problem solving is the thesis of technocrats (Freire 1973), which is underpinned by the empirico-scientific approach to research. This could be related to the problem solving approach utilised by the 'nursing process', which reduces human beings (for whom nurses care) into components with areas that require action, whether the problem is physical or psychological. Freire's (1973) theory of problematising is based around groups reflecting on reality and thus generating a critical consciousness which empowers them to alter social reality as it is imposed. The need for collaboration is vital as there is the possibility for cessation of reflective activity if attempted alone, because the realisation of being oppressed may add to the oppression one is already under.

Radical pedagogy was taken up by Carr and Kemmis (1986) for the education of teachers, so that the 'practice-theory' gap could be addressed as well as the instigation of a more collaborative approach to education and curriculum. Their position was to argue for the inclusion of school com-munities, principals, teachers, students and researchers in the process of educational reform. The pedagogical aims of critical theory for education and educational research (or for any professional discipline) are that it will enable the transformation of current educational practices to ones which are collaborative and participatory. From this position, Carr and Kemmis (1986) say that critical education '...is not research on or about education, it is research in and for education'. Consequently solving everyday problems is possible using critical theory, as oppressive social conditions are highlighted and

41

awareness of repressive ways of knowing and understanding the world are exposed. Thus, different ways of implementing research and education can be conceived by educators, students, practitioners and society.

Ascertaining nursing knowledge

In the United States of America (USA) from the 1950s onwards, nursing theories were formulated in order to distinguish nursing from medicine and other disciplines. Nursing theories were predominantly derived from personal knowledge of nursing and knowledge from other disciplines, such as psychology. By the 1970s schools of nursing were required to implement a conceptual framework for curricula to ensure accreditation (Meleis 1985). Gradually, logical positivism began to influence nursing research and shape theories of nursing (Cull-Wilby & Pepin 1987) which have, as a result reproduced some of the dominant ideologies of that time.

There has been movement in the thinking of theorists from interpersonal, systems and existential concepts toward holist perspectives in the past few years. Each has provided new knowledge for nursing, but no one perspective provides a complete framework for research, practice and pedagogy. Nor are these theories inclusive in being able to critique socio-historically structured knowledge and underlying ideologies.

Nursing theorists have soundly critiqued the empirical/scientific paradigm as being the only epistemology on which to base nursing theory (Carper 1978, Brown 1989, Pearson 1989, Thompson 1987). These critiques are based on the reality of nursing, which is one of human phenomena. The utilisation of the empirical paradigm alone, excludes subjective experience and meaning, and as the scientific method is supposedly 'value-free', and objective, it produces facts and 'provable' hypotheses. Carper's (1978) paper set the scene for change in theorising nursing knowledge. Carper analysed the patterns of knowing in nursing, which were categorised as

1 empirics, the science of nursing
2 esthetics, the art of nursing
3 the component of a personal knowledge in nursing
4 ethics, the component of moral knowledge in nursing

She indicated that none of these components alone can form the basis of nursing knowledge, and that they are not mutually exclusive. All are interrelated and need to be researched or developed inclusively to form a body of knowledge for nursing (Holter 1988). Furthermore, Winch (1993) raised criticisms about the use of the interpretative paradigm for the construction of nursing knowledge. She argued that the specificity of the context in which the research occurs, means that findings are not generalisable because there is no discussion about the broader social or political context.

Tacit knowledge has been explored by Benner (1984) and Benner and Wrubel (1989) by theorising about clinical practice, and explicating expert nursing practice. However, Holmes (1991) rightly points out that there are inherent problems in both of these works because the question about what constitutes 'expert' practice has not been answered. Meerabeau (1992) critiqued the ability of research to be able to apply adequately a methodology which will uncover tacit knowledge that practitioners have, simply because questionnaires would be unsuitable, although informal interviews and participant observation may be helpful. Two recent studies conducted in Australia (Street 1992, Lawler 1991) have added considerable weight to the argument for tapping the tacit knowledge of clinical nurses. Lawler (1991) articulated nursing knowledge which has never been covered in formal curricula, uncovering the aesthetic and ethical practices which abound in nursing practice.

Nursing research is now being conducted utilising many different methodologies such as critical ethnography (Street 1992), hermeneutical-dialectical methodology (Hedin 1987), poststructuralism (van der Reit 1993), feminist methodology (Leach 1993), critical theory using action research as the methodology (O'Brien 1993) and grounded theory (Lawler 1991). Nurses are now incorporating research methodologies which suit the particular questions being asked. The variety of methodologies enables a more comprehensive look at nursing and brings to light knowledge which the utilisation of only one research paradigm would not uncover.

Reflective processes are viewed as a way of uncovering knowledge in nursing because of the need to describe what nursing is. Nurse scholars are working to articulate and legitimate knowledge relating to nursing so that nursing knowledge will become recognised within the health care system. Writers such as Pearson (1989) and Gray and Forsstrom (1991) advocate theorising nursing from a position which is grounded in nursing practice. This links into Schön's (1983) theory of reflection-on-action, or reflecting back over events to identify practices and generate theories from these. There is a problem with this kind of knowledge as pointed out by Carr and Kemmis (1986) that although '...it may be true that consciousness "defines reality", it is equally true that reality may systematically distort consciousness'. With this form of theorising there needs to be a means by which self understandings and irrational beliefs and contradictory practices are distinguished. Collaborative discourse is a means by which critical self reflection on practice and theorising can be achieved.

More recently nurse academics from the USA have begun to incorporate critical theory in their writing (Allen 1990a, 1990b, Holter 1988, Thompson 1985, 1987). Overall there is a general exploration of how critical theory would answer nursing's need for a philosophy to underpin research, practice and pedagogy. Thompson (1987) wrote that critical scholarship was aimed at defining a pattern of thought and action which challenged the power relations encountered in the social reality of nursing. She discussed ways in which control and domination of nursing are exercised through distorted communication, as she wrote that '...language functions to reproduce relations of domination'. She raised the issue of pre-reflective practices which make unquestioning assumptions about the world, ensuring social control and domination. Her article explained that nurses have been able to name, analyse and critique the sources of institutionalised power relations and conditions and to protest these. She is one of the few nursing scholars in the USA who has included discussion of Habermas' later works on communication and the importance of language as being a means of domination and control. Thompson noted the similarity of critical theory to radical feminism whereby both encourage consciousness raising through critique and the use of language.

Another nurse academic from the United States who has also 'discovered' Habermas' critical theory and his later works on communicative action, is Allen (1990a). Nursing literature from the USA rarely mentions the work of scholars who emanate from a Marxist/socialist background. For example, Bevis and Murray (1990) wrote on hegemony in relation to a 'curriculum revolution', but did not state the historical background to the word (which is Gramscian in origin), or even whence their definition of hegemony came. According to Holmes (1993) when authors from the United States discuss critical theory as a research methodology 'there is a reluctance to openly state the political ideology on which it [critical theory] is founded'.

Critical theory and curricula in Australia

In Australia, the positivist model has been, and to a large extent still is, the predominant model for nursing practice, education and research. This trend is changing, as many Australian nursing curricula are now using American theorists' models of nursing on which to base their pedagogy and practice.

Habermas and Freire appear to be the main philosophers referred to in Australian nursing literature centred on critical theory, at this point in time (Holmes 1991, Cox et al 1991, O'Brien 1993, Cameron & Fassett 1993, Retsas 1993). In Australia, there appears to be a more concerted effort to examine critical theory for nursing, with an explosion of writing and conferences centred on it. Aspects of critical theory have also been broadly adopted in some curricula for nurse education. The promises of critical theory for nursing were discussed by Hickson (1990) when she argued for an understanding that nursing practice is socially and politically constructed, and as such, can be transformed. She described the changes which have already taken place in nursing, for example the transfer of nurse education from the hospitals to the tertiary sector and the implementation of phenomenological research to ascertain patients' experience of illness. However, as Bruni (1989 cited by Hickson 1990) points out, the discourse of nursing is related only to those changes which are perceived to occur within nursing, detached and isolated from the social, economic and political structures of institutions in which nursing is practised.

A cautionary note is included in Hickson's (1990) paper, relating to the belief that when hegemony and reification are identified in nursing institutions, nurses can 'automatically...reconstruct our social worlds, resist domination and no longer participate in maintaining the conditions of our own domination or the domination of others'. Hickson also noted that critical theory does not provide a 'recipe' for how these actions can be taken and it could be argued therefore that this is an inadequacy of critical theory. However, Carr and Kemmis (1986) point out that Habermas, in his writing on critical theory, did not give a 'recipe' of how his theory was to be put into practise. They detailed 'action research' as a method for research in education.

One way that critical theory was adopted in nursing was through pedagogy. Perry and Moss's (1989) article outlined a different way of thinking about curriculum (post Tyler) and included a discussion on the need for reflective processes to encourage transformative action, whereby the structures and traditions of nursing domination become overt. They outlined the process utilised in Deakin University's (1988) nurse education program, whereby the student is envisaged as being able to creatively and constructively transform clinical practice. This was to be undertaken through an innovative curriculum based upon Habermas' knowledge constitutive interests, so that various ways of knowing were utilised in the curriculum and educational process. This curriculum was to be process driven rather than objectives based, and students were encouraged to gain knowledge of nursing in many and varied ways (not all of which could be measured through behavioural objectives).

Brown (1989) puts forward a similar approach to that of Perry and Moss (1987), giving a very clear, incisive discussion on technical, practical and emancipatory knowledge and the role this knowledge will play in nurse education, thus attempting to educate nurses as practitioner-researchers with the ability to theorise their practice. She wrote of the reflexive partnership between theory and practice implying that this is a way for nurses to emancipate themselves and the discipline. Although Smyth is an academic in teacher education, he too has written on the subject of critical theory for nursing (1986). He said that by theorising about the social, cultural and political nature of their work, nurses can develop a language and an understanding of nursing which will ultimately lead to change, altering the constraints imposed on it. This is what a critical theory curriculum is about: a search for meaning. However, does this really have any impact on nursing practice or the understanding nurses have about how to change their environment?

Reflective practice is a tool of a critical approach to theory and practice which is utilised in nursing curricula. Writers such as Horsfall (1990) require students to reflect upon their experience of practice in debriefing sessions. Unfortunately in her paper, she has not encouraged nurses to to keep a written journal of their reflections for further, later reflection. Reflective processes are, according to Habermas (1972), a means to emancipating self, but there needs to be a 'critical' person to help uncover aspects of 'false consciousness', as often an individual may not be able to perceive power relationships unless these are initially pointed out. Horsfall acknowledges that debriefing, with its inherent reflective processes, is a form of stress management for students. She wrote that the aim of debriefing '...is to empower students by developing new understandings and/or skills'. This is a beginning to emancipatory practices but there still needs to be written reflection in order for rituals, myths and everyday practices to be reviewed critically at a later date. A point made by Goulet in the introduction to Freire (1973) is that action cannot be instituted without critical reflection, and that '...theory and introspection in the absence of collective social action is escapist idealism or wishful thinking'.

Nursing scholars in the United States have led the field in nursing theories in the past thirty years. However their theories were driven by the need to write curricula for nurse education programs. These theories unfortunately made no attempt to include any social analysis in their conceptual frameworks. In other words nursing theorists wrote theories which were used to underpin curricula, and were predominantly based on systems philosophies (Neuman 1982, Rogers 1970, King 1981). The need for nursing to have its own 'body' of knowledge was regarded as the means by which nursing could become a fully fledged profession. In recent years nurse academics in the United States have shifted their thinking from these original nursing theories, to look at curriculum development incorporating phenomenological or interpretative stances and latterly critical theory.

Analysis of curricula

To determine if critical theory has penetrated curriculum development and design in Australia, a letter was sent to 37 tertiary nurse education institutions by the author. The letter requested a copy of curriculum documents if any aspects of critical theory, reflective processes, knowledge constitutive interests, praxis or transformative action were included. Nine (23%) nurse education institutions responded by sending copies of their undergraduate nursing curriculum documents for perusal. It must be noted that these documents were sent in 1992 and many may have been changed or updated since that time. Nine documents are a small sample and may not be representative, although some aspects identified in those nine may be evident in documents not tendered. The author recognises that outcomes suggested by pedagogies referred to in the documents may not be the actual outcomes of nursing programs, because individual nurse educators interpret curriculum according to their own nursing and teaching philosophy.

The curriculum documents sent for perusal inferred that aspects of critical theory were included, however it is clear that the meaning of 'reflection' used in some of these documents is quite different to the meaning used in critical theory. The use of reflective practice in many of the curriculum documents relates to reflection on practice in order to improve self understanding which will lead to improved practise. Moreover, in one document, reflection is the final stage in a problem solving approach to patient care. In some documents knowledge of nursing is that knowledge which is derived from experience. The implication is that through this form of reflection, practice is perceived in an unconstrained and rational way, and that individual nurses are then able to shape their practice world, while at the same time practice shapes their perceptions. This form of reflection and the knowledge derived from it, is very limited in its capacity to place practice and the environment in which it occurs, in a social, historical and economic context.

All nine curriculum documents included objectives which are related to the Australasian Nurse Registering Authorities Conference (ANRAC) competencies (now known as the ANCI competencies), and the reflective components of each of the objectives comprise reflection on personal experiences which leads to the identification of values and beliefs held by the student. I would argue that this form of reflection is different from the reflective processes in critical theory and therefore, it is remiss of nursing institutions not to clearly state their understanding of reflection or to quote the ANRAC definition of reflection. The ANRAC reflective practice competency relates to self evaluation—not practising in areas outside of competency, being able to identify educational needs for self and others or valuing research. None of these areas relates in any way to critical theory and its explication of reflective processes. Therefore, knowledge gained from reflection is not about raising consciousness of restrictive or hegemonic practices or structures, but a means to generate personal practical knowledge (this is a desired outcome, but it needs to be clearly understood that this form of reflection is different from critical reflective processes). This is reminiscent of Schön's (1983) theory of reflection in and on action to increase knowledge of practice, rather than in the Habermasian sense of reflective processes which enable the formation of emancipatory knowledge.

Each of the curriculum documents made statements about turning out a competent, safe nursing practitioner who is able to make nursing diagnoses and clinical judgements, and implement the nursing process in practice. This is an interesting example of the difference between training for a particular profession and place of work rather than striving to develop an educated person. An argument could be presented that students are moulded into the correct product for the health care system, with the 'correct' values and knowledge base to perform according to expectations. The Habermasian idea of reflective processes needs to be incorporated with action to bring about change or committed action (Speedy 1990). Davies (1991) suggested that nurse education programs with a traditional focus devote more time to the practical aspects of nursing than to theory and that more reflection is required to bridge the practice-theory gap. However, if one engages in critical theorising then a practice-theory gap is not perceived, because practice and theory are in a dialectical relationship, whereby one does not occur without the other. The above analysis points to reflection or reflective processes being directed only at nursing practice and the means by which nursing theory and practice are integrated. In the Habermasian sense of reflective processes, it would be expected that students would also reflect on nursing practice and how it relates to theory, dialectically, rather than in the one way, linear fashion that appears to be espoused in all curricula reviewed. Reflection appears in most documents as a means of improving practice and personal knowledge of practice.

Only one of the documents implemented a process oriented curriculum. All other documents included behavioural objectives which students had to meet. These objectives included ANRAC competencies which tended to focus curricula on outcomes of student learning rather than the processes by which students gain knowledge of nursing. Stenhouse (1975) argued that '...the process model of curriculum...is more appropriate than the objectives model in the areas of the curriculum which centre on knowledge and understanding. The objectives model appears more suited to curricula areas which emphasize information and skills'. The overarching objectives of the curricula were to exit safe, competent practitioners, meaning that students would be able to practise legally, safely and competently. They would be able to use technologies and techniques for caring for clients' physical well being. Unfortunately improving practice was the extent to which political action or raised consciousness was directed. These documents did not overtly mention any of the criteria, except reflective practice, required in a critical theory curriculum.

One curriculum document examined indicated that Neuman's systems model has been adapted to explicate the philosophy of the school of nursing, as well as providing a 'pedagogical device' on which to base the curriculum. Another school of nursing included many nursing theories (Roy, King and Neuman) to underpin individual units of study. I would argue that nursing theories decontextualise the nurse, the person, the environment and health. For example, references by American nurse theorists to the environment in which nursing takes place is devoid of any other health care workers, only the nurse is discussed; nor is there any inclusion or discussion of social and historical data about the environment. Nursing is indicated as taking place in a vacuum. Additionally, the patient is often a different person when admitted to a health institution environment, simply because in Western society, people are socialised into the 'sick role' which encourages dependence and passivity. The patient is not their normal independent self in areas of decision making and personal autonomy (Bruni 1991).

Perceived ideologies immanent in curricula

Ideology refers to the social constraint or redefinition of individual desires and intent by external agencies (Giroux 1981, Apple 1990). This occurs through social structures (for example educational institutions) which produce (or reproduce) society and individual action. Ideology critique was argued by Marx as being the way for humanity to liberate itself from political oppression and imposed ways of thinking and acting. In focusing on ideology critique, critical theory attends to those forms of social life which subjugate people while at the same time serving the interests of those who would dominate (Carr & Kemmis 1986).

In analysing the curriculum documents, a number of themes became apparent. These were not overtly expressed, but were inherent in the statements and pedagogical practices outlined. Tertiary institutions (in this instance the reference is to schools of nursing), function as distributors of the ideological values and knowledge that they want nurses to possess. The culture of nursing is reproduced through nursing courses in ways other than through the overt curriculum. Pedagogical practices and resources shape learning to reproduce desired attributes.

Apple (1990), throughout his book 'Ideology and curriculum', discusses the close relationship between teaching practices and curriculum with the formation of consciousness and the socialisation of students into what is 'required' by society and the professional group they will join. Therefore, he views teaching as a political activity because of the overt and covert knowledge taught, the selection of content taught, the criteria and modes of student assessment and the evaluation techniques utilised to determine the effectiveness of teaching and learning. The socialising influence that educational programs can have on students is to inculcate them with the idea that '...knowing why is not as important as knowing how' (Davies 1991). According to Pitts (1985), the overt curriculum relates to knowledge and skills required by nurses to practise competently, whereas the covert curriculum inculcates values and attitudes which ensures the status quo in the socialisation of nurses. His ideas about the 'covert' curriculum, are similar to the phrase 'hidden curriculum' in teacher education parlance. Pitts contended that the socialisation of students is not confined to the overt curriculum; that the power relationship educators have with students ensures students' socialisation into accepting authority and hierarchical relationships, thus maintaining nurses' position of low status.

Ideology of the status quo

Curriculum development and implementation can have an enormous effect on nursing students' knowledge, values and attitudes. Curriculum based on behavioural objectives supports the maintenance of society as it presently exists, because of the separation of this form of knowledge inculcation from historical or critical analyses. The theoretical implications of behavioural frameworks are that the values inherent in these theories are covert and unstated, and knowledge is objectified (since prior experience and learning by the student does not intervene in the learning process), thus ensuring society is maintained in its present form. The environment in which objective reality is preferred to subjective experience, teaches conformity and adoption of the values of the educators or those with authority.

Although many curricula articulated pedagogical practices which were intended to emancipate and uncover meaning in nursing practice, they have in fact continued to socialise nursing students to conform to the status quo. Structures of teaching have not changed, therefore hierarchical relationships continue to dominate in the teacher-student relationship. Allen (1990b) wrote that nursing education needs to look at the structures in which it operates as well as the dialogue incorporated in the teaching/learning process. Dialogue includes issues of 'power, control and conformity' which impinge on education through the accreditation processes of nursing education. Giroux (1981) addresses educative practices as creating students who offer no resistance to the work practices and structures to which they graduate. He stated that 'corporate sanctioned personality traits include: punctuality, proper level of subordination, intellectual over-affective modes of response, respect for external rewards, and orderly work habits'.

Clinton (1993) wrote a powerful critique of reflective practices, where personal reflection is seen as an effective means by which to improve nursing practice. He critiques Schön's (1983) theory of reflection-in-action whereby the power and control that a professional has over a client is even greater through the implementation of this theory. According to Clinton, reflection-in-action through the use of theories in action, reduces the client's privacy, 'making interventions more deeply penetrating, even for those who wish to resist the efforts of the practitioner rather than to arrive at an agreed agenda for change'. This practice ensures the client comes even more under the control of the practitioner. Therefore, practitioners are able to define reality for their clients albeit in an open and mutually sharing relationship. His hypothesis is derived from Bourdieu's (cited in Clinton 1993) view that the professional fulfils the 'conservation and development of professional ideologies'. This means that although a practitioner engages the client in open dialogue, the internalised codes or ideologies of the particular profession are part of the sub-conscious identity of the professional, and therefore impact on the content and the way in which encounters occur. As nurses we:

> are embedded in our personal histories and in the specific histories relating to the contexts in which we work. We are also influenced by the histories which constitute medical domination, oppression by race, gender and economic means and by the construction of nursing in the past. These legacies are often unknown and more often unacknowledged, yet no nursing act is carried out in isolation [from these] (Street 1991).

Reflection by itself does not enable a practitioner to understand the impact that the above influences can have on the social context in which client-nurse interactions take place. Habits and routines are self imposed constraints and, because of the lack of personal understanding, situations and practices are seen as immutable. Consequently, reflection on theories in use (Schön cited by Clinton 1993) as a means to transform nursing practice, can only be achieved to the extent to which a practitioner is cognisant of influences which shape individual nursing practice.

Cox et al (1991) have noted that reflecting by oneself can be traumatic because of the difficulty in 'sustaining surfacing and transcending what may be our own distorted self-understandings, asking ourselves difficult, often self-exposing questions, facing the difficult answers to such questions, and, perhaps most particularly keeping our vision directed towards new possibilities for understanding and action'. Although nurse education needs to address all of these, in order for future practitioners to be able to practise in a reflective manner, the previously noted limitations of Schön's theory need to be kept in mind when considering the inclusion of his notions of reflective practices in nursing curricula. The possibility arises that what the student is critically reflecting on, is '...vacuous, ahistorical, one-sided and ideologically laden' (Apple 1990). The result for Apple is that students see knowledge as a social construct but fail to see '...*why* a particular form of social collectivity exists, *how* it is maintained and *who* benefits from it'. The reflective process, in the critical theory sense, is expected to lead to emancipatory knowledge which enable people to 'see' the ritual practices and hegemony which govern their work, and therefore actually 'see' the real workings of institutions in both their positive and negative lights. Illumination of the contradictions enables nurses to 'see' other ways of practising nursing and new ways of structuring their work and environment (Apple 1990).

Continuing dialogue and research with nurses and other health worker groups may in the future lead to a reshaping of health institutions which will break down the barriers of structural hegemonic practices to enable nurses to practise in an emancipated sphere free from oppression. For this to occur, nursing needs to be politicised and this can begin with the curriculum, whereby conscious attention to actively politicising the nature of teaching and learning, may in the future impact on nurses. Holmes (1991) says that to not do so gives 'nurses the impression that nursing is apolitical, that politics is to do with governments and institutions rather than with individuals, that they have nothing to say that is politically significant, that they are politically powerless, and that they are safe to remain in a state of political naivety'. Nursing education and theory needs to become political to equip future nurses to face the unfolding realities of their chosen field, in the rapidly changing health care sphere. To many nurses the reality of being able to assert control over work practices and the institutions in which they work is nonsensical. Hegemony is such that nurses remain and will continue to remain 'captives' of their environment and socialisation unless they become an 'organic' intellectual as described by Gramsci (1971), actively working, thinking and writing about their practice. Furthermore, Street (1992) writes that emancipatory knowledge and change 'takes a commitment to ideology critique and negotiated collaborative strategies for change and takes time'.

Science, rationalism and positivism

Thompson (1987) critiqued liberal nursing curricula in the USA as being consistent with and reproducing male, white, middle-class culture. This is inculcated through 'a positivist frame of reference concerning science, functionalism as a frame of reference concerning the social world, pro-fessionalism as an ideology that legitimizes class divisions in the social world, deontological and utilitarian ethical theory as frameworks for social ethics, and if progressive, liberal feminist content as a way of addressing the changing role of women'. She insisted that critical theory should be included in nursing curricula, in a positive, expansive environment.

Leddy and Pepper (1985) wrote that because '...nursing is a science and the nursing process is based on logic and scientific method', therefore ipso facto, the nursing process helps to professionalise nursing practice. The nursing process is also seen as a means to scientise (Lawler 1991) and legitimate nursing knowledge. Lawler described the scientising of nursing through the nursing process as 'assessing patient's needs using nursing histories (a term adapted from medicine), writing a plan of care (documentation is stressed), im-plementing that care and then evaluating it. More recently, another step was added—making nursing diagnoses (another term from medicine)'. She equated taking a nursing history, with the Foucaldian term 'nursing gaze' which she said 'poses a danger of subjecting the patient...to unnecessary surveillance'. Unfortunately, teaching the nursing process detracts from nursing students' ability to think about the care they give, because of the linear process that is followed in order to 'solve' problems. In particular the NANDA approach gives students a recipe or formula for solving the problems encountered in nursing practice (for example Gordon 1982). Hiraki (1992) made the point that in nursing texts there is an assumption that a translation can be made from caring to problem solving activities. Mason (1993) noted that there is an 'increasing recognition of the inappropriateness of generalising personal as well as technical aspects of care into mechanistic problem solving'. Problem solving approaches in nurse education supposedly teach students skills or a series of methods to enable them to take responsibility for their own learning. However, if the above arguments against the nursing process are accepted, there are implications for future curriculum design and pedagogical outcomes.

Pitts (1985) cited a study by Olesen and Whittaker (1965) whereby knowledge and values held by students may be implicitly replaced by those which conform more closely to those of the educator, through objectives based curriculum. Bevis (1990) stated that in the objectives model, both teacher and student are dominated and oppressed by the objectives and the 'authoritarian assumptions underlying the model'. She outlined the way in which this occurs; the teacher decides on the objectives to be met, selects the content to meet the objectives, designs the format for delivering the content, and implements the means of evaluation to determine if the objectives have been met. Bevis argued that in objectives based curricula there are many attitudes and values which are difficult to teach and evaluate. Among these are the qualities of an educated person, such as:

> critical thinking; creativity, flexibility; emancipation from oppressive and/ or conformist thinking; critical social consciousness; caring; ethical and moral commitment; insight; foresight; anticipatory inventiveness; originality; flexible strategizing; style; personal power; its acquisition, use, and sharing; a sense of the significant; the ability to cut cleanly to the core of issues; vision of the assumptions underlying issues and the assumptions underlying assumptions; the ability to engage in dialogue rather than polemics; skilled use of intuition; commitment to fraternal/sororital colleagueship and friendship; a sense of social, professional, and personal responsibility; and a continuing search for meaning.

In summary, Schools of Nursing through their curricula, are graduating students who have been socialised through a different social or cultural context (universities) but conform to the traditional mould of nurse.

Conclusion

The main criteria of the nine curricula analysed, were to inculcate new nursing recruits with the knowledge, attitudes and skills which would allow them to work safely within the hospital setting.

It was apparent from the curriculum documents studied, that there are many variations and interpretations of what constitutes critical theory. Analysis of the documents emphasised that critical theory has not impacted on curriculum development in a major way. The analysis showed clearly that academics designing these documents have largely incorporated the language of critical theory, in particular reflection, without incorporating the epistemological basis of critical theory. Emphasis is still on the attainment of the technical/instrumental skills of old, which can be easily taught and measured. The outcomes emphasise behaviours, skills and practices which fit within the health care system. There is a need to develop curricula which includes education in the history of nursing, the role of women and nurses in society, as well a critical analyses of the structures in which nursing occurs. The most pressing need is for nurse scholars to critically look at the ideologies underlying curricula and begin to think about undergraduate nurse education with a view to change the educational processes which currently promotes the status quo.

Habermasian critical theory is able to provide nursing with guiding principles to enable the exploration of how nurses know what they know, a grounding for research and the search for new knowledge, as well as a basis for curriculum development for the education of nurses for the 21st century.

REFERENCES

Allen D G 1990a Critical social theory and nursing education. In: Curriculum revolution: redefining the student-teacher relationship. National League for Nursing, New York

Allen D G 1990b The curriculum revolution: radical re-visioning of nursing education. Journal of Nursing Education 29(7):312-316

Apple M 1990 Ideology and curriculum, 2nd edn. Routledge Chapman Hall, New York

Benner P 1984 From novice to expert: excellence and power in clinical nursing practice. Addison-Wesley, Menlo Park

Benner P, Wrubel J 1989 The primacy of caring. Addison-Wesley, Menlo Park

Bevis E 1990 Has the revolution become the new religion? In: Curriculum revolution: redefining the student-teacher relationship. National League for Nursing, New York

Bevis E, Murray J 1990 The essence of the curriculum revolution: emancipatory teaching. Journal of Nursing Education 29(7):326-331

Brown J 1989 Emancipation through praxis: the reflexive relationship between theory and practice. In: Koch T (ed) Theory and practice: an evolving relationship. Conference proceedings, National Nursing Theory Conference. South Australian College of Advanced Education, Adelaide

Bruni N 1991 Nursing knowledge: processes of production. In: Gray G, Pratt R (eds) Towards a discipline of nursing. Churchill Livingstone, Melbourne

Cameron J, Fassett D 1993 The reflective practitioner and the development of a Bachelor of Nursing course (the practice-theory relationship; an experiential course? Conference proceedings, Critical theory, feminism and nursing. Quality Health Forums/Faculty Health Sciences, Griffith University, Gold Coast

Carper B 1978 Fundamental patterns of knowing in nursing. Advances in Nursing Science 1(1):13-23

Carr W, Kemmis S 1986 Becoming critical: knowing through action research. Deakin University, Victoria

Clinton M 1993 On reflection: towards a critique of reflective practice as a strategy for the development of nursing practice. Australian Journal of Mental Health Nursing 2(4):162-169

Cox H, Hickson P, Taylor B 1991 Exploring reflection: knowing and constructing practice. In: Gray G, Pratt R (eds) Towards a discipline of nursing. Churchill Livingstone, Melbourne

Cull-Wilby B, Pepin J 1987 Towards a coexistence of paradigms in nursing knowledge development. Journal of Advanced Nursing 12(4):515-521

Davies E 1991 The relationship between theory and practice in the educative process. In: Gray G, Pratt R (eds) Towards a discipline of nursing. Churchill Livingstone, Melbourne

Deakin University School of Nursing 1988 Diploma of Nursing Curriculum. Deakin University, Victoria

Descartes R [1637] 1986 Meditations on first philosophy. Cottingham J (trans). Cambridge University Press, Cambridge

Freire P 1972 Pedagogy of the oppressed. Penguin Books, Hammondsworth

Freire P 1973 Education for critical consciousness. Sheed Ward, London

Giroux H 1981 Ideology culture and the process of schooling. Temple University Press, Philadelphia

Giroux H 1983 Theory and resistance in education: A pedagogy for the opposition. Bergin & Garvey, Massachusetts

Gordon M 1982 Manual of nursing diagnosis. McGraw Hill, New York

Gramsci A 1971 Selections from prison notebooks. Hoare Q, Smith G (trans). Lawrence Wishart, London

Gray J, Forsstrum S 1991 Generating theory from practice: the reflective technique. In: Gray G, Pratt R (eds) Towards a discipline of nursing. Churchill Livingstone, Melbourne

Habermas J 1972 Knowledge and human interests. Shapiro J (trans). Heinemann, London

Hedin B 1987 Nursing education and social constraints: an indepth analysis. International Journal of Nursing Studies 24(3):261-270

Held D 1980 Introduction to critical theory Horkheimer to Habermas. University of California Press, Los Angeles

Hickson P 1990 The promises of critical theory. Conference proceedings Embodiment empowerment emancipation conference, La Trobe University, Melbourne

Hiraki A 1992 Tradition rationality and power in introductory nursing textbooks: a critical hermeneutics study. Advances in Nursing Science 14(3):1-12

Holmes C 1991 Theory: where are we going and what have we missed along the way? In: Gray G, Pratt R (eds) Towards a discipline of nursing. Churchill Livingstone, Melbourne

Holmes C 1993 Praxis: a case study in the depoliticization of methods in nursing research. Scholarly Inquiry for Nursing Practice: An International Journal 7(1):3-10

Holter I M 1988 Critical theory: a foundation for the development of nursing theories. Scholarly Inquiry for Nursing Practice 2(3):223-232

Horsfall J 1990 Clinical placement: prebriefing and debriefing as teaching strategies. The Australian Journal of Advanced Nursing 8(1):3-7

Hume D [1739] 1969 A treatise of human nature. Penguin, Hammondsworth

Kant I [1781] 1929 Critique of pure reason. Kemp Smith N (trans). MacMillen Education, London

King I 1981 A theory for nursing: a systems concepts process. John Wiley, New York

Lawler J 1991 Behind the screens: nursing somology and the problem of the body. Churchill Livingstone, Melbourne

Leach S 1993 Feminist research moral perspectives and nurse education. Conference proceedings, Critical theory, feminism and nursing. Quality Health Forums/ Faculty Health Sciences, Griffith University, Gold Coast

Leddy S, Pepper M 1985 Conceptual bases of professional nursing. J B Lippincott, London

Mason E A 1993 Nursing practice outside scientific positivist models. Conference proceedings, Critical theory, feminism and nursing. Quality Health Forums/ Faculty Health Sciences, Griffith University, Gold Coast

Meerabeau L 1992 Tacit nursing knowledge: an untapped resource or a methodological headache? Journal of Advanced Nursing 17:108-112

Meleis A (1985) Theoretical nursing: development and progress. J B Lippincott, Philadelphia

Neuman B 1982 The Neuman systems model: applications to nursing education and practice. Appleton Century Crofts, New York

O'Brien B 1993 An exploration of structure process and outcomes: nursing in four wards. Conference proceedings, Critical theory, feminism and nursing. Quality Health Forums/Faculty Health Sciences, Griffith University, Gold Coast

Pearson A 1989 Translating rhetoric into practice: theory in action. In: Koch T (ed) Theory and practise: an evolving relationship. Conference proceedings, National Nursing Theory Conference. South Australian College of Advanced Education, Adelaide

Perry J, Moss C 1989 Generating alternatives in nursing: turning curriculum into a living process. The Australian Journal of Advanced Nursing 6(2):35-40

Pitts T 1985 The covert curriculum what does nursing education really teach? Nursing Outlook 33(1):37-42

Pusey M 1987 Jurgen Habermas. Ellis Horwood, Sussex

Retsas A 1993 Religion caring and the body: toward a critical theory appraisal. Conference proceedings, Critical theory, feminism and nursing. Quality Health Forums/Faculty Health Sciences, Griffith University, Gold Coast

Rogers M 1970 An introduction to the theoretical basis of nursing. F A Davis, Philadelphia

Schön D 1983 The reflective practitioner: how professionals think in action. Basic Books, New York

Smyth WJ 1986 Leadership and pedagogy. Deakin University, Victoria

Speedy S 1990 Nursing theory and nursing education: ships that pass in the night? Conference proceedings, National Nursing Education Conference. La Trobe University, Melbourne

Stenhouse L 1975 An introduction to curriculum research and development. Heinemann, London

Street A 1991 From image to action: reflection in nursing practice. Deakin University, Victoria

Street A 1992 Inside nursing: a critical ethnography of clinical nursing practice. State University of New York Press, New York

Thompson J L 1985 Practical discourse in nursing: going beyond empiricism and historicism. Advances in Nursing Science 7(4):59-71

Thompson J L 1987 Critical scholarship: the critique of domination in nursing. Advances in Nursing Science 10(1):27-38

van der Reit P 1993 Domestic violence and patient's perceptions of nursing discourse. Conference proceedings, Critical theory, feminism and nursing. Quality Health Forums/Faculty Health Sciences, Griffith University, Gold Coast

Winch S 1993 Constructing nursing knowledge implications of critical theory for nursing epistemology. Conference proceedings, Critical theory, feminism and nursing. Quality Health Forums/Faculty Health Sciences, Griffith University, Gold Coast

4

The emergence of a scholarly tradition in nursing

LINDA WORRALL-CARTER

Nursing is an art; and if it is to be made an art, it requires as exclusive a devotion, as hard a preparation, as any painter's or sculptor's work; for what is the having to do with dead canvas or cold marble, compared with the living body...it is one of the Fine Arts; I had almost said the finest of Fine Arts (Florence Nightingale in Donahue 1985).

Introduction

As an activity, nursing is probably as old as human existence itself. But as a formal, structured and scientific practice, modern nursing is remarkably recent, generally tracing its history to the work of Florence Nightingale in the mid 1850s. As recent literature has shown (Chaska 1990, Meleis 1991) nursing has continued to evolve and develop at an ever-increasing rate, so that now, in the closing years of the twentieth century, it is making a strong bid for acceptance as a fully-fledged profession.

One of the corollaries of this rapid professionalisation has been increased attention to systematic and disciplined nursing education, first in the hospital sector, but more recently in universities. Throughout Australia, as elsewhere in the world, programs of nurse education have been established in the higher education sector. This has impacted not only on the type of students being attracted to the field, but also on the curriculum, teaching approaches, assessment practices and general intellectual culture of the courses. It has also meant that those responsible for designing, managing and teaching such programs have had to embrace many of the norms and standards that prevail elsewhere in the university sector.

Of course, as academics come to be recruited from among graduates from such programs, it is likely that they will have relatively little difficulty in adapting to the expectations and mores of higher education, as these will be familiar to them. But in the initial stages, when almost all of the faculty are drawn from among the ranks of the hospital trained, and few hold higher degrees in nursing or indeed in any other field, academic conventions may seem strange and unfamiliar.

Central to the Western concept of the university is the notion of scholarship, and accordingly it is this which nurse academics will need to understand and to incorporate into their world view. The purpose of this chapter, therefore, is to explore what is meant by 'scholarship'—both traditionally and currently—and to examine what this means in terms of nurse education. The chapter argues that, although there are certain discrepancies between nursing and traditional forms of scholarship, emerging notions of scholarship are not entirely incompatible with the values and aspirations of most nurse academics; therefore, nurses may find it easier to become more scholarly in their practice. The chapter concludes with some recommendations about ways in which to encourage scholarship in nursing.

What is scholarship?

Scholarship can be defined succinctly as the acquisition of knowledge through study. The gathering of information, synthesising of new ideas and generating of new meanings all constitute scholarship. Most commonly when one thinks of a scholar, one calls to mind a person who is learned and intellectual, someone who is cultured, literate and studious. Traditionally scholarship is fundamental to the culture of the university. Becher (1989), Clark (1987), Harman (1989) and a number of others have all given attention to the issue of academic culture. Clark (1989), for instance, found that common values and beliefs were shared, and that for many research was the first priority. Indeed, the rewards system tends to reflect and reinforce the strong orientation towards the pursuit of new knowledge, based on the grounds of promoting academics for research and published scholarship.

Although some people clearly view scholarship as little more than a role, one among many performed by academics, for others it is a more far-reaching and overarching commitment to intellectual endeavour. May et al (1982) claim that scholarliness includes such things as scepticism, risk-taking with ideas, creativity, and taking the role of the critic. Whereas, Meleis (1992) suggests that the scholar is able to generate questions as well as answers, has a sense of history, is committed to the development of knowledge in the discipline, has a passion for excellence and a sense of integrity. Others describe it as a way of being; Armiger (1974), for instance, describes it as involving morality and commitment, and demanding involvement of the whole person, 'not only the intellectual and imaginative faculties alone'. In this paper scholarship will be referred to as encompassing these various aspects, but will concentrate specifically on the focus of research as this is the area which nurses need to develop in order to promote scholarship within the discipline.

What do scholars do?

Basically, scholars conceptualise, theorise, inquire, analyse, reflect, critique and evaluate. These skills are used to develop ideas, and then to communicate them to others. This they do through a variety of forms, but principally through writing and publishing. The publishing of articles in refereed journals and writing of books in relation to an academic's speciality are particularly valued. It appears that the rate of publication is linked to productivity, yet consideration should also be given to quality. Pelikan (1983) claims that the quality and impact of published work are difficult to assess, therefore quantitative methods of evaluating scholarship such as the number of books and articles in refereed journals tend to be used. But Allen (1990) argues that this method could be biased, as a controversial but poorly written article may attract many critical citations, whereas a well written article in a field with few scholars may rarely be cited. This latter is often the position for nurse educators in Australia, since scholarly activity is only just beginning to flourish.

Another common measure of scholarly productivity is not so much output (in terms of either quality or quantity of publications) but input; in other words, the number and size of research grants obtained. Managing to attract substantial research grants, and being the initiator of research and chief investigator will typically attain more kudos than merely being part of a research project. In this regard, too, nurse academics are at a disadvantage. They confront a vicious cycle: in order to obtain research funding, usually it is necessary to have a research record, and in order to develop a research record they must have attracted some research funding. For nurses, this 'Catch 22' situation is exacerbated by their workloads; they are commonly struggling to succeed in higher education with competing demands such as being in a new environment and trying to establish an identity for nursing. They are also in the position of attempting to gain higher degrees, being oriented to teaching rather than research, and of constantly developing new curricula, as well as trying to establish research and publication records.

The need for scholarship

It can be argued that the relationship between scholarship and nursing should not be seen as a one-way process, and nursing has as much to offer scholarship as vice versa. This is further discussed under a section on relating nursing to new concepts of scholarship. However, nursing has embraced the notion of scholarship for various reasons, such as establishing an identity as a discipline within the university; furthering the profession (for example, the practice of nursing) by drawing on and utilising clinical knowledge; and ensuring that there are nurse scholars who will continue the pursuit of new knowledge in the future.

Establishing an identity as a discipline

There are a multitude of factors which have shaped nursing. These include obvious ones, such as the women's movement, but also more subtle influences, such as the multicultural nature of Australian society. Many nurse academics have obtained their postgraduate degrees in North America and in other parts of the world, bringing with them a history and influence which contribute to the development of a nursing culture within Australia. A recent report by Anderson (1993) for the Department of Employment, Education and Training on sources of Australian academics' qualifications, highlights a longstanding practice of making academic appointments which favour non-Australians. Thus, they are recruited because they are non-Australian and because their academic qualification has been obtained overseas. The statistics show that 19% of university academics obtained their highest qualification from the United Kingdom and 13% from North America. Foreign recruits account for one quarter of all university academics, which on the one hand encourages cross-fertilisation between countries but on the other hand can lead to the favouring of or adopting trends which are occurring in the United States of America (USA) or the United Kingdom. Much of the literature cited in this chapter is from North America and we can learn from their experience, but we should not lose sight of the need to develop our own identity for the discipline and our own vision for where nursing is heading in the future.

The discipline of nursing has grown most significantly over the last 20 years, and the two main factors which have promoted the discipline have been the development of nursing knowledge and the move of nurse education into the higher education sector. Meleis (1991) claims that theory provides disciplines with the means to articulate their foci, in other words theory is the foundation on which disciplines are based. Smyth (1986) argues that knowledge needs to be available for critique and contestation, therefore it should be publicly disclosed and available to be scrutinised and tested by others. Thus, scholarship combines theory which is based on research, and practice. It needs to be grounded in theory, documented accurately and available to other disciplines in order that nursing knowledge is validated. The second aspect which has promoted the discipline has been the move into higher education. However, this has been made more complicated by changes which were occurring in the higher education system itself. From 1957 to 1990, tertiary education in Australia constituted a two-tiered system—colleges of advanced education (CAEs) and universities—and when nursing transferred into higher education most schools entered the colleges. In 1991, the binary system was abolished and a Unified National System created. By amalgamating colleges to form universities or amalgamating colleges with existing universities, most schools of nursing entered the universities. This meant that many nurse educators had first to make the transition from hospital to CAEs which were predominantly teaching based, and then make a further move into the university, which had differing values including, in many cases, a predominantly research focus. Nurse academics have now established themselves in higher education and are beginning to produce scholarly work. They are questioning current practices and issues in nursing, and beginning to demonstrate to other disciplines that nursing can claim to be a discipline in its own right, and therefore worthy of being in the university.

Furthering the profession

Scholarship is not only fundamental to the development of nursing as a discipline, it underpins the whole nature of being in the higher education sector. Thus, it is of paramount importance that nurses develop norms and tools of scholarliness which they can use to further the practice of nursing. An infrastructure promoting nurse research has been implemented by professional organisations such as Royal College of Nursing, Australia and the Australian Nursing Federation. Nurse leaders in both the hospitals and the universities have begun to promote research in various forms, whether through collaborative or individual projects. A study by Sellick et al (1993) investigated how many hospitals in Victoria had a research policy. They found that 25% of the hospitals had nursing research policies, 45% expected nurses to be involved in research, 31% had nursing positions with primary research functions, 31% had nursing research committees and 50% provided some research education. Therefore, in many cases there is a commitment from the hospitals to pursue research in clinical practice, although as these statistics indicate, more hospitals should have a research policy and should not only encourage nurses to be involved, but ensure that there is adequate support.

Clinical scholarship is defined by Palmer (1986) as 'that knowledge derived from the analysis and synthesis of observations of clients and patients'. This type of scholarship is becoming more widespread, whether in established research centres in hospitals or as a part of the staff development programs run within hospitals. Development of research programs in hospitals and the establishment of research co-ordinators and research teams, contributes to a growing awareness of research and its application in practice. MacKay et al (1991) describe the development of such a program in Western Australia, and more recently Williams et al (1993) have outlined how 'fun' projects can increase awareness in such a program. These projects encourage nurses to learn more about the research process and they can be involved at any stage of the project. The areas chosen for promoting research are in prominent places (for example next to the canteen), they are inviting, the questionnaires take no more than ten minutes to complete and a prize is often offered on completion of the project. Rapid feedback is also given through hospital memos, newsletters and short reports, and should the program identify a knowledge deficit in staff then an educational program follows the project. By whatever approach it is implemented, clinical scholarship should be seen as an integral part of nursing scholarship.

Ensuring the supply of nurse scholars

The third and final reason why nursing should actively embrace the notion of scholarship relates to the previous two. If nursing is to strengthen its claims to disciplinary status, and consolidate its position as a recognised profession, then scholarship will need to become an integral part of the culture of nursing. Of course not all nurses will want to become scholars in the conventional sense of the term, just as not all doctors, lawyers, architects or accountants are scholars. But there is a distinct need for nurses to develop a writing culture and a scholarly record as well as developing into a community of scholars. The scholarship profile should not only include those issues which relate to clinical practice but also those which are foundational to educational practices, and those which underpin nursing as a discipline. As these elements progressively take hold, new generations of nurse scholars will arise to supplement and replace those already acting in this role. Nursing will further legitimise its claim to parity of esteem with other, longer established fields of scholarly endeavour.

Difficulties in establishing scholarship

Despite the compelling arguments in favour of developing a higher profile for scholarship in nursing, when examining the activities, qualities and characteristics traditionally associated with scholars and with scholarship in the university, it is evident that many—perhaps most—nurses do not easily fit the mould. In the sections that follow, several possible reasons for this are examined, before a consideration of how emerging notions of scholarship may provide a better 'fit' between scholarship and nursing.

Nursing is new to academe

The first and most obvious difficulty for nurses in embracing scholarship is that as a field, nursing is relatively new to academe. In Australia, it is only in the last decade that nursing has been within the university and only in the last few years that schools of nursing attached to the hospitals ceased to operate altogether. The socialisation process into academe helps to develop the associated skills for scholarship and in the past these skills have been significantly lacking in nurses. It is not surprising that many nurses experience something of a culture shock when embarking on their first experience with reading, conceptualising, philosophising and then writing, as most of them have only a limited academic background, and likewise lack role models. A longitudinal study by Donoghue et al (1994) on the impact of graduate education on the profession, found that students consistently had problems with professional writing, and those few who produced work of a publishable standard lacked the confidence to publish. However, the number of papers presented by nurses at conferences had increased, which was attributed to nurses preferring to disseminate knowledge by use of their verbal skills. Another study (Lewis & Barraclough 1993) into the expectations held by higher degree students on returning to study in universities, identified particular issues of concern to nurses enrolled in both a School of Education and a School of Health. These included:

- balancing the competing demands of home, work and study
- moving from clinical practice into higher education

- feeling the need for more structure, such as help with the asking of questions and dealing with content, and requiring closer direction and feedback from the supervisor
- lack of advanced written communication skills.

From the perspective of supervisors in both Schools, the students were highly motivated but needed more personal support in order to cope with the relative lack of research experience, and the juggling of commitments. They felt students needed to develop a sustained commitment to a single research project, and would often require help to overcome problems of bureaucracy, such as gaining access to hospitals for research projects. Often the research proposal would not be sanctioned if it was not viewed as favourable (for example the use of clinical decision making for nurses in critical care) which may have been due to medical influence on the hospital ethics committee.

Nursing is a practice-based field

A second consideration is the relatively applied, practice-based nature of nursing, as many nurses are simply not inclined towards scholarly work. This was identified as far back as 1927 by Grey, who pointed out that there are different types of people oriented to work: those who were primarily practical minded manual workers, or 'thing thinkers' as she called them; and 'idea thinkers' or ideationists—those who enjoyed research and study. The former were practical and very effective workers who provided high quality care to patients, but because they were practically oriented, rarely became scholars. The reason for this is possibly that the 'practical' nurse may experience the need to be active, as discussed by Armiger (1974) who alludes to the constant need for nurses to be 'doing things' and argues that they often experience a discomfort in just 'being'. Thus there is a need for nurses to learn the skills of reflection, and of taking quieter moments for the contemplation which invites creativity. The nature of scholarship does not include merely critiquing the work of others, researching a topic and writing up the results. It requires an intrinsic motivation to want to immerse oneself in the literature, to collect and work with the data and to write up the findings and disseminate these in various ways. It could be argued that not all nurses are suited to full scholarly work, which may include research, but this does not preclude them from assisting others in some way or from becoming involved in other forms of scholarship such as the giving of conference papers.

Furthermore, largely because of the practical focus of the field itself, nurse education has historically been more concerned with passing on 'craft' knowledge than with abstract theory. To the extent that many current nurse academics have considerable background experience in the hospital-based system of nurse education, and that they selected the career of nurse education because of their aptitude for teaching, both they and the field as a whole may find an emphasis on scholarship to be uncomfortable and even unwelcome.

When examining the practice disciplines, such as nursing and chiropractic which are new to academe there appears to be a tension for many academics. This is because they are grappling with the multiple expectations of gaining qualifications, teaching, and being engaged in new aspects of scholarship such as research and publications. Harman (1989) argues that practice-based disciplines share the traditional university culture with its commitment to scholarship and intellectual life, while on the other hand, they are necessarily involved with the transmission of vocational skills and attitudes for professional practice. Contrary to what Harman found, there is evidence in the nursing literature (Fawcett 1979, Pittman 1982) that many nurse academics have not entirely adopted the values of higher education and continue to have a preference for teaching above scholarship including research. This is not altogether surprising as the love of teaching was often the first reason for nurses turning to nurse education. The problem with valuing teaching above scholarship is that it not only disadvantages the nurse academic in promotion and tenure, but perhaps more importantly it disadvantages the profession as a whole. It is important that the devaluing of scholarship does not continue and that there is a change in 'valuing' and establishment of a scholarly research culture. The recognition of what scholarly activities include also needs to be broadened.

Not only is nursing a practice-based field, but it is also claims to be a 'caring' profession. Many people who were originally drawn into nursing were attracted by its tradition of concern for people. When nurse education was conducted in the hospitals, and later in the colleges of advanced education, this 'concern for people' could still be expressed primarily through the teaching role, especially in the clinical setting. To the extent that scholarship is more preoccupied with abstractions than with the experience and plight of real people, many nurse educators may find uncomfortable, even problematic, the necessity of bridging the gap between a concern for people and a concern with ideas.

Nursing is predominantly an oral culture

Since time immemorial, nurses have had to rely on gaining information orally. Not only have they had to listen carefully to what their patients are telling them, but they have had to communicate and work with other team members. This has included the tradition of 'handing over' patients with an overview of their condition at change of shifts. Against this background, it is little wonder that much nursing knowledge has been acquired informally, on-the-job, through oral communication. In recent years, however, the dominance of oral forms of communication has been challenged, partly by the need for more extensive documentation in the clinical areas, and partly through the emergence of a professional literature and the expectation that nurses, like other professionals will 'keep up with the literature'. Of course these two forms of written discourse place quite different demands on the literary skills of nurses. The collection of data from patients, or the compilation of case notes, involves a much less fully developed written culture than the ability to read (or indeed to contribute to) the professional literature. While it is to be expected that nurse academics, who are themselves the products of higher education institutions, will be able to deal more comfortably with the writing demands of academic life, there are those who have entered academe from hospital-based programs. These nurses may lack the 'academic literacy' that their students either already possess or are expected to develop during the course of their undergraduate studies.

Nursing has traditionally been dominated by women

In 1983, Cass et al explored the phenomenon of women in academe. While things may have improved markedly over the intervening decade or more, the fact remains that women in academe are still systematically disadvantaged compared to their male colleagues. Since nursing has traditionally been dominated by women (though this, too, is changing), nurse academics are subject to the same kinds of disadvantages and challenges that confront women academics generally.

It is hard to believe that entering the 19th century women were still continuing to disguise themselves as men whilst endeavouring to become well known and accomplished scholars. Examples of these early female scholars are George Elliot, George Sand and Currer Bell (Woolf 1929). The idea of women in those times 'having a voice' and daring to write and publish seemed preposterous, and thus it has taken women decades to become fully part of the academic community. Even now, the statistics are not altogether favourable. Taylor (1993) reports that only 10% of women academics are above senior lecturer level, 19% are senior lecturers, 39% are lecturers and 51% are below lecturer level. The figures are equally as poor for tenure and promotion. Allen (1990) states that 1 in 16 university academics is a full-time tenured woman, whereas 1 in 2 university academics is a full-time tenured man. Women continue to be in the lower ranks of academic employment and are taking longer to reach senior positions. She claims that this is because of lack of support (or even active discouragement) from superiors, as well as women being disadvantaged in access to informal networks which can provide a valuable source of information about employment. A study by Anderson (1993) found that more women than men had Masters degrees and the reverse was true of doctorates. Women are entering postgraduate studies significantly more than in the past. A report by the Department of Employment, Education and Training (1990) stated that 34% of enrolments in doctorates were women. So it can be seen that more women are undertaking doctoral programs and accordingly raising the profile of women in academe.

Factors such as the unfamiliarity with scholarship and the competing demands of domestic responsibilities including child care, are far from the only influences at work in shaping women's roles and experiences in academe. There are other subtle pressures at work, including women's values, and how they relate to others. Belenky et al (1986) argue that women have different ways of operating from men. These have been called 'different ways of knowing' and they include valuing connection, relationships and caring. All of these are values with which nurses are indoctrinated during their training and with which they operate in the hospital. As men often value achievement and separateness, there are differences which can sometimes lead women academics to feel undervalued. These findings were confirmed in a recent study in New Zealand by Lee and Fleming (1993). They interviewed 23 female academics to see what they did and did not like in the way men operated in the university, and identified women as operating differently when interacting with others. These included: listening to students and colleagues—giving them time at expense of their work; feeling less confident about new and challenging situations; tending to be modest; learning to balance and juggle competing demands; remaining silent in meetings rather than engaging in confrontation and argument; and being motivated towards teaching more than research, due to teaching being a participatory activity whereas research is a more solitary one.

Thus women use different skills when interacting with others, and they appear to favour teaching due to its being a more social activity. Likewise, a study by Pease (1993) who looked at the work roles adopted by males and females at universities in the USA, identified women as commonly being employed in areas of teaching which was parallel to the traditional mother/wife role. He goes on to say that 'teaching, like motherwork, is general, diffuse, inclusive and applied. Research, like fatherwork, is specialized, specific, segmental, and basic. Teachers and moms must be joans-of-all-specialities...The business of research, however, is specialization. Men specialize; women go into general practice'. This highlights the lack of value associated with teaching; women have occupied not only the lower ranks in the university but have also tended to accept a heavier teaching workload. For example the role of tutor or associate lecturer is predominantly to teach, and the higher one goes towards a professorial level the more research and administrative duties there are. Cass et al (1983) describe women as being in the university basically as teachers, taking the heavier role of teaching to serve the research and teaching demands of the male academics.

As nurses now constitute the largest contingent of females in academe, as a discipline, nursing has a role to play in the future of women in academe and scholarship. Although it is not an easy task, nurses are traditionally praised for their tenacity and overall commitment to their work. These characteristics should bear fruit for women in higher education, as well as for the discipline of nursing. At the same time there needs to be a change in the way universities define scholarship, to enable a broadening of the boundaries of scholarship to include other areas such as teaching, community work and clinical practice.

Changing conceptions of scholarship

As previously mentioned, in the majority of universities the major emphasis for advancement is on research, which is seen as the first and most essential form of scholarly activity. Although some credit is given to teaching, for the most part there is a substantial if not total preoccupation with the more esoteric forms of knowledge production and dissemination, through inquiry, critique and publication. While there is no doubt that these are vital aspects of the scholar's role, there are strong reasons for extending and broadening the notion of scholarship to include academics who not only conduct research and publish, but also convey their knowledge to students or apply what they have learned in often quite complex 'real world settings'. One person who has argued very strongly for this broader vision of scholarship is Ernest Boyer (1990) of the Carnegie Foundation for the Advancement of Teaching.

Boyer argues that knowledge is not developed in such a linear manner, that theory leads to practice and vice versa, and that teaching shapes both theory and practice. This points to a more comprehensive view of scholarship, one which includes teaching, research and service. For nursing there is also a need for service in both the hospital and the community to be taken into consideration, and progress has been made in the development of the connection between research and professional practice. This suggested change in the dimensions of scholarship indicates that the work of academic faculty needs to be redefined, so that it reflects more realistically the full range of academic and civic mandates. Boyer accepts that the work of the scholar includes original research but he argues that it is being able to step back from that research, and build bridges and see connections between theory and practice that is important. To describe his vision, Boyer talks about four concepts of scholarship: the scholarship of discovery, the scholarship of integration, the scholarship of application and the scholarship of teaching. In the next part of this chapter which draws freely and without specific acknowledgment on Boyer's work, each of these four will be addressed individually.

The 'scholarship of discovery' is classed as the development of knowledge and the freedom of inquiry which contributes to the intellectual climate of the university. This is probably the closest to the traditional notion of a scholar as a researcher, with publications as the primary yardstick by which scholarly productivity is measured. Traditionally, the type of research academics engage in is also of importance (for example scientific), as well as issues such as whether the research has been supported by a grant, and whether the academic is the primary researcher or assistant. There also appears to be a need for regular launching of new research projects and the development of publications on a regular basis. Boyer argues that this is very difficult for most scholars, as creativity 'doesn't work that way'—in other words according to demand—and often requires inspiration and sustained time out for writing. Boyer's solution is to broaden the range of writing to include not only articles in refereed journals and scholarly books, but also the writing of textbooks and writing for non-specialists 'as it requires a deep and thorough knowledge and keen literary skills to make complex ideas understood by a large audience'. Therefore all of these activities should be classed as scholarly endeavours.

Turning to the 'scholarship of integration' (which is related to the scholarship of discovery as it involves having to do the research first), the scholarship of integration underscores the need for scholars to give meaning to isolated facts, and encourages them to put these findings in perspective by making connections across disciplines. Boyer describes this as having the effect of illuminating data in a revealing way as it seeks to interpret, draw together and bring new insights from original research. He argues that carrying out research in a multidisciplinary area is not worth any less than discipline specific scholarship, indeed it may even be more valuable as it forces new knowledge to be developed at boundaries where fields and disciplines converge. This type of scholarship can be acknowledged in the designing of new courses and curricula, in the development of cross-disciplinary seminars, and in the use of television.

The 'scholarship of application' asks how knowledge can be applied to consequential problems. It is recognised that service (like teaching) is routinely praised but accorded little attention. One of the problems with service not being valued in the university is that it can inevitably force a devaluing by the profession. Boyer argues that service needs to be taken seriously as 'it is demanding work which requires vigour and accountability associated with research activities'. Service can include activities such as being on campus and on outside committees, which need to be connected to the academics special field of knowledge, and it can also be carried out through consultation, technical assistance, policy analysis and program evaluation.

Lastly, the 'scholarship of teaching' alludes to the fact that teaching was primarily the focus of scholarship until the mid 19th century. Since then, there has been the development of the PhD, and the emphasis previously on undergraduate education—which was predominantly teaching—is now on graduate education and research. Boyer argues that it is futile to talk about improving the quality of teaching if, in the end, faculty are not given recognition for the time they spend with students. Unfortunately it is assumed that all faculty can teach, which is why it is not rewarded. Yet in practice there are relatively few great teachers. Those that do exist are remarkable because they are rare; 'they create a common ground of intellectual commitment, stimulate active not passive learning, and encourage critical creative thinkers—which stimulates students to go on learning long after their college days are over'. Teaching, then, both educates and entices future scholars, and those who teach must be well informed and steeped in the knowledge of their fields. They should not only utilise lectures but also encourage reading, classroom discussion, comments and questions. Thus teaching can be well regarded only if academics are widely read and intellectually engaged.

While acknowledging that in practice all four categories are inextricably linked with each other, and that they interact, Boyer argues that it is important to tease apart and examine them as individual, intellectual functions before grouping them together and classifying them as 'academic work'. Thus other forms of scholarship such as teaching, integration and application need to be fully acknowledged and treated on an equal footing with the scholarship of discovery. He concludes that there is a need for scholars who not only skilfully explore the frontiers of knowledge but also integrate ideas, connect thought to action and inspire students.

Relating nursing to new conceptions of scholarship

There can be little doubt that nursing as a field has made very rapid progress in the past few years. Looking at the present status and extent of nursing education in Australia, it is hard to believe that a mere decade ago—much less in some cases—nurse education was entirely a matter for hospitals and their associated training schools. Nursing now has many of the trappings of a fully-fledged profession, including its own literature base (and scholarly journals), its own professional associations, its own scholarly conferences, and university level preparation including the availability of higher degrees. Progressively, graduates and programs are taking their place in the ranks of academe. With formal preparation in established approaches to research and scholarly inquiry, they are enjoying professional acceptance and recognition, not only in the field of nursing but more broadly across the university. Thus, in a very real sense, scholarship in nursing is increasingly a reality rather than a distant hope. In addition to this movement, which might be described as 'nursing embracing scholarship', there is another significant development, which might be described as 'scholarship embracing nursing'. By this it is meant that, in recent years, scholarship itself is being broadened and redefined in ways that are congruent with many of the fundamental values of nursing. In particular, the acceptance of forms of inquiry that are grounded in practice, or the recognition of forms of scholarship other than traditional 'research' have both allowed nursing to establish itself as a 'scholarly' activity.

Practice-based inquiry

Kelly (1992) in her paper on the question of nursing scholarship speculates as to what constitutes a scholarly person. She asks: 'Does the completion of a graduate or undergraduate degree make a scholarly person? Does the continuation of learning by whatever legitimate means compromise scholarship? Or should the term be reserved for nurses actively engaged in research and subsequent publication of findings?'. It is my view that scholarly activity should be carried out not only by those nurses in academe but also by those at the interface of clinical practice, and that all nurses can contribute to scholarship within nursing. It is not exclusively for nurse academics involved in research and publication. Thus, the pursuit of new knowledge should not be restricted to those who work solely in a university. It is the role and responsibility of all nurses, and many are finding that they are taking on the role of a scholar whether through gaining further qualifications or whilst carrying out research in a hospital. The notion of scholarship is not completely foreign to nurses or nursing and can be embraced by all in order to further develop the discipline of nursing.

A broader conception of scholarship

A community of scholars can be developed regardless of whether they work in hospital or university. I agree with Leininger (1974), who stated over 20 years ago that the hallmark of nursing scholarship 'and the true scholar of nursing is known by the substantive contributions which the nurse makes to the practice of nursing, teaching, research, the literature, society, and to other disciplines regarding nursing'. So whether the scholar is a nurse-practitioner, nurse-researcher, nurse-teacher, nurse-administrator, or in other roles, she or he will earn their reputation as a scholar for their substantive knowledge and special insights about nursing and their ability to communicate this knowledge by a variety of media to others.

From the foregoing, it is evident that nursing and scholarship are not as far apart as perhaps they were in the past. Not only are nurses and nurse academics increasingly comfortable with and competent at 'conventional' scholarship, but scholarship itself is undergoing a radical reorientation that makes it more consonant with the values underlying both nursing and nurse education. In this section of the chapter, attention will be focused on the steps that can be taken—by the profession, by schools and faculties in nursing, and by nurse academics themselves—to further strengthen and enhance scholarship in nursing.

Professional level

First, there needs to be promotion of scholarship at the overall level of the nursing profession. In a sense this has already begun by relocating Royal College of Nursing, Australia in Canberra. This will allow it to function alongside other professional bodies and put forward policies and the position of nursing in public policy decision making debates. Likewise, the National Review of Nurse Education (Reid 1994) is a form of scholarship on nursing, and examining educational issues and practices with a view to change is imperative for growth. One other way of promoting nursing is by the development of research centres in both the university and the hospital. The use of professors who are joint appointees can facilitate the promotion of research in the form of ongoing projects, and the sharing of expertise, as well as fostering collaboration between the university and the hospital staff. It would be impossible for one individual to do this alone, and she or he would need the support of the staff development units within the hospitals. There have been recent developments of this kind, with the establishment of professors in nursing based at a university but also holding a prominent position within the hospital. This, too, has not been without its problems. Barclay (1994) reports that the main obstacles came from people who had a vested interest in maintaining the status quo and from those who were not willing or open to learning or change, including both nursing and medical staff. However, the collaboration between health and education has resulted in a major increase in applied research, and the development of these research centres and encouraging clinical research is a major feat for nursing.

Another way of promoting nursing would be the establishment of endowed chairs. In the USA approximately 40 have been established within the last decade (Fitzpatrick & Carnegie 1991). Endowed chairs are highly prestigious. They are usually named after the benefactor, and are only awarded to the most distinguished academics, who are then able to carry on their own research. In Australia, there are approximately 18 fully or partially funded chairs, which are government funded and consist of both clinical and community chairs (James 1993). They represent a move in the right direction for nurses promoting scholarship in sectors other than the university.

At the level of discipline, scholarship involves developing knowledge, disseminating this knowledge and utilising it in various ways. The development of knowledge, as discussed previously, is important in the establishment of a discipline and one way of extending this is by the development of doctoral programs in nursing. There have already been approximately twelve institutions who have established doctoral programs within Australia (James 1993). Post-doctoral research will eventually be carried out by nurse academics which will allow for continued questioning of underlying practices and principles on which the discipline is based.

Of equal importance is how this knowledge is distributed. The development of scholarly journals and publications in nursing serves the needs of a community of scholars which includes various clinical specialties. Publications are one avenue of distributing this knowledge, another is giving papers at conferences, both nursing and multidisciplinary. The third aspect of utilising knowledge can be carried out by promoting nursing amongst other disciplines. This will allow for nurses to gain credibility through encouraging other disciplines to utilise nursing work, and ultimately draw on nursing expertise. Promoting this awareness can be in the form of publishing in other professional journals and offering courses to other disciplines—which may benefit both parties by establishing cross-disciplinary scholarship including research and publications, development of seminars, networking and mentorship.

Level of faculty

At the level of faculty there may be a need for restructuring of faculty time and workloads. Despite Fawcett's (1979) view, that those who are committed to research will make time for it, many are too busy to be able to think or have time to produce work of a scholarly nature (Armiger 1974, Freund 1990). Whether or not time is an issue, it is certainly true that many nurse academics are unfamiliar with the research process and are in need of assistance on a number of levels. One other way of providing this assistance is to have groups of faculty working together on research projects. This provides benefits which are twofold; they are able to share expertise amongst the group, and if it is done in collaboration with the hospital or with another discipline it can make those necessary connections which Boyer (1990) describes as part of the scholarship of integration. Becoming involved in research at a junior level can provide a means of learning the research process. Another is in the form of mentoring.

The benefits of mentoring have been documented widely both in literature on women in higher education (Bolton 1980, Smith 1992, Whittle 1989) and in the nursing literature (Fields 1991, Meleis 1992, May et al 1982). The notion of mentorship and sponsorship is essential for the development of a scholarly approach in nurses. Zey (1984) gives four characteristics of the mentor: the role of teacher (giving advice, guidance); counsellor (providing psychological support and acting as a confidence builder); intervener (providing access to resources and protection); and sponsor (facilitating promotions either directly or indirectly). The use of mentors can assist in the socialisation role and promote integration expediently, especially if they are familiar with the culture and networks of higher education. Some of the literature (Allen 1990, Fitzpatrick 1987) indicates that women are less likely to acquire mentors and have less access to formal networks, so the use of mentorship, whether it is someone from the same discipline and gender or not, will be of significant benefit. Whilst on the subject of networking, it may be worth pointing out that many nurse academics are coming to realise that time spent on networking with others is crucial to their own professional development and to the furthering of their career. Thus, it is important to develop a strong communication network through institutional activities, professional and discipline-based societies, the use of electronic mail and other sources.

Lastly, faculty evaluation needs to reflect the embryonic stage of nursing as a discipline. Some universities are continuing to waive the standard criteria for personal promotion and tenure for nurse academics, others are not. The issue is a sensitive one. On the one hand, in order to gain credibility in the eyes of other disciplines, many nurse academics agree that they should be considered for promotion and tenure on the same basis as others. On the other hand, nurses are under incredible pressure to gain qualifications, carry out additional research (by obtaining research grants) and to publish, while at the same time teaching well, and carrying heavy clinical workloads and administrative duties. It is not surprising that they often feel the combination is too much to cope with, and that they are unable to compete on the same grounds as other more established disciplines.

Individual level

Finally, on an individual level there will need to be the development of new skills such as critical and reflective thinking, and writing skills. For many, their first encounter of requiring to learn these skills is often in their experience of gaining further qualifications, in which case their supervisors may need to give substantial assistance early on. Once past this stage, and embarking on publishing, nurses should try to learn from others and publish alongside someone already familiar with the processes of scholarship. Gradually nurses should aim to become sole authors of published articles and books, and eventually apply for research grants. One way to become familiar with research is to become involved by being a research assistant. This is illustrated by Johnson et al (1992) who recounted their first year as doctoral students, and how being involved as research assistants with their faculty mentors helped them to develop an understanding of what it was like to carry out research, experiencing both the challenges and difficulties. They also emphasised the importance of selecting the topic for doctoral research and how this was linked to an area of expertise. Thus nurses need to think about their career trajectory and specialise in one area, rather than being generalists as many are. The development of experts or 'gurus' in various areas of nursing is vital to the establishing of and future of nurse scholars and can be promoted by the use of mentoring, which was discussed in the previous section. However, each individual can also begin to develop a personal portfolio which includes a curriculum vitae outlining all personal and professional commitments, a section on field work, publications, peer reviews, student evaluations and unsolicited letters of commendation. This can be a tool for encouraging nurses to think about their own career, and set personal and professional goals, and can be used for promotional or evaluation purposes. Another part of the scholarship process is to learn to present to others, to debate ideas and to defend knowledge orally. This can be carried out at research colloquia and at conferences. These forums for discussion, however, must be conducive to learning. As Armiger (1974) emphasises, seminars should provide a climate congenial to scholarship and should not be a forum for personal display, power struggles, petty jealousies, or pedantry.

Nurses need to consider all aspects of scholarship, and once they have developed an area of expertise they can act as a consultant, become involved in policy development and strengthen ties with their professional area. For example if their speciality is in a clinical area they need to collaborate with the field, keep up to date with current issues and maintain a standard of expertise. Using opportunities such as sabbatical leave are important; as Franklin (1980) illustrates it can allow for taking 'time out', for travelling, for widening networks and for developing new channels of thought. These experiences can then be shared with others in the form of seminars and writing.

Conclusion

If we take a historical perspective it can be seen that nursing is not altogether unfamiliar with scholarship. The seeds were sewn as far back as 1852 when Florence Nightingale began documenting her thoughts on religion and women in society. When she returned from the Crimean war, she continued with her writing and published her *Notes on Nursing* (1859) on the value of nursing training, and she carried on to write a plethora of policies and publications. Since then nurses have made great strides in defining their own discipline, and are creating their own identity within the university setting.

Currently there are many changes occurring in higher education, including changes in the concept of scholarship. The traditional view of scholarship as related only to research and publications is now being challenged; additional aspects including service—whether on outside community committees or in clinical practice—are altering the views of scholarship, perhaps in favour of nursing. It has been illustrated in this chapter and through the nursing literature cited, that nurses are making substantial progress towards embracing the notion of scholarship. They are doing this not only through discovering new knowledge and examining old practices, values and beliefs but, perhaps more strikingly, also through helping to redefine the very essence of what we mean by scholarship.

REFERENCES

Allen F 1990 Academic women in Australian universities. Monograph no. 4. AGPS, Canberra

Anderson D 1993 Sources of Australian academics' qualifications. Department of Employment, Education and Training. AGPS, Canberra

Armiger B 1974 Scholarship in nursing. Nursing Outlook 22(3):160-164

Barclay L 1994 Role of clinical chairs in promoting research. Paper presented to First Nursing Academic International Congress, University of Canberra

Becher T 1989 Academic tribes and territories: intellectual inquiry and the cultures of disciplines. The Society for Research into Higher Education. Open University Press, Milton Keynes

Belenky M, Clinchy B, Goldberger N, Tarule J 1986 Women's ways of knowing: the development of self, voice, and mind. Basic Books, New York

Bolton E 1980 Conceptual analysis of the mentor relationship in the career development of women. Adult Education 30:195-207

Boyer E 1990 Scholarship reconsidered: priorities of the professoriate. The Carnegie Foundation for the Advancement of Teaching. Princeton University Press, New Jersey

Cass B, Dawson M, Temple D, Wills S, Winkler A 1983 Why so few? Women academics in Australian universities. Sydney University Press, Sydney

Chaska N (ed) 1990 The nursing profession: turning points. C V Mosby, St Louis

Clark B 1987 The academic life, small worlds, different worlds. The Carnegie Foundation for the Advancement of Teaching. Princeton University Press, New Jersey

Clark B 1989 The academic life, small worlds, different worlds. Educational researcher 18(5):4-8

Department of Employment, Education and Training 1990 Postgraduate Students (Higher Education Series) Report no 5, Canberra

Donahue M P 1985 Nursing. The finest art. C V Mosby, St Louis, p 469

Donoghue J, Duffield C, Pelletier D 1994 The impact of graduate education on the individual and the profession. Paper presented to First Nursing Academic International Congress, University of Canberra

Fawcett J 1979 Integrating research into the faculty workload. Nursing Outlook 27(4):259-262

Fields W 1991 Mentoring in nursing: a historical approach. Nursing Outlook 39(6):257-261

Fitzpatrick J 1987 Toward the socialisation of scholars and scientists. Nurse Educator 12(3):23-25

Fitzpatrick J, Carnegie M 1991 Endowed chairs in nursing. Nursing Outlook 39(5):218-221

Franklin V 1980 The sabbatical leave. Nursing Outlook 28:109-111

Freund C 1990 Faculty workload standards: assuring teaching, service, and scholarship. Nurse Educator 15(3):8-13

Grey G 1927 Stimulating scholarship. American Journal of Nursing 27:331-335

Harman K 1989 Professional versus academic values: cultural ambivalence in university professional schools in Australia. Higher Education 18:491-509

James J 1993 Personal communication from Secretary of Australian Council of Deans of Nursing

Johnson R, Moorhead S, Daly J 1992 Scholarship and socialisation: reflections on the first year of doctoral study. Journal of Nursing Education 31(6):280-282

Kelly L 1992 The question of nursing scholarship. Reflections 18(4):30

Lee J, Fleming N 1993 The Lincoln women in academia case study. Conference paper presented at Higher Education Research and Development Society of Australasia, University of New South Wales

Leininger M 1974 Scholars, scholarship and nursing scholarship. Image 6:5-14

Lewis R, Barraclough S 1993 The experience of higher degree supervision in the professions. Paper presented at Higher Education Research and Development Society of Australasia. Making a difference: postgraduate research supervision at RMIT

MacKay R, Cruickshank J, Matsuno K 1991 Developing a hospital research program. The Australian Journal of Advanced Nursing 8(2):10-14

May K, Meleis A, Winstead-Fry P 1982 Mentorship for scholarliness: opportunities and dilemmas. Nursing Outlook 30:22-28

Meleis A 1991 Theoretical nursing: development and progress, 2nd edn. Lippincott, Philadelphia

Meleis A 1992 On the way to scholarship: from master's to doctoral. Journal of Professional Nursing 8(6):328-334

Nightingale F 1859 Notes on nursing. Harrison, London

Palmer I 1986 The emergence of clinical scholarship as a professional imperative. Journal of Professional Nursing 2(5):318-325

Pease J 1993 Professor mom: woman's work in a man's world. Sociological Forum 8(1):133-139

Pelikan J 1983 Scholarship and its survival. The Carnegie Foundation for the Advancement of Teaching. Princeton University Press, New Jersey

Pittman E 1982 The role of the nurse administrator and nurse educator. Part 1 evaluation study of the Bachelor of Applied Science, Advanced Nursing Course, Lincoln Institute of Health Sciences, College of Nursing, Australia

Reid J (Chair, Steering Committee) 1994 Nursing education in Australian universities. Report of the National Review of Nurse Education in the Higher Education Sector—1994 and beyond. AGPS, Canberra

Sellick K, McKinley S, Botti M, Kingsland S, Behan J 1993 How many hospitals have a research policy? A Victorian survey. The Australian Journal of Advanced Nursing 10(4):20-25

Smith A 1992 Women in university teaching. Womens Studies Journal 8:101-128

Smyth J 1986 The reflective practitioner in nurse education. Keynote address to Second National Nursing Education Seminar, South Australian College of Advanced Education

Taylor G 1993 Female academics. Department of Employment, Education and Training, Higher Education Series Report no 18

Whittle J 1989 Women in tertiary education. Research and Development in Higher Education 12:68-74

Williams A, Poroch D, McIntosh W 1993 Fun projects: increasing awareness of nursing research in hospitals. The Australian Journal of Advanced Nursing 11(1):14-18

Woolf V 1929 A room of one's own. Reprinted 1977, Grafton Books, London

Zey M 1984 The mentor connection. Dow Jones Irwin, Illinois

5

Journey of the nurse practitioner to scholar

LYN COULON, LESLEY M. WILKES

> Two roads diverged in a wood, and I—
> I took the one less travelled by,
> And that has made all the difference.
> (Robert Frost, *The road not taken*)

Introduction

The discipline of nursing will only define and extend its domains when nurse practitioners become scholars. These scholars will not only describe, analyse and theorise nursing from a practice perspective, but they will also propagate this knowledge through documenting and translating it for and to others. The authors' premise is that the discipline of nursing will grow through a purposeful pursuit, discovery and assertion of nursing knowledge which empowers nurse practitioners and liberates the profession.

Nurses travel many different roads on their journey to scholarliness. One such journey along an untrodden road is the focus of this discourse. The central purpose of this chapter is to portray how scholars may be educated in a university program. The authors propose that the exploration of current nursing scholarship, critical reflection on practice and sharing of knowledge are crucial in nurse practitioners' journeys towards scholarliness.

Becoming a scholar: developing scholarliness

Scholars, both nurses and others, have espoused scholarliness as having a number of characteristics (Armiger 1974, Meleis et al 1980, Palmer 1986,

Boyer 1990, Meleis 1992). In the nursing literature there appears some consistency. Armiger (1974) suggests that scholarliness includes a persistence, dedication, flexibility and willingness to weigh all sides of an argument. Further, she contends that scholarliness is the pursuit of excellence, not only in research but in all aspects of the scholar's life. A scholar must demonstrate proficiency, mastery of systematised knowledge and excellence in performance (Meleis et al 1980). Similarly, Bullough (1985) perceives that the properties of scholarliness include high intellectual ability, persistence, independence, integrity and self-discipline. They are learned and are the result of vigorous effort and a continuing quest for excellence.

As highlighted by these authors, the scholar must be creative not only in exploring fundamental questions but also in encouraging their pursuit by others. The propositions of these nurse scholars are captured in the portrait of scholarliness depicted by Meleis in 1992 when she stated that a scholar is a person who is

> able to see the questions as parts of the whole of the discipline. A scholar has a sense of history, a vision of the whole, a commitment to a discipline, and an understanding of how scientific work is related to the discipline's mission and to humanity as a whole. A scholar has a lifelong commitment to the development of knowledge in the discipline and therefore is always engaged in a systematic program for knowledge development...A scholar has a passion for excellence and a sense of integrity.

Scholarliness in nursing is not to be seen as separate from practice. Often clinical scholarliness is seen as disparate to academic scholarliness (e.g. Palmer 1986). However, as McClymont (1987) advocates, the link between theoretical learning and practice is essential. Clinical expertise is as important a characteristic of scholarliness in nursing as is research and learned writing. As Boyer (1990) suggests, scholarliness of its members is the heart of what a profession is all about. Nursing is practice, theory and philosophy intertwined and as such scholarliness must be formed from discovery (research), integration (connections across disciplines), application (practice) and teaching (Boyer 1990). If a profession is to become a discipline and achieve scholarliness it should recognise the diverse talents of all its members.

To achieve true scholarliness a nurse must bridge the gap between nursing action and nursing thought (Palmer 1986). There needs to be an interlinking between science, health science, art and the humanities. The scholarliness that a nurse has is ever changing. Its characteristics change in relation to each other. In a sense each characteristic forms a pattern in a kaleidoscope of scholarliness. As the nurse travels along the road to scholarliness, different characteristics are emphasised and become the dominant pattern at different times within the kaleidoscope. The movement and changing patterns evolve spontaneously (Chaska 1990). In this search for scholarliness there is an infinity of thought and beliefs that can converge to crystallise a momentary vision. At one moment the central pattern important for the nurse scholar may be clinical excellence, at the next research, at another both.

Whilst scholarliness is characterised by a number of traits, in order to become a scholar one needs to transcend these. The scholar uses these traits of scholarliness to develop wisdom and thus become a 'learned person'. The authors postulate that to become this scholar the nurse needs to become a critical and creative thinker.

Critical and creative thinking: an essential element

Critical thinking can be defined as a composite of attitudes, knowledge and skills that include:

1   attitudes of inquiry that involve an ability to recognise the existence of problems and an acceptance of the general need for evidence in support of what is asserted to be true
2   knowledge of the nature of valid inferences, abstractions and generalisations in which the weight or accuracy of different kinds of evidence are logically determined
3   skill in employing and applying the above attitudes and knowledge (Watson & Glaser 1964).

For critical thinking to proceed, significant questions need to be posed in order to capture accurate relevant answers. Taking time to analyse one's decision-making process by using critical thinking skills is considered an important tool that may also assist in making morally appropriate decisions in clinical practice (Thompson & Thompson 1990). Time to think critically is imperative for defining and describing what is nursing. In the discipline of nursing are we asking the right questions? (Russell 1991). Further, does the average nurse clinician know and use the skills of critical thinking? Indeed, what is critical thinking and how can it best be enhanced for nurses undertaking university education?

When faced with a task, or problem of higher order complexity, a blending of multiple skills is required; in turn this necessarily involves higher cognitive functioning. Matthews and Gaul (1979) have identified that critical thinking encompasses 'the cognitive skills of comprehension, application, analysis, synthesis and evaluation thinking'. Bandman and Bandman (1988) wrote:

...The role of critical thinking in nursing means movement from freedom of expression to an enriched freedom or reasoned restraint...It consists in sharpening the distinctions between certainty, near certainty and degrees of uncertainty. A nurse learns to discriminate by understanding and observing criteria.

Interwoven within these processes is the nurse's own ability and motivation not only to raise the right questions, but also to challenge forthcoming answers, always seeking the best solution. Argument is thus central to critical thinking (Blair 1985).

Whilst scholarliness develops from critical thinking, to extend this dimension further creativity must be encouraged. Edward de Bono (1992), a leading authority in the field of creative thinking and originator of the term 'lateral thinking', believes that the lack of fresh constructive thinking is the vital ingredient missing in the way many businesses and people tackle the problems of the 1990s. Yinger's (1980) premise is that the creative aspects of thinking enable the production of ideas and alternatives, while the critical aspects permit the testing and evaluation of the product of creative thinking.

Chinn (1984) suggests a separation between creativity and scholarliness postulating that there must be a balance between the two. We contend that creativity is the essence of scholarliness. Creativity is that 'stab in the dark', that 'leap in the imagination' which allows the scholar to be different. Without creativity, critical thinking can become rigid and compliant in a process devoid of flexibility and willingness to diverge from the espoused path. Creativity often means having the courage to go off the track, to journey 'the less travelled road'. The challenge for the teacher is to assist students to identify cues along the road, to transcend the characteristics of scholarliness to become scholars.

In the journey described in the following pages the authors guided a group of students along an untrodden road. The journey took the form of a special course unit which provided the students with a unique opportunity to explore nursing knowledge, what it is and what it is not. The students were encouraged to extend the frontiers of science, art and nursing located in their clinical practice and in the literature. The teachers endeavoured to assist the students' passage and the students' critical and creative thinking, inspiring them to transcend the patterns of their kaleidoscope of scholarliness.

The journey

'Nursing and Knowing', a two hour per week, fourteen week course unit in the Master of Nursing program at Australian Catholic University (NSW), was the vehicle for the journey of discovery. It was a journey by reading, writing and debate designed to enable students to observe and reflect on their life experiences and the readings used during the course, and to explore the conceptualisation of answers to the following questions:

1　What is knowing?
2　What is critical thinking?
3　Is nursing an art, a science, both or neither?
4　What is nursing in Australia today?
5　What factors affect the ways nurses know?

From the beginning the authors, as the two main facilitators in the weekly class meetings, aimed to create a climate in which scholarliness was rigorously pursued and supported, and one which sustained the development of individual progress. This climate was achieved through a formula of sharing in an open classroom which encouraged flexibility, debate, analysis, synthesis of ideas, reflection on readings and observations from practice. The intent was to nurture and develop keen scholars committed to lifelong learning using processes of discovery, organisation of ideas and the transmission of knowledge resulting from client-oriented nursing practice (Palmer 1986).

The program provided foundations in logic, thinking, reasoning, critical thinking, and creative thinking. Central to this proposition was our expectation that students would not only explore, discover and acquire new nursing knowledge, but would also conceive, test and impart its wisdom.

The class environment was one of flexibility where neither teacher nor students would dominate, but rather where a shared relationship of push/pull would be employed to encourage, stimulate and tease minds in the search for 'knowing'. Just because it had 'always been done that way', never sufficed when we were searching in the swampy lowland (Street 1990), seeking to improve and apply clinical strategies to health care problems. Such strategies, as suggested by the students, were viewed not only for possible outcome, but also for their potential. An important principle here was that the free floating of ideas was encouraged. Through the greyness of not knowing, the students were encouraged to think only from a positive and ideal perspective, to traverse a range of alternative solutions, to take these back to the clinical area, to discuss options with colleagues seeking even minimal improvement and to keep bringing them back for further discussion. In this way a history of ideas was captured in the students' journals.

Improvement of any kind, whether in writing, verbalising or reasoning, was encouraged and recognised as a hallmark of success, no matter how small the improvement (de Bono 1992). We believe this approach stimulated minds and imagination to push back the frontiers, whilst experiencing the joys of learning and in the process accelerated creativity. This is exemplified in an extract from a student's journal, four weeks into the course:

> as the group developed people are far less concerned with proving they know everything about a particular topic, far less worried about being exposed, about being wrong about something...an atmosphere of sharing what you think, even if not convinced that you are absolutely right about something and so much the better the atmosphere for critical thinking (S3).

And another student at about the same time:

> We have quickly gone past the idea that we must prove something or that there should be any pretence and we all seem to be getting on and simply sharing the knowledge and opinions that we have. It seems that we are getting a lot out of it. I am, in that I am being asked to verify my beliefs and thoughts, and I enjoy it (S4).

[(S1-S7) indicates a particular student in the group].

The itinerary

The journey was designed to embrace a range of issues and problems which would stimulate discussion and provide a bridge between the nurse clinicians and the academics. Six of the seven students were clinicians having specialisations such as intensive therapy, coronary care, gerontology and palliative care. The seventh student was a nurse academic who had extensive clinical experience in intensive therapy. Both authors were the teachers in the unit and worked as a Siamese pair, rather than separately in the classroom. Another lecturer, a philosopher, provided expert input and stimulus for early discussions on the construct of 'knowledge'.

Three essential elements enabled the journey. These were: readings from the nursing literature, reflective journalling and open debate in the classroom.

The readings

The readings were selected by the teachers to initiate a focus for each week's class deliberation. The weekly topics were organised to provide a progression in the exploration and development of the students' nursing knowing. These topics, in chronological order, were:

- Introduction to reflective journalling
- What is it to know?
- What is it to know, think, and understand?
- Critical thinking in a search for nursing knowledge
- Critical thinking, creativity and research
- Nursing an art, a science, both or neither?
- Perspective on ways of knowing in nursing
- The feminist perspective on knowing and its influence on knowing in nursing
- Formal and personal knowing, intuition
- Reflective practice: a way of knowing
- Ritual and tradition in forming nursing knowledge
- The image of nursing and the challenge to know
- Caring: is it the essence of nursing?
- Two Australian studies on nursing.

From the structured readings the students' various ideologies and nursing philosophies were examined through the vehicle of language. On occasions, the meanings inherent within the words took on a game-like quality where quickness and surprise added dimensions of fun. Similarly, storytelling related to nursing problems was encouraged and analysed. We found that this mode of inquiry provided ground rules for innovative thinking. We also called on the students' observations, reflection, questioning of assumptions, assessment, evaluation, feelings and vision (Bandman & Bandman 1988).

Reflective journalling

Reflective journalling was an essential component on this journey to scholarliness. It was introduced in the first week of the semester and the students were provided with a number of readings on the topic including Holly (1984). Her description of journalling was cited as a model that students could choose to follow. She described a journal as 'the structured, descriptive notes of the log and the free flowing impressionistic meandering of the diary'.

Reflection has been postulated as helpful to the learning process since Dewey (1938) recognised that all genuine education comes through experience, although 'this does not necessarily mean that all experiences are genuinely or equally educative. For some, experiences are miseducative'.

Various approaches to reflection and its part in learning have been discussed in the literature. Friere (1972, 1974) emphasised that the relevance of reflection is more apparent when action follows thought. Mezirow (1981) described a model of reflective learning with seven levels of reflection from awareness to deep theorising. Argyris (1982) related reflection to a problem solving process which may be moderated by socialisation factors. Schön (1983) refers to the 'reflection in action' of professionals, which takes the form of 'on the spot surfacing, criticising, restructuring and testing of intuitive understandings of experience phenomena'.

Schön (1983) suggested that professionals use sample cases from experience to determine their actions rather than technical knowledge. Benner (1984) supported this premise in nursing practice in her study of novice and expert nurses. She stated that the expert nurse tends to use concrete past experience (paradigms) as a basis of practice, whilst the novice uses context free rules to determine practice.

The model of the learning cycle described by Kolb (1984) incorporates reflective observation as the second of its four sequential elements, while Jarvis (1987), among others, has developed a fundamentally similar but more complex model. Boud et al (1985a) noted that learning through reflection must be, ultimately, a personal and individual process. They (Boud et al 1985b) described a model of learning which emphasised the emotive aspects of reflection. Kemmis (1985) added a political dimension to the social and ideological dimensions of the reflective process and Jarvis (1987) maintained that people reflect through language and utilise memory from previous experience. We contend that reflection is an essential partner in the development of critical and creative thinking.

Journalling can bridge the gap between theory and practice (Smyth 1986, Cowan 1991, Emden 1991) and enhance the development of skills in nursing (Lyte & Thompson 1990, McGaugherty 1991, Cooper 1992). Allen et al (1989) postulate that by writing to learn, application, analysis and synthesis are encouraged. These are believed to be important components in critical thinking. There is no place for vagueness or ambiguity in critical thinking. Clearly articulated ideas are sought and probed, a technique which enables clarification of reasoning. This development of critical thinking skills is an indispensable component of education, and a trait of an educated person (Glaser 1985) and the scholar.

The ideas of reflection and its place in the learning process are often complex. The basic premise is that an extension of a person's conceptions will be encouraged if he/she focuses on an experience, writes about it, and re-evaluates the experience from the writing. Experience in the context of the Unit 'Nursing and Knowing' included readings, classroom debate and nursing practice.

Boud and Walker (1991) maintain that group processes help in the essential stage of revaluation and attending to feelings. Kemmis and McTaggert (1988) suggest that if journals are to be effectively used to encourage reflection the process must have the following characteristics:

- all participants must keep a journal
- a time must be set aside to do silent uninterrupted sustained writing
- all writing must be shared with the other participants
- time must be set aside in the teaching program to allow feedback on shared journal writings
- a structured and supportive atmosphere for journal writing.

Open debate

Open debate, a vital component of 'Nursing and Knowing', was consistent with suggestions in the literature and was reinforced in previous experience in using reflective journalling with students in a nursing program (Batts & Wilkes 1993). In this previous project the researchers felt that there had not been enough time spent in the classroom debating critical issues emanating from the journals.

Argument as open debate was also seen as an essential element in promoting critical thinking (Blair 1985). The students pursued the anatomy of argument using recommended readings and other strategies, with the class session structured to enable dissection of propositions. From clinical experience and observation of relationships among health practitioners we found substantial evidence that many nurse practitioners employed argument without structuring premises that supported or led to justifiable conclusions.

The journey experience

The students were asked to keep a journal for the fourteen weeks of the Unit. In the first class it was emphasised that initially the students may need just to write down their thoughts as they emerged and in this way the reflective process would develop over time.

In the early weeks when the discussions and readings were orientated to the philosophical meaning of knowledge, the students' entries in their journals ranged from indications of being overwhelmed to being wakened to questioning and challenge. For example, one student wrote in her first journal entry: 'The session with [the philosopher] was overwhelming to me at the start—I thought "what have I got myself into". Knowledge what is it? I wouldn't have a clue after this session. The session generated interesting comments and interaction between the group. I look forward to the continuation of the unit'. (S1)

And the same student during the week after the first lecture:

Reading 'Understanding Human Knowledge in General' (Chisholm 1966) confirmed my thoughts about do we ever know anything or do we just think we do. While reading this article I [a palliative care nurse] thought that if I have not been terminally ill, how do I know how to deal with people who are terminally ill, do you have to experience something to know about it? (S1)

These ideas of uncertainty were confirmed by others in the group. The kindling of critical thought was seen in some students' reflections concerning the reading cited above: 'Many thoughts and feelings were generated as I read this paper. I felt that there was no end to the circles that were spiralling backwards in search of where the knowledge came from'. (S7)

Another student after the second session:

Nurses need to do nursing, which will lead to the development of evidence about nursing from which we will develop nursing knowledge [comment of teacher during class]. This seems a logical and reasonable way to go about 'getting' nursing knowledge which we can later attempt to relate to our greater question of 'what is knowledge?' Overall this week I am feeling more confident about this idea of knowing and reflection. The process of this writing aids in reflection which helps clarify the ideas and beliefs I have about knowing. (S2)

The emotive aspects of the journalling process espoused by Boud et al (1985a) are portrayed in this last exemplar and with other students it was clearly seen as important. The next exemplar emphasises how the class environment can often have a long lasting effect on our associations with learning:

The course started last week in one of the 'education' classrooms [primary science room]. I don't especially like this room—it somewhat reminds me of a schoolroom—this is where the students do their pracs and make things. It sort of conjures up negative thoughts about school activities which I don't ever remember embracing with any enthusiasm...I did move school a lot. I wonder if my superficial feeling and approach to education is tied up with all this? (S4)

However in the last entry in this student's journal in week 14: 'To end I am now used to the classroom and no longer have the same assertions as in the beginning. Today the clock is gone!' (S4)

Using the readings as a focus for class discussion, the journey during weeks 3 and 4 was directed to a discourse on critical thinking. The students read a number of articles and extracts from books. Selected readings were utilised to explain the concept of critical thinking, for example extracts from Barry and Rudinow (1990) and Meleis' (1991) chapter on knowledge; whilst others, such as the research article by Kunnel et al (1988), tempted the students to employ critical thinking. At this stage the teachers needed to push, probe and pull the students to encourage them to relate to each other's knowledge, explore their ideas and question assumptions. 'Both myself and...[S4]...thought the article on temperature was boring but...[S5]...thought it good'. (S1)

Another student: 'Once again I learnt especially from...[the teacher]...to critically evaluate and there is some merit in the research...[article cited above]...Even though I found it of little value to me the probing questions made me look carefully at it'. (S4)

The students were neither self-starting nor in many cases sufficiently critical of their reasoning. However, the class activities and readings did challenge them to question the nature of critical thinking. For example: 'The discussions and readings of this week I really enjoyed. I thought a lot about critical thinking and what it meant and how I achieved it. I agree that it does involve reflection and arguing with myself and others to reach the validity of what has been stated'. (S6)

The article by Thayer (1991) discussing the place of 'gut experience' in nursing knowledge stimulated the students to argue. Some students agreed and some didn't. At this stage the students were asked to relate the readings to their own way of learning. They had examined Barry and Rudinow's (1990) chapter on argument and were invited to participate in a structured, surprise debate during class. Most students commented on the usefulness of this strategy and found they were cued to think more objectively when reading and to look critically at reasoning within argument. As one student commented:

Debating the topic...[nursing is a trade not a profession].. was hard as I didn't agree with the side I was on. However some points raised were good— I tended to attack and point whereas the 'winner' used premise and conclusions. The point was that people were swayed by the argument that they believe, or has convinced them, not one that they have lost. (S5)

In the following week the topic for consideration was nursing as an art or science. This is 'the big question' constantly debated over time. The students differed often in their opinion and at this stage were commencing to argue their point of view. The group had become more cohesive and the 'quiet ones' had become just as vocal as the rest. The students conjured up arguments and questioned what was written in the literature. O'Brien's (1990) article on a discourse of whether nursing was an art, craft or science was a stimulus for much reflection by the students. Many of the students' reflections were concerned with their clinical work and these reflections often showed creative thought. One nurse related her story of a dying patient and of encouraging him and his wife to spend the night together and have a candle-lit dinner. She summed up her feelings as: 'When looking at the art in nursing there are many ways and different situations when nurses have been artistic—ways outside the normal routine of patient care?' (S7)

Another student working in Accident and Emergency said, 'Even in casualty, where the mostly scientific prevails, I feel that some amount of artistic thinking occurs as well?' (S3) However this same student later in the week:

I've being trying to think of ways nursing is an art in the emergency department. Nursing as a science is easy. As an art though it is quite a lot harder, although I'm sure that we must do that. Perhaps by just being around, and occasionally even supplying beds for patients to come in even if we know that they really have not just had a huge haemo-chuck that they had said they had. That's not much. The more I think about the more I think how sterile the place is. (S3)

This student used critical analysis to blend her expanding knowledge to explore the meaning of her work.

One student came to the conclusion at this stage that it didn't matter, 'nursing was nursing' and this student postulated: 'There may be components of either or both...[art/science]...of these that nursing has taken along the way and now used but what makes nursing exclusively nursing is not a science or an art. That's my last word on the subject...for the moment?' (S5)

Week 6 provided exploration and extension of the literature on ways of knowing. This had been touched on before but the focus was the classical work of Carper (1978) on patterns of knowing in nursing. This extended the science/art argument from the previous week. As well, the effect of research philosophy on knowledge growth in nursing was explored using articles related to paradigms of research. The class discussion was much more relaxed and the students were not solely orientated to the readings. They initiated the probing of broader questions and they pushed and teased the teachers and each other. Clarification of the term 'discipline' was also sought. This question stemmed from the students' dipping into Gray and Pratt (1991).

The students contended that they saw 'discipline' as a set of rules that must be obeyed. They believed nurses needed to strive not for discipline but professionalism. The academics seemed to be striving for both but their conceptions were different. One teacher referred the class to Meleis' (1991) definition of 'discipline' as 'a unique perspective, distinct way of viewing all phenomena within a particular field'. Meleis argued that 'discipline' includes the content, processes, and theories developed to describe and explain the various roles of nurses. Whilst not trying to undermine the students' ideas, the direction to other meanings prompted action with the students commenting that it would be beneficial to examine Meleis further. Would this have happened in the early weeks? The students were seeking out truth, content, theories and processes from their learning to answer questions from their practice experience. Their knowledge and the urge to know were growing.

Pushing into week 7 the students were apparently surprised to see readings related to feminism. Many comments indicated an indifference to the topic before the stimulus to read was initiated. For example:

Feminism: why have they given us this rubbish to read. I don't think I am any different to my brothers...I don't feel oppressed. Is it my personality, my expertise, my professional knowledge? What is this journalling saying about me, I am more confused about what is knowing and knowledge. I hope this confusion leads to more. Confusion? Knowledge? (S1)

Another student: 'The readings on the feminist approach have been quite challenging...How is the feminist perspective different to anyone's interpretation of experience—it is entirely individual. Everyone (gender aside) must interpret their experiences as they see them'. (S2)

By now the students were questioning their own frameworks and often providing reflections on their truths even if these were different to what they were reading. With their increasing exposure to scholarly readings and discussion the students were beginning to critique their own writings and reflect on their reflections.

From feminism a natural path in this journey was to revisit different ways of knowing and how these are expressed, particularly in nursing. Revisiting reflection was used to orientate the students more thoughtfully to the process, give them a broader perspective and explore it as a way of knowing particularly in relation to nursing in action. Schön's (1983) work on 'reflection in action' for the professional, and excerpts from Gray and Pratt (1991), formed the basis of this exploration. As well, the place of intuition was explicated and the works of Benner and Tanner (1987) and Rew (1987) were used to stimulate a re-exploration of this 'gut-feeling' concept. The students' journals posed many questions at this stage. For example:

How can we acquire 'artful practice'?...I cannot recognise theory that directs my practice. Has Clarke (1986) got the right idea that theory comes from practice? (S2)

INTUITION—do I think there is such a thing or not. Was I swayed by the arguments in the articles I read? I have always been a firm believer that there was no such thing as intuition in nursing practice...I think that nurses should distance themselves from this quickly? (S5)

Whilst the last nurse questioned the concept of intuition, others related to it in very definite terms and this not only was made clear in their journals but was also evident in their arguments in class time, as illustrated in excerpts from two nurses' journals:

A lot of the ideas about nurses using intuition are very relevant to me and made me stop and look at why and how I regard myself as an expert and how that reflects my way of working...I think there is a rationale behind intuitive judgement. I cannot always put an easy rationale to why I do things but I believe it is based on a whole heap of learned associations. (S6)

And:

After reading the article [by Rew] I feel relieved that my 'gut-feeling' or 'feelings of dread' are recognised as valid. Can I put a name to these feelings? Patterns or similarity recognition, commonsense understanding, skilled knowledge, sense of salience or deliberate rationality—I'm not sure...but it's reassuring that these feelings should not be dismissed or devalued by others...I need to explore these feelings more and try to decide that I recognise the problem. (S1)

These two nurses, experts in their practice field, were becoming scholarly by theorising from their practice and seeing the importance of translating their ways of knowing for themselves and others.

During the next phase of the journey the students searched for other factors that helped them to form nursing knowledge. The place of ritual and tradition was prospected by reading Walsh and Ford's (1989) book which speculated that nurses tended to use rituals rather than research findings for their actions. This book further instigated the students questioning whether nursing is a practice discipline and, if so, what is meant by it. Some deliberations from the students at this point illustrate this:

> Clinicians probably formulate theories without realising it and in an informal way. Research should be generated from practice to build on the theory of nursing and to guide practice...A practice discipline has a unique body of knowledge aimed at improving the outcomes of practice as needs are identified from practice? (S2)

And: 'I believe that nursing is a practice discipline and although this encompasses how beliefs about nursing have arisen from our practice it is not static as our beliefs and practices are constantly changing. We are critically analysing and shaping our ideas on nursing knowledge'. (S6)

'Nursing is a practice discipline because it is the gaining of knowledge through learning certain skills related to the practice area or clinical area in which we work.. Our practice is the beliefs, skill, methods we learn/acquire along the way'. (S4)

Whilst the students' ideas were different they each illustrated an integration of reading, analysis and theorising. These were seen as essential to their growth as critical and creative thinkers and as emerging scholars.

The image of nurses as 'doing' rather than 'thinking' was canvassed and the students were challenged to decide what would be needed to change this image. Most students argued that a change was needed and some proposed changes to education, more research and better clinical pathways. The students' premise was based on the view that members of the general public do not see nursing as a profession and that this is a fundamental obstacle to changing the image.

Caring as the essence of nursing was discussed to allow the students to see whether this concept had influenced their conception of knowledge related to nursing. In their reflections that week most students discussed their conceptualisation of caring in nursing: 'Caring is respect for the patient as a person, encouraging individuality and involvement of patient participation in what he/she wants to achieve and helping him/her to work towards it'. (S6)

And: 'I don't know how caring in nursing is different to that of doctors, physios and other health professionals. Maybe it's the time nurses spend with their patients, the sharing of their pain, loss and recovery or maybe nurses are just different people to other health professionals'. (S1)

And: 'caring can represent both art and science'. (S7)

Finally, two books which explored nursing in Australia (Lawler 1991, Street 1992) were prescribed to enable the students to explore the concepts visited during the journey within a native context. These authors described nursing from a practice and sociological perspective; Lawler as a nurse, Street as a sociologist. For the students these readings produced mixed reactions and feelings. At this stage of the journey their capacity to effectively initiate professional opinion backed up by argument was evident. Many arguments

89

were generated from the students' personal philosophies of nursing practice. The books served the purpose of opening and stimulating questions for the students. Again, the students were becoming more scholarly.

Journey's end or a beginning

At the conclusion of the fourteen weeks the teachers and students reflected on the process and the outcomes. From the teachers' perspective it had been a journey of uncertainty at times, which caused both authors to question whether they were on the right road. As the semester drew to a close the students invited the two teachers to provide their reflections on the Unit. One teacher wrote:

> For me the teaching moment in our sessions was always the next question...There were no boundaries to learning only horizons for both you as students and we as facilitators...Between our meetings I often reflected on your significant contribution and enjoyment in our sessions. This motivated me to work harder. I often wondered if you were conscious of your wealth of clinical knowledge and expertise... As the semester progressed I felt the joy that a teacher knows when challenged by the students' advanced questions and newly formed developing frames of reference.

And the other teacher: 'When I met the group I felt that we would be travelling a long path...I believe that you and I learnt not only about nursing but ourselves. I know I learnt a lot about the reality of nursing. I really feel that we all need more time to be able to do this reflecting'.

The students' reflections on the journey often mirrored that of the teachers but were expressed in differing ways: 'It made me think about nursing...It made me critical in my thinking and reading'. (S1)

> It challenged my perceptions of nursing...gave me the authority to challenge authors about their work...strengthened my beliefs in nursing and my commitment to the profession? (S2)
>
> It was enjoyable and valuable in my professional growth...It gave me the opportunity to express and discuss ideas and issues. It helped me to think and learn. (S3)
>
> It gave me an appreciation of the breadth of nursing literature...I need to rethink many things. (S4)
>
> The focus of the course has been that one needs to approach things with an open, yet critical mind...It shouldn't be just open and critical to areas of nursing theory or philosophy, but it should be open and critical in all aspects of life in order to live life to the fullest and get the most out of every encounter...I have learnt to look at things in a different way...in a better way...so that I get the most out of what I am thinking. (S5)
>
> It challenged me to research...I became more aware of critically analysing what I read...It made me look at nursing and where it is going. (S6)

At the beginning I wondered why we were doing the course. But I was amazed at how much information and enjoyment I got out of it. Critical thinking has always being difficult for me but reading the articles and discussing them made it seem easy. (S7)

Finally one student summed all our thoughts: 'I think I am more positive about where I'm at and where I want to be—That is where I am—nursing!'(S1)

From the students' words we learn that they are not at the end of their journey. Rather, their confidence to be critical and to challenge their ideas about nursing has provided the impetus to sustain their momentum along other roads to scholarliness.

Conclusions

The journey described here reflects one aspect of the changing patterns of the kaleidoscope which is scholarliness. The wisdom emerging in the students was creative. They were appreciating and striving for the clarity, thoroughness and precision of thought and analysis which typifies the nurse scholar (Johnson et al 1992). As teachers the challenge remains to enable students to become more creative, to tread alone or with others along the next 'less travelled' road. The students learned to bridge the gap between theory, practice and philosophy permitting them to become intertwined. They built links between the sciences, humanities and arts in nursing whilst observing that there is a uniqueness in nursing which beckons and awaits the scholar.

Whilst there is no exact formula or recipe for scholarliness and nor should there be, others engaged in educating nurses could be encouraged to develop a culture of exploration and debate as described in this chapter. To achieve this teachers need to generate in their students a sense that there is another 'right' often around the corner. For example, when Newton developed his Laws of Motion he was 'right'. Later, Einstein showed that Newton's theory could be questioned. Now, Hawkins has queried Einstein.

In guiding students along the educational journey our intention was to tease minds to think critically and creatively for nursing. Our vision as teachers provides for an empowered future for nursing. We envisage a future in which nurse scholars take the roads less travelled to wisdom and this will make 'the difference' in the pursuit of knowledge for the enhancement of nursing as a discipline and a profession.

ACKNOWLEDGMENT

The authors wish to thank the Australian Catholic University NSW Master of Nursing class of 1993 for sharing the reflections from their journals. The helpful suggestions received from Tim O'Hearn and Marianne Wallis are greatly appreciated. We also extend our thanks to Michael Jones and Chantal Coulon for their persistence in pursuing the literature.

REFERENCES

Allen D G, Bowers B, Diekelmann N 1989 Writing to learn: reconceptualisation of thinking and writing in the nursing curriculum. Journal of Nursing Education 28(1):6-11

Argyris C 1982 Reasoning, learning and action. Jossey Bass, San Francisco

Armiger B 1974 Scholarship in nursing. Nursing Outlook 22(3):162-163

Bandman L, Bandman E 1988 Critical thinking in nursing. Appleton & Lange, Norwalk

Barry V, Rudinow J 1990 Invitation to critical thinking, 2nd edn. Holt, Rinehart & Winston, Fort Worth

Batts J E, Wilkes L M 1993 Reflective journalling in science teaching. In: Bain J, Lietzow E, Ross B (eds) Promoting teaching in higher education. Griffith University, Brisbane

Benner P 1984 From novice to expert: excellence and power in clinical practice. Addison Wesley, Menlo Park, California

Benner P, Tanner C 1987 How expert nurses use intuition. American Journal of Nursing (January): 23-31

Blair J 1985 Some challenges for critical thinking. In: Bandman L, Bandman B (eds) Critical thinking in nursing. Appleton & Lange, Norwalk

Boud D J, Keogh R, Walker D (eds) 1985a Reflection: turning experience into learning. Kogan Page, London

Boud D J, Keogh R, Walker D 1985b Promoting reflection in learning: a model. In: Boud D J, Keogh R, Walker D (eds) Reflection: turning experience into learning. Kogan Page, London

Boud D J, Walker D 1991 Experience and learning: reflection at work. Deakin University, Geelong

Boyer E L 1990 Scholarship reconsidered: priorities of the professoriate. The Carnegie Foundation for the Advancement of Teaching, New Jersey

Bullough B 1985 The deanship and the promoting of scholarship in nursing. Journal of Professional Nursing (January-February): 22,65

Carper B A 1978 Fundamental patterns in knowing. Nursing Advances in Nursing Science 1(1):13-24

Chaska N L 1990 The kaleidoscope of nursing. In: Chaska N L (ed) The nursing profession: turning points. C V Mosby, St. Louis

Chinn P L 1984 The editor's role—creativity and scholarship. Advances in Nursing Science 7(1):vi-viii

Chisholm R 1966 Theory of knowledge. Prentice Hall, Englewood Cliffs, New Jersey

Clarke M 1986 Action and reflection: practice and theory of nursing. Journal of Advanced Nursing 11:3-11

Cooper S S 1992 Methods of teaching revisited experimental diaries and learning logs. Journal of Continuing Education in Nursing 13(6):32-34

Cowan J 1991 Attitude and assessment in nurse education. Journal of Advanced Nursing 17:473-479

de Bono E 1992 Serious creativity. Fontana, London

Dewey J 1938 Experience and education. Collier Books, New York

Emden C 1991 Becoming a reflective practitioner. In: Gray G, Pratt R (eds) Towards a discipline of nursing. Churchill Livingstone, Melbourne

Friere P 1972 Pedagogy of the oppressed. Penguin, Harmondsworth

Friere P 1974 Education: the practice of freedom. Writers and Readers, London

Frost R 1969 The road not taken. In: Robert Frost: selected poems. Penguin, London

Glaser E 1985 Critical thinking: education for responsible citizenship in a democracy. Phi Kappa Phi Journal 65:(1)24-27

Gray G, Pratt R (eds) 1991 Towards a discipline of nursing. Churchill Livingstone, Melbourne

Holly M L 1984 Keeping a personal-professional journal. Deakin University, Geelong

Jarvis P 1987 Adult learning in the social context. Croom Helm, New York

Johnson R A, Moorehead S A, Daly J M 1992 Scholarship and socialisation: reflection on the first year of doctoral study. Journal of Nursing Education 31(6):280-282

Kemmis S 1985 Action research and the politics of reflection. In: Boud D J, Keogh R, Walker D (eds) 1985 Reflection: turning experience into learning. Kogan Page, London

Kemmis S, McTaggert R 1988 The action research planner, 3rd edn. Deakin University Press, Geelong

Kolb D A 1984 Experiential learning. Prentice Hall, New Jersey

Kunnel M, O'Brien C, Munro B, Medoff-Cooper B 1988 Comparison of rectal, femoral, axillary and skin-to-mattress temperature in stable neonates. Nursing Research 37(3):162-164, 189

Lawler J 1991 Behind the screens: nursing, somology and the problem of the body. Churchill Livingstone, Melbourne

Lyte V J, Thompson I G 1990 The diary as a formative teaching and learning aid incorporating means of evaluation and renegotiation of clinical objectives. Nurse Education 10:228-232

McClymont A 1987 Scholarship in practice: some examples from health visiting. Recent Advances in Nursing 18:168-176

McGaugherty D 1991 The use of a teaching model to promote reflection and the experiential integration of theory and practice in first year nurses: an action research study. Journal of Advanced Nursing 16:534-543

Matthews C, Gaul A 1979 Nursing diagnosis from the perspective of concept attainment and critical thinking. Advances in Nursing Science 2(11):17-26

Meleis A I, Wilson H S, Chater S 1980 Towards scholarliness in doctoral dissertation: an analytical model. Research in Nursing and Health 3:115-124

Meleis A 1991 Theoretical nursing, 2nd edn. Lippincott Company, New York

Meleis A 1992 On the way to scholarship: from masters to doctorate. Journal of Professional Nursing 8(6):328-334

Mezirow D 1981 A critical theory of adult learning and education. Adult Education 32(1):3-24

Palmer I S 1986 The emergence of clinical scholarship as a professional imperative. Journal of Professional Nursing 2(5):318-325

O'Brien B 1990 Nursing craft, science and art. In: Conference proceedings: dreams, deliberations and discoveries: Nursing research in action. Royal Adelaide Hospital, Adelaide, 306-312

Rew L 1987 Nursing intuition: too powerful and too valuable to ignore. Nursing 87(July):43-45

Russell L 1991 Are we asking the right questions? In: Gray G, Pratt R (eds) Towards a discipline of nursing. Churchill Livingstone, Melbourne

Schön D 1983 The reflective practitioner: how professionals think in action. Basic Books, New York

Smyth J 1986 Reflection in action. Deakin University Press, Geelong

Street A 1990 Nursing practice: high, hard ground, messy swamps and the pathways in between. Deakin University Press, Geelong

Street A 1992 Inside nursing: a critical ethnography of clinical nursing practice. State University of New York Press, Albany

Thayer M 1991 Let it begin with me. Paediatric Nursing 17(5):504-505

Thompson J E, Thompson H D 1990 Applying the decision making model: case study 1 Neonatal Network 9(October)(3):75-77

Walsh J, Ford P 1989 Nursing rituals, research and rationale for actions. Heinemann Nursing, London

Watson G, Glaser E 1964 Critical thinking appraisal manual. Harcourt, Brace and World, New York

Yinger R 1980 Can we really teach them to think? In: Young R (ed) Fostering critical thinking. Jossey Bass, San Fransisco

6

Can faculty practice be scholarly?

HELEN MILLICAN

Staying in practice

I have to admit to moonlighting. This has nothing to do with not paying the rent, making moonshine whisky or unfortunately, having romantic encounters under a moonlit sky. It has to do with the fact that during the early stages of my role as a nursing academic I worked some weekend hospital shifts to maintain contact with and expertise in the clinical area. This form of faculty practice is described in the literature as moonlighting (Nahas 1990, Keithley & Uebele 1989, Stainton et al 1989). This is because the clinical practice is a staff nurse position which has been arranged independently outside the academic role, with no formal administrative or institutional support from the university. My moonlighting did not lead to visits from the rent collector or the alcohol licensing board, but some aspects of it were negative. It was while working to address these negative aspects that the material for this chapter on the scholarly aspects of faculty practice began to develop.

With a clinical background in neurosurgical and high dependency medical-surgical nursing, I found my weekend clinical shifts to be personally and professionally valuable. The patient caseload provided rewarding interactions with patients, their families and ward staff, and I gained satisfaction from feeling that I might have made some small difference for them. The clinical practice provided an active and refreshing counterbalance to weektime academic activities, as well as enhancing my teaching with current ideas and information about the clinical area.

The moonlighting form of clinical practice has no formal links to the academic role, merely having the status of a second job. The literature indicates that this form of practice is quite common, particularly in schools of nursing where there are no formal faculty practice arrangements in place (Joachim 1988, Just et al 1989). I was unhappy to continue my clinical role under these informal circumstances for several reasons. Firstly, the academic role is demanding of time and energy, and additional weekend shifts make for a very long week with little time for family or recreational activities. Secondly, the requirement to maintain professional links and clinical expertise is an expected part of the academic role, yet, at that time, the only way I was achieving this was by undertaking additional outside employment. Therefore, for organisational and professional reasons it was important to find some other arrangement, such as a supernumerary clinical position during the working week which could be sustained, and which would be formally recognised by the university as a normal, and hopefully scholarly, part of my academic role.

In order for the clinical experience to support my academic and theoretical development the arrangement would need to permit a focus on issues other than direct care delivery, an approach to practice which could not occur while being part of a ward roster. Algase (1986) suggests that for faculty practice to advance the discipline of nursing it must have as an outcome the goal of moving the faculty member beyond mere acquisition and maintenance of skills.

This chapter provides an outline of some organisational models of faculty practice and the three main types of faculty practice roles. Some of the assumptions underlying the nature of faculty practice are then briefly discussed. My two formal excursions into faculty practice are described with details of the politics and pragmatics of getting in and getting started, and the value of the use of interpretive reflection-on-action and critical reflection-in-action approaches for developing the role. It was the important understandings and learnings which occurred during these practice experiences which provide the basis for my argument that faculty practice is a valuable form of scholarship for knowledge development in the discipline of nursing. As such, faculty practice needs to gain more formal recognition and reward within the university environment.

Models of faculty practice

There are several different models or organisational structures through which faculty practice arrangements can be formalised.

Unification model

This is where the faculty of nursing and the practice area come under a single administrative structure, and where the director of nursing is also the dean of the faculty. The aim is to establish roles which encompass service, education and research. There is no arrangement like this currently in Australia, while several exist in the United States of America, with Rush University and University of Rochester as moderately successful examples (Pearson 1988). The organisational, structural and cultural changes required to move to this model are enormous. Most reports indicate that it definitely results in closer theory-practice links and a higher involvement in research, but the organisation and administrative issues can be cumbersome and difficult to manage. Therefore measures of its success have occasionally been guarded (Kelly et al 1990).

Collaborative model

This is where there are separate organisational structures for the college and the clinical area, but they function interdependently and educators and clinicians hold dual appointments in education and service. The most common form of these are joint appointments, such as those at Deakin University (Crane 1989), the University of South Australia (Emden 1986, Geoghegan et al 1993), the University of Tasmania and Western Institute of Technology (Cooper 1988).

Joint appointments work reasonably well if there is organisational recognition of the dual role, the dangers lying with possible unmanaged workloads and certain role conflicts (Acorn 1991, Steele 1991). It is interesting to note that the Deakin University appointments as lecturer/clinician or clinician/lecturer reflect certain weightings of clinical practice involvement. The first involves about 20% time with a clinical case load, the second approximately 50% each way, although these proportions can vary. The requirement that the practice involves direct patient care via a case load, although supernumerary in the 20% case, is rather limiting on the possibilities which faculty practice can offer.

Integration model

In this model the university develops its own independent health care service, and faculty members provide direct and indirect patient care in conjunction with their role as teachers. The administrative support here is similar to that of a collaborative model. Barger and Bridges (1990) and Barger et al (1993) found that colleges with nursing clinics fostered theory-practice links and increased scholarly output. In Australia it is likely that the development of poly health clinics by some universities, which include the provision of nursing services, will be seen in the next few years.

Private practice model

This is where faculty have arrangements to access a clinical area for practice. The arrangement between the university and the hospital may include student teaching, and occasionally payment for services. The two faculty practice experiences described below follow this model.

Staff nurse role

This is where faculty gain clinical positions outside their working hours or during holiday and summer breaks or by moonlighting.

These models reflect organisational structures within which faculty practice may occur. Within these models Just et al (1989) have drawn on the various definitions of faculty practice to identify three main roles for academics undertaking faculty practice: the nurse-researcher, the nurse-clinician and the nurse-consultant. These three roles provide a framework within which almost any involvement in the practice area by nurse academics can be described as faculty practice. Each role aims to improve patient care and enhance scholarly development and this chapter provides examples of the latter two roles.

There are some assumptions which limit views of what faculty practice can achieve. For example, based on the commonly held belief that 'those that can't practice, teach' (Carter 1987, Street 1992), there is an assumption that the main purpose of faculty practice must be to upgrade forgotten clinical skills. Whether this belief about nurse educators had any validity in the past or still has in the present, one unfortunate outcome is the rather limited view it may lend faculty practice. Algase (1986) points out that this limited view is difficult to support academically or economically. Using faculty practice as a means of acquiring and maintaining skills alone, detracts from the possibilities it provides for furthering theoretical and practical knowledge for the academic and clinicians involved.

Another perception about faculty practice is that it is only of value for the faculty member, not for the clinical area. Certainly most of the discussion in the literature about this role occurs amongst academics. It is refreshing therefore to read the views of McClure (1987), Director of Nursing at a medical centre and one of the few non-academic writers in this field. She notes that many benefits accrued to her centre as a result of faculty practice arrangements. Hospital staff, who were able to share their practice setting with faculty members with extensive expertise, gained considerably in their knowledge and understanding of their field of practice. McClure felt sure that the two-way flow of ideas and information between faculty and hospital staff contributed significantly to the better preparation of students.

Kramer and Schmalenberg (1979) and Moorhouse (1992) ascribe much of the reality shock new graduates experience to the collision between the educational values of the university, to which they have been socialised, and the service provision values of the hospital. Parker (1994) also comments on the oppositions of concepts which reinforce the education-service gap when she mentions the binary divisions underpinning the term 'faculty practice,' where the university faculty produces pure, abstract and generalised knowledge, and the practice setting deals with applied, concrete knowledge within localised contexts. She suggests that in view of current structural, economic and work force issues which have the potential to divide the profession again, it is time to move beyond the dualistic mode of understanding faculty practice to an approach which encourages collaboration in practice.

Faculty practice as a nurse-clinician

My first formal faculty practice arrangment was as a nurse-clinician within the private practice model. The experience of this role provided background for the development of a second role as nurse-consultant during the subsequent year.

The first placement was as a staff nurse in a city trauma unit for two weeks during summer semester break. The timing of this practice was important as it contributed to a positive experience. At the university during this time of year there are many administrative and academic matters requiring attention in preparation for the coming academic year, but teaching and student contact loads are low. By working to get ahead with preparation and co-ordination work, and with the university department Chairperson freeing me from a few of the administrative activities which occur during this period, I was relatively free of other academic responsibilities for the two weeks of practice, and needed to return to the office on only two days each week. The resulting focused attention and energy enhanced the benefits gained and the enjoyment of the experience.

Written permission was obtained from the hospital Director of Nursing and the Chairperson of the university School of Nursing, and salary and insurance cover was continued by the university. Although supernumerary to the ward roster I negotiated with the charge nurse to work some of those shifts where staff numbers were slightly lower. Perhaps this was simply a need to feel useful, a case of old habits dying hard, but it did help increase my level of participation in patient care.

My purpose for this experience was primarily to take a patient case load to upgrade and improve my clinical knowledge, decision making and skill level. In addition, because this particular unit had separate funding and a less hierarchical management structure than that of other areas in the hospital, I was interested in finding out about the management of the unit and the role of the charge nurse in its funding, resource planning, staffing and professional development decisions.

I enjoyed this period of practice with its change of pace from academe. I was made to feel very welcome by the charge nurse and ward staff, and this proved a crucial factor as it enabled me to feel quite comfortable with the patients, staff and ward environment within a few days. At the end of each shift I made notes about the events of the day. As the days passed my jottings changed from recounting events to being more focused on aspects or themes I was noticing. For example, the different attitudes to health and wellness between older and younger patients, and their responses to and reflections, or lack of them, on their accidents and trauma. I also observed the charge nurse's democratic style of leadership and appreciated the extent to which it enabled nursing staff to participate in ward decisions and planning.

My journalling was done at the end of each day, using only one side of the page to allow for further jottings, insights and interpretations as I reviewed my observations of events. This process is consistent with the reflections on actions described by Holly (1987), Schön (1983), and Carr and Kemmis (1986). I took an interpretive approach when reviewing my own and others' actions. I sought to understand the meaning of these by taking into account the timing and context of each situation. An interpretive approach seeks to generate knowledge which promotes self-awareness. Deriving from the work of Heidegger (1962), and the symbolic interactionism of Mead (1934) and Blumer (1969), it aims to minimise distortions when gaining an understanding of a particular event by attempting to view the world from the perspective of the other person or persons involved. To do this their interactions with, and the influence of, contextual factors are taken into account when reflecting on an event.

During my first formal faculty practice experience I was pleasantly surprised to find the ease with which I re-acquired or slipped back into what Helen Cox (1991) delightfully describes as the confident 'fluidity of practice'. This is the ability to deal with and calmly co-ordinate nursing care in an environment that is largely unstructured and frequently unpredictable. Cox believed that it is the fluidity of practice which allows us to shift our focus out from ourselves so that we can really see the people for whom we are caring. She felt it was an essential element of practice which nurses often take for granted and do not value. During this period of faculty practice my speed of care delivery was occasionally slower than that of the local ward staff, but I was happy to find that I was able to comfortably maintain an outward focus even when dealing with unfamiliar issues or trauma unit emergencies.

The experience of this fluidity in practice and the ideas which surfaced from the reflection-on-action process strongly influenced my choices when arranging a second faculty practice situation the following year.

Developing a nurse-consultant faculty practice role

In retrospect, the transition from a nurse-clinician role with a patient care focus to a nurse-consultant role with a focus on broader service delivery issues may seem a natural development. At the time however, the exact manner in which to approach the second faculty practice placement was not clear. My first placement had found me comfortable with a patient case load, and the interpretation of my journal had raised interesting issues and created some new understandings. However I felt my faculty practice role could be extended and deepened by exploring the possibilities and challenges which exist within a practice setting, and then being able to follow through and act upon an issue identified through journalling. This meant setting up a practice situation which permitted flexibility of timing and focus, for it was not possible to anticipate exactly where this process would lead.

Following discussions with the charge nurse of a neurosurgical ward, a proposal was drawn up which set out some guidelines for my practice. Some general aims were set down, and the timing was to be approximately one half day per week, the day and time to be renegotiated between us each week. The proposal was approved by hospital and university administrations who at this time were working to formalise a faculty practice program. This program fell within the framework of a private practice model and was initially aimed at improving patient care and developing and maintaining skills. Later developments of this program reflected broader collaborative goals including the enhancement of professional development and the advancement of the discipline of nursing. Under this program academic staff retained super-numerary status with salary and insurance covered by the university.

My first few weeks in the neurosurgical ward involved full day shifts with a patient case load. Although I knew the ward well from teaching pre-registration students there, these shifts allowed me to settle in, get to know the staff and experience the ward routine. From my ward experience and my early journal entries it became apparent very quickly that one of the difficulties experienced in this ward was the lack of experienced staff to guide the first year graduate nurses, several of whom were on their first rotations. Only two of the five associate charge nurse positions were currently filled, there were two second year registered nurses and eight first year graduate nurses. The remainder of the staff was made up of hospital student nurses in their final year of studies, and two enrolled nurses.

Using the Dreyfus model, Benner (1984) has suggested that the best guidance for novice nurses comes from nurses who are one level ahead in their development, such as an advanced beginner. There were only two nurses in the ward at this level, and few others with expertise in the neurosurgical nursing specialty. Not surprisingly, the charge nurse had found that the graduates were having some difficulties with defining their registered nurse roles. The first year nurses were undertaking a one year graduate nurse transition program which was supporting them well, but there were still some difficulties in knowing how to take responsibility and accountability for their actions, and particularly in following through on the outcomes of their care. The graduates were still in transition from student role to that of registered nurse.

The following three weeks involved working as a buddy for a morning shift with a graduate identified by the charge nurse. My aim during this time was to provide role modelling, support and guidance as necessary. Perry (1988) emphasises the importance of modelling expert practice to improve graduates' belief in their capacity to achieve. I had some concerns about my role as some of the graduates had studied at the university, and although I had not previously been their clinical teacher, they knew me through my lecturing role. It was possible that they, and I, could confuse the buddy role with that of being a clinical teacher. I believed that perpetuating such a teacher-student relationship would not promote their role development. It is interesting to note here that some writers take the view that faculty practice should not include the supervision of students in the clinical area (McClure 1987, Kuhn 1982). However, these writers also tend to see faculty practice as being limited to the maintainance or updating of clinical skills.

The feedback from the graduates and the charge nurse about the days as buddy was mainly positive, and I found it useful to be able to see novice university and hospital prepared graduates in action. They particulary needed support in the clinical decision making cycle, specifically in pulling together the details they obtained from their assessments and making sense of them for care planning, delivery and follow through. My work during this period was supported by using Thomas et al's (1991) information on the differences between expert and novice decision making. Each week I worked with a graduate to create specific problem solving strategies in relation to our assigned patients, and then later discussed with them how these strategies might be generalised to other situations.

After three weeks I had only spent time with three of the eight new graduates. I was keen to continue working with the graduates, and felt sure that there must be a way of spending some rewarding time with more of them than I was achieving through buddying. It was time to review my goals and objectives with the charge nurse. We decided I would conduct some group sessions for the first and second year graduate nurses during double shift time in the early afternoon. The charge nurse organised for as many as possible to attend, and at most sessions there were 5 or 6 nurses.

Since there were few role models close to their level of experience available in the ward, I wanted to create a situation where the graduates began working on developing the following aspects of their beginning practice:

1   creating a strong peer support group which was focused on progressing their learning and professional development
2   clarifying their ideas of the qualities which a registered nurse with one or two years of experience might have, in contrast to those they would expect from an expert nurse with many years of experience
3   using this support and information to set some goals for their own and the group's ongoing development.

Using reflection-in-action with first year graduate nurses

At this time I realised I had moved from a reflection-on-action approach to critical reflection-in-action (Fay 1987, Smyth 1986). I had begun sharing my journal notes with a university colleague as well as with the charge nurse. Schön (1983) mentions the need to talk with others in order to uncover the obvious issues that we cannot see ourselves. By using reflection in and on action to discover what lies below the surface we extend ourselves and our knowledge of the discipline. Cox (1991) found reflection-in-action during her faculty practice caused her to encounter some sudden realisations of what was happening whilst in the midst of action. As a result she was able to immediately change her behaviour. Similarly during this period with the graduate nurses, I had a real sense of thinking and acting on my feet, as I worked with them through some of the difficulties they were encountering in developing their new roles. My realisations occurred while in action, and during subsequent reflections on the events, when my understanding was deepened and sometimes changed.

Although the graduates were on friendly terms, they actually knew very little about each other so the first group session involved some 'getting to know you' processes. One process involved identifying the qualities and strengths they brought to their nursing in this ward, and sharing these with the group. Some links were made at that point for various members to help others with particular issues, where special expertise had been identified. Other non-ward sources of support were also discussed briefly at this time. Moorhouse (1992) noticed that some new graduates tend to choose inappropriate role models. Since this group were working mainly with their peers, it was important to guide them in identifying and valuing each other's strengths, and to emulate these where appropriate.

Subsequent discussion during the first session centred around noting the differences they had observed between the practice of novice and experienced nurses, in order for them to have some closer and more realistic goals for their stage of development and to guide them as they extended their professional roles. Attempting to become an expert practitioner immediately was unrealistic and unattainable in the short term. Although the graduates had noticed the differences in levels of practice and were able to describe them quite accurately, few of them had previously thought about this in relation to their own level of professional development.

The second session began with further group work processes to strengthen their supportive peer group links. The graduates were then asked to write down problems they were experiencing in their practice. To ensure that this process remained productive and did not disintegrate into just another 'gripe' session (Moorhouse 1992), the identification and rating of the problems took the form of a Beckhard analysis (Beckhard & Harris 1987). All their problems, large and small, were brought forward and acknowledged. They were then ranked by the group, firstly for importance, and then for ease of solution. A whiteboard was used for the ranking process. Many problems had been raised, but a clustering of those rated as most important by the group were:

- increased levels of responsibility related to the lack of experienced staff and their own limited experience
- complex, sometimes confusing and inefficient communication channels within the hospital
- patterns of patient allocation which sometimes created stressful workloads
- documentation, including their own lack of skills and the inadequate notes made by other nurses
- long handovers which did not always provide enough information about patient needs
- charts being away from the bedside for handovers and checking.

During the next session the problems were reviewed and the group was guided to choose one or two from the 'important and easy' group (rather than the 'important and difficult' group) with which to begin work. It was important for the task to be manageable and achievable for this their first exercise in group problem solving, yet it should still be seen as being sufficiently important to justify their efforts.

The problems chosen related to increasing the availability of charts at the bedside and enhancing the effectiveness of handovers. Initially the graduates tended to feel that they were unlikely to be able to achieve change. Ensuing discussion then related to the process of researching why something was being done, how else it could be done, and then working for change if that was still believed to be necessary. The possibility of trialling new processes for short periods such as one month was raised, and avenues for accessing and communicating with other ward staff such as addressing the next staff meeting, use of a bulletin board and suggestion box were identified. Some beginning tasks were identified and assigned to the group and, as my period of faculty practice was soon to end, some ongoing processes for change were discussed.

The problems raised by the graduates were mainly organisational in nature, and their initial reluctance to work for change may reflect in part their strong need to fit in with a pre-existing culture. The need to fit in provides some explanation for the tradition in nursing of the 'gripe' session, which is thought by many nurses to be a way of debriefing their stresses. While these sessions may relieve some stress through sharing experiences, they can actually work to perpetuate the existing culture, beliefs and behaviours. Without structure or guidance such sessions do little to create the changes and improvements in nursing practice which could lead to less stressful working structures and environments (Moorhouse 1992, Street 1992, Wolf 1988).

When discussing the group sessions with the charge nurse we both believed that by working to achieve some small change and improvement in their practice, as begun during the group sessions, the graduates would begin to experience their roles as registered nurses more fully, and it would ease their transition from student to novice practitioner. Once I had completed my faculty practice period, this group continued with these issues until they changed wards for their next graduate year clinical rotation. Rotating rosters and clinical placements had made it difficult to sustain continuity with the graduates throughout the time I was working with them. Fortunately the ward staffing situation is now much improved, but the lack of experienced staff meant that I relied heavily on the charge nurse to take over some of this role when my time was completed.

Reflection-in-action: some scholarly insights

My work with the first year graduate nurses was intended to facilitate their introduction to organisational and professional processes and thereby enhance their role development. However, what really concerned me during the sessions with the graduates was their frequent focus on what I will call survival issues. During one of the sessions I asked the group to add up how many times that day they had spent time on things such as searching for equipment, finding out about ward and/or hospital procedures and protocol, and generally attending to other orientation and familiarisation level functions. It was quickly very clear that a large proportion of their time and energy was going towards this level of function, the group estimating that this could be as high as two thirds on some days. Two themes from my journals had alerted me to pursue this issue.

Firstly, when listing their problems none of the graduates mentioned areas of their nursing practice which they felt needed to be extended or deepened. The problems they raised were external and organisational, not related to a growth in personal practice as I had expected. Secondly, several graduates seemed to be relating change of environment to the process of learning. That is, they equated adapting to change and adjusting to the newness of a ward with the process of learning about nursing practice. Both hospital and university graduates spoke in these terms. Judith Perry's study (1985, 1987) suggests that our educational processes create a culture of learning where clinical mobility is the norm. This mobility does not permit a depth of practice development. Students become adept at learning to fit in and survive in different environments where they are able to function without being too seriously deterred by their lack of familiarity with the local milieu. Once the environment becomes familiar, and the student, or graduate, becomes comfortable, it begins to feel to them as though they are no longer learning and it is at this point that they believe they should be moving on. The graduates in our group who had been through previous clinical rotations believed that it took two or three months to become familiar enough in one area to begin feeling comfortable about working there.

Therefore frequent clinical rotations such as those in some graduate year programs perpetuate this situation. It seems likely that just at the very point of comfort when it might be possible for the graduate to begin advancing to the next level of practice, the next clinical rotation occurs. Benner (1984) considered that novice nurses are often given too much variety which prevents them from concentrating on and becoming competent in one area. It is very difficult to advance levels of expertise when the graduate is frequently unsettled by new and unfamiliar environments. In fact, existing learning is often temporarily forgotten while graduates are busy adapting to new situations, and this may retard their progression overall, affecting their confidence in their ability to cope and develop as a competent nurse.

The survival issue was what interested and challenged me most during this period of faculty practice. In nursing education we talk about using reflective practice to deepen our expertise and explore our potential as carers, but we create learning situations which teach adaptability in survival level skills and an expectation of mobility. Although there are no easy answers to this issue, we need to continue considering ways of structuring learning which would enable students to extend beyond this level of practice. Recent changes to the graduate program at this hospital have meant that students now have one rotation during their first year, with the option of one change on their request.

On reflection, my faculty practice and subsequent working through some of these ideas has deepened of my knowledge of the discipline of nursing. These experiences have influenced my approach to curriculum issues, my own teaching and the preparation of other clinical teachers, and the structuring of clinical practicum for the students. It has been a very scholary experience indeed.

Implications of faculty practice for nursing scholarship

Surveys of staff involved in faculty practice have found that most academics consider faculty practice to be a scholarly activity (Starck et al 1991). In addition, many believe that participation in faculty practice at various times during their academic life increased their scholarly productivity (Starck et al 1991, Steele 1991). Starck also discovered a significant number of academics who were still engaged in informal forms of faculty practice such as the moonlighting model, although others, such as Kuhn (1982) argue that moonlighting should not be regarded as a form of faulty practice. Barger et al (1990, 1993) found that more schools of nursing with access to their own nursing clinics had formalised practice arrangements than did schools without such clinics. In addition, faculty practice was more likely to be a criterion for promotion but not for tenure in these schools. Cook and Finelli (1988) describe how the development of a scholarly faculty practice plan was a means of revitalisation for their school of nursing and enabled exploration of new partnerships between nursing service and education.

This section provides discussion of aspects of academic life which promote the development of scholarly faculty practice. There are two main aspects. The first is a review of those criteria related to the setting up of a private practice arrangement such as the one above, which contributed most strongly to its success. The second aspect relates to some suggested changes in the structure and outlook of nursing faculties which may enhance the acceptance and development of faculty practice at an organisational level.

Some criteria to promote scholarly faculty practice

My experience of faculty practice enriched me personally and professionally, and this flowed onto my classroom and clinical teaching. It expanded my own and others' views on how we might develop more creative, thoughtful and productive links with the clinical area. It has opened channels of informal and formal communication within the clinical area, and provided a sound base from which to establish more creative clinical experiences for students. The experience has guided some curriculum changes particularly at pre-registration level, and ideas for further study and projects have been stimulated.

When setting up our arrangement the charge nurse and I realised that we needed an approach which had flexible time frames and allowed for creative exploration of issues which might arise. The faculty practice program being established at that time between the hospital and the university permitted this flexibility and creativity. The criteria we used were similar to those set out by Polifroni and Schmalenberg (1985) when describing the conditions which permitted the development of their nurse-consultancy roles, namely:

1   It was important to have the approval and legitimisation of both hospital and university at Director of Nursing and Chairperson or Dean level
2   It was important to have positional authority, resulting from the academic's own experience and expertise and from the hospital administration and charge nurse, to increase acceptance by clinical staff
3   Flexibility and creativity were fostered by leaving the exact details for the nature and times of the placement to the discretion of the charge nurse and the academic, with room for revision and change as either felt the need
4   As the role developed clear benefits for the academic, the charge nurse, the ward, hospital and the university needed to continue to be seen. Frequent reviews of progress achieved this
5   Non-interference by hospital or university administration with the process. In particular, faculty should not be asked to evaluate the clinical area as this would change the whole nature and ethics of the relationship.

A detailed report of the experience was made to both administrations at the completion of the period. The Charge Nurse and I were able to increase our understanding of the nature of the discipline of nursing. This sense of collegial and scholarly sharing may not have happened so easily if the role had been more structured or had an income generating focus.

Improving formal recognition of faculty practice in academia

Emden and Young (1987) state that nursing should develop its own unique research traditions. Similarly, nursing faculties need to arrange their managerial traditions, including faculty practice, to suit the needs of the profession. Nursing is a relative late comer to the university environment. Into this very different environment with its largely empirical, academic, elitist and paternalistic traditions nursing brings a history and culture which can place it at great disadvantage. The background of apprenticeship style training, the traditional subservience to the medical profession, and a largely female population are at odds with the university culture. Considerable change is required in order for nursing to fit in, and the question is with whom or where should these changes take place?

Low participation by academic staff members in faculty practice is reported by several writers (Just et al 1989), and a survey by Bellinger (1985) found that a majority of schools had no policy on faculty practice at all. Most writers mention lack of time as a reason for non-involvement as well as the failure to count faculty practice as criterion for meeting tenure. Curtis (1980) suggests that part of this may be because faculty practice is difficult to evaluate, particularly when compared to research and publication, the traditional measures for promotion and tenure at university.

Rather than change or adapt completely to the existing university traditions, it is appropriate for nursing to take a pro-active role in creating and setting in place new traditions which will serve it best within the university and the professional milieux. It is inappropriate for nursing to take on board structures, management styles and scholarly processes which pre-exist in other unrelated disciplines and which are not relevant for a practice based discipline. For example, the models of university life which might work for the faculties of philosophy or history are inappropriate for professional faculties such as engineering, education or nursing.

Management structures in a professional school such as nursing which permit staff to redesign their roles from year to year would promote individual professional development and a responsiveness to the rapidly changing social and economic environment within which the university operates. In this way the role would reflect the proportion of the areas of teaching, practice, research and community activities on which the academic is focusing at that time, rather than some arbitrary proportioning of time set down by selection, promotion or workload guidelines. This permits rotation of responsibilities, and formalises recognition of areas which might not otherwise be counted for workload purposes. It reduces the risk of role conflict, overloading and burn-out by promoting the ability of the staff member to rotate and develop in each of the areas viewed as important for promotion and tenure, yet without the need to be performing in all of them at any one time. It would also foster a sense of newness and freshness of purpose every few years as staff change their roles to suit their current level of academic development and the current needs and projected goals of the organisation. A rotational system encourages the perception of each of these roles with equality, rather than seeing pure research as the highest form of scholarship, part of the old elitist paradigm. It can provide formalised opportunities for younger staff to develop roles in areas other than classroom teaching, while allowing more senior staff to experience classroom teaching again.

Yeatman (1993) discusses the need to set up equity oriented change processes in education faculties, where a large number of the students are female, in order to achieve equality for women in the gendered university culture. This includes actively initiating, formalising and legitimising management processes for women and for non-empirically based forms of scholarship. In nursing it is necessary to take these steps too. Speedy (1990) describes some consciousness raising and collegiality activities which could be organised by management to address issues such as gender roles and responsibilities and academic competition. Her suggestions are based on a premise that some of the perceived disadvantages for nursing faculty in the wider university may be turned around by exploring their basis and finding ways of changing or working around them. In this way the changes we make can have impact on the way we organise and provide rewards for our work both within the nursing faculty and the wider university.

Conclusion

In our report to the hospital and the university the charge nurse wrote:

> The experience provided us with the opportunity for a cross-fertilisation of ideas. Preparation of reports and other papers from this experience are good for expanding the experience and expertise of staff in this ward. It has provided further means of recognition for myself and the ward for undertaking the exploration of new ideas. The interactions between Helen and the newer ward staff provided them with challenges and the opportunity to enhance their professional role development.

Our experience was that faculty practice can do much more than merely upgrade skills, or bridge the theory-practice gap. It can lead to a deeper understanding of the theory and processes of nursing, and, more importantly, contribute to changes and shifts in these. We found that nursing knowledge derives from practice, but is also extended with the interplay of theoretical perspectives, practice processes and wider philosophical and societal influences and knowledge.

'A professional discipline's knowledge base is associated with the realm of practice...The generation of this body of knowledge will involve both scholars and practitioners' (Gray & Pratt 1991). Fawcett and Carino (1989) identified two hallmarks of success in contemporary nursing practice as the establishment of links between nursing education and nursing service, and the recognition of clinical scholarship as a professional imperative. Speedy (1989) also believes that an interplay of theory and practice are highly desirable. Faculty practice which is flexible and creative can bring academics and clinicians together and add to our knowledge of nursing by forming the basis for more formal research, consultancies and collaborations, and thereby enhancing knowledge development within the discipline.

When stepping into the university culture, it is important to shed those aspects of our own nursing culture which no longer serve us. Just as important is the need to influence and change those aspects of the university hegemony which do not further our development by creating structures and systems which embody nursing philosophies and values. Formalising organisational processes for the recognition of faculty practice as a scholarly activity within schools of nursing is one essential step to gaining recognition and reward for it within the wider university milieu.

ACKNOWLEDGEMENT

I am indebted to the support and encouragement I received from Katy Fielding and Ruth Denson, the two charge nurses with whom I collaborated during these experiences. Without their willingness to share their intellect and expertise none of this would have been possible.

REFERENCES

Acorn S 1991 Relationship of role conflict and role ambiguity to selected job dimensions among joint appointees. Journal of Professional Nursing 7(4):221-227

Algase D L 1986 Faculty practice: a means to advance the discipline of nursing. Journal of Nursing Education 25(2):74-76

Barger S E, Bridges W C 1990 An assessment of academic nursing centres. Nurse Educator 15(2):31-36

Barger S E, Nugent K E, Bridges W C 1993 Schools with nursing centres: a 5-year follow-up study. Journal of Professional Nursing 9(1):7-13

Beckhard R, Harris R 1987 Organizational transitions: managing complex change, 2nd edn. Addison-Wesley, Massachusetts

Bellinger K 1985 Faculty practice policy. Journal of Nursing Education 24:214-216

Benner P 1984 From novice to expert: excellence and power in clinical nursing practice. Addison-Wesley, California

Blumer H 1969 Symbolic interactionism: perspective and method. Prentice Hall, New Jersey

Carr W, Kemmis S 1986 Becoming critical: knowing through action research. Deakin University, Victoria

Carter M A 1987 Professional practice: those that can't practice, teach. Journal of Professional Nursing 3(3):131

Cook S S, Finelli L 1988 Faculty practice: a new perspective on academic competence. Journal of Professional Nursing 4(1):23-29

Cooper D 1988 My experience of being a joint appointee. Bridging the gap! between nursing theory and practice. Conference Proceedings, Deakin University, Geelong, Victoria

Cox H 1991 Exploring clinical practice: a journey of critical reflection. Embodiment, Emancipation and Empowerment. Conference Proceedings, November, Melbourne

Crane S 1989 Joint appointments: the Deakin experience. The Australian Journal of Advanced Nursing 6(3):21-25

Curtis M 1980 Evaluating the clinical performance of faculty: fact or fantasy. Cognitive dissonnance: interpreting and implementing faculty practice plans in nursing education, National League for Nursing, New York

Emden C 1986 Joint appointment: an Australian study illuminates world views. The Australian Journal of Advanced Nursing. 3(4):30-41

Emden C, Young W 1987 Theory development in nursing: Australian nurses advance global debate. The Australian Journal of Advanced Nursing 4(3):22-40

Fawcett J, Carino C 1989 Hallmarks of success in nursing practice. Advances in Nursing Science 11(4):1-8

Fay B 1987 Critical social science: liberation and its limits. Polity Press, Oxford

Geoghehan M, Haebich E, Bartel A 1993 Innovative collaborative practice. Shaping Nursing Theory and Practice. Second National Conference Monograph 2, La Trobe University, Department of Nursing, Melbourne

Gray G, Pratt R 1991 Towards a discipline of nursing. Churchill Livingstone, Melbourne

Heidegger M 1962 Being and time. Harper & Row, New York

Holly M L 1987 Keeping a personal-professional journal. Deakin University, Victoria

Joachim G 1988 Faculty practice: dilemmas and solutions. Journal of Advanced Nursing 13:410-415

Just G, Adams E, DeYoung S 1989 Faculty practice: nurse educators' views and proposed models. Journal of Nursing Education 28(4):161-167

Keithley J K, Uebele J A 1989 Faculty practice: issues and applications for perioperative nurses. AORN Journal 50(3):587-594

Kelly K, Maas M, Maske J 1990 Adjunct executive appointment for faculty. Journal of Nursing Administration 20(10):35-42

Kramer M, Schmalenberg C 1979 Reality shock: the voices of experience. Nursing Resources, Massachusetts

Kuhn J 1982 An experience with a joint appointment. American Journal of Nursing 82:1570-1571

McClure M 1987 Faculty practice: new definitions, new opportunities. Nursing Outlook 35(4):162-166

Mead G H 1934 Mind, self and society: from the standpoint of a social behaviourist. University of Chicago, Illinois

Moorhouse C 1992 Registered nurse: the first year of professional practice. La Trobe University Press, Victoria

Nahas V L 1990 Faculty practice: keeping up with change. The Lamp 47(1):26-27

Parker J M 1994 Collaboration in practice: the concept of faculty practice. The First International Congress of Collaboration in Nursing: Working Together To Achieve Academic Excellence, keynote address, University of Canberra, Canberra, ACT

Pearson A 1988 What is unification? Bridging the gap! between nursing theory and practice. Conference Proceedings, Deakin University, Geelong, Victoria

Perry J 1985 Theory and practice in the induction of five graduate nurses: a reflexive critique. Masters Thesis, Massey University, New Zealand

Perry J 1987 Creating our own image. NZ Nursing Journal 80(2):10-13

Perry M 1988 Preceptorship in clinical nursing education: a social learning theory approach. The Australian Journal of Advanced Nursing 5(3):19-25

Polifroni E C, Schmalenberg C 1985 Faculty practice that works: we call it clinical consultancy. Nursing Outlook 33(5):229-230

Schon D 1983 The reflective practitioner: how professionals think in action. Basic Books, New York

Smyth W J 1986 Reflection-in action. Deakin University, Victoria

Speedy S 1989 Theory-practice debate: setting the scene. The Australian Journal of Advanced Nursing 6(3):12-20

Speedy S 1990 Nursing faculty development: from principles to practice. Royal College of Nursing Australia Monograph Series, Melbourne

Stainton M C, Rankin J A, Calkin J D 1989 The development of a practising nursing faculty. Journal of Advanced Nursing 14:20-26

Starck P L, Walker G C, Bohannan P A 1991 Nursing faculty practice in the Houston linkage model: administrative and faculty perspectives. Nurse Educator 16(5):23-28

Steele R L 1991 Attitudes about faculty practice, perceptions of role and role strain. Journal of Nursing Education 30(1):15-22

Street A F 1992 Inside nursing: a critical ethnography of clinical nursing practice. State University of New York Press, Albany

Thomas S A, Wearing A J, Bennett M J 1991 Clinical decision making for nurses and health professionals. Saunders Bailliere Tindall, Sydney

Wolf Z R 1988 Nurses' work: the sacred and the profane. University of Pennsylvania Press, Philadelphia

Yeatman A 1993 The gendered management of equity-oriented change in higher education. In: Baker D, Fogarty M (eds) A gendered culture: educational management in the nineties. Victoria University of Technology, St. Albans, Victoria

FURTHER READING

Barger S E, Bridges W C 1987 Nursing faculty practice: institutional and individual facilitators and inhibitors. Journal of Professional Nursing 3(6):338-346

Barger S E, Nugent K E, Bridges W C 1992 Nursing faculty practice: an organisational perspective. Journal of Professional Nursing 8(5):263-270

Borttorff J 1986 Degree graduates: reflections one year on. The Australian Journal of Advanced Nursing 3(2):33-45

Carlson l, Crawford N, Contrades S 1989 Nursing student novice to expert: Benner's research applied to education. Journal of Nursing Education 28(4):188-190

Choudry U K 1992 Faculty practice competencies: nurse educators' perceptions. The Canadian Journal of Nursing Research 24(30):5-17

Dufault M A 1990 Personal and work-milieu resources as variables associated with role mastery in the novice nurse. The Journal of Continuing Education in Nursing 21(2):73-78

Gardner G 1989 An action research project to investigate the transition support needs of a group of nurse graduates, Masters Thesis, Monash University, Melbourne

Hamilton J, Kiefer M 1986 Survival skills for the new nurse. Lippincott, Sydney

Harvey J 1988 Life's not easy when you're first through a course, but ... The Australian Journal of Advanced Nursing 5(4):19-21

Herr K A 1989 Faculty practice as a requirement for promotion and tenure: receptivity, risk and threats perceived. Journal of Nursing Education 28(8):347-353

Keen M F, Dear M R 1983 Mastery of role transition: clinical teaching strategies. Journal of Nursing Education 22(5):183-186

Klaich K 1990 Transitions in professional identity of nurses enrolled in graduate education programs. Holistic Nursing Practice 4(3):17-24

Lambert C E, Lambert V A 1988 Faculty practice: unifier of nursing education and nursing service. Journal of Professional Nursing 4(5):345-355

Williamson N B, McDonough J E, Boettcher J H 1990 Nursing faculty practice: from theory to reality. Journal of Professional Nursing 6(1):11-20

7

Scholarship in nursing practice

JENNIFER GREENWOOD

Introduction

According to the Shorter Oxford Dictionary (1983), scholarship is '...an attitude of a scholar' and a scholar is someone who is 'learned'...! These definitions are singularly unhelpful for what, precisely, does the attribute of scholarship entail or reflect (or, what precisely do 'learned' individuals do)? In this chapter I will attempt to elucidate the nature of scholarship, particularly as this relates to nursing; I will show that it is reflective of certain values and skills which manifest in a rigorous and open criticality to all sorts of insights, irrespective of their source. By this I mean that scholarship in nursing requires the careful and systematic examination of the validity of insights derived from both formal science and from experience.

Nursing is a practice. So also are nursing education, nursing management and nursing research and, as practices, are deserving of the most valid theoretical bases. The most humane and effective nursing care, education, management and research is a function of scholarship; this is because rational humanity is a function of scholarship.

The values and skills reflective of scholarship for and in nursing practice are acquired or learned although, clearly, innate intellectual acuity will influence the degree of scholarship to which individuals might reasonably aspire. The nature of these values and skills and their acquisitive processes will be the focus of this chapter; I will argue that scholarship *for* practice finds expression in theoretical reasoning and scholarship *in* practice, in practical reasoning. And further, that theoretical reasoning involves both inductive and hypothetico-deductive manipulation of propositions, derived from a range of sciences and experiences, at differing levels of inclusiveness and awareness. Theoretical reasoning enables the practitioner to describe, explain and predict, more accurately and adequately, the practical nursing realities she has or will experience. By the same token, practical reasoning which involves only hypothetico-deductive manipulation of situationally salient propositions, again derived from a range of sciences and experiences, at differing levels of inclusiveness and awareness, enables the practitioner to control and produce the practical nursing realities she considers desirable.

In addition, I will argue that the quality of the theoretical and practical reasonings of nurses are, in turn, a function of both the validity of their salient norm and fact-stating propositional contents and the cognitive skills with which they are manipulated. This will entail an examination of:

a nursing as a social practice
b the nature of representations (concepts) and their acquisitive processes
c the nature and levels of theory
d theoretical and practical reasoning.

Salient implications for the development of nursing scholarship will be discussed as they arise in these analyses. The chapter will terminate in a description of the roles of nursing education, nursing research and, to a much lesser extent, nursing management in the development and promotion of scholarship for and in practice.

Nursing as social practice

Nursing as social practice implies two things. Firstly, that as a social practice what nurses believe about nursing either explicitly or, more probably, implicitly is constitutive of nursing and, secondly, that it is directed to the achievement of change rather than to truth or knowledge (however construed).

Social practices do not exist independently of the knowledge of the actors involved in them; nurses could not nurse or, indeed, even recognise instances of nursing if they did not 'know' it, at some level. Social practices are constructed and sustained by the observation of certain social rules which are 'known' to obtain in any given social situation by all the actors involved. What this implies is that people interacting in social situations understand, at some level, the meaning(s) of the situations and the meaning(s) of the rules which both constitute and sustain them. The 'rules' of nursing (and, therefore, nursing itself), for example, exist only when nurses interact in certain, anticipated ways which probably, inter alia, expedite discharge of workload (Melia 1981, Seed 1991, Moorhouse 1992).

People both encounter 'objects' in the world and experience those 'objects' subjectively; for example, we can recognise an object of experience such as our first-born and we can 'experience' that object through intense feelings of joy. It is the combination of such objective and subjective representations which constitutes the meaning of experiential 'objects' of whatever kind. The intellectual manipulation of mental or internal representations of both types of experience allow human beings to act on, as well as in, their worlds (Sanford 1984). I will return to this subsequently.

114

Nursing as a practice (or practical activity) is directed towards change; it is distinguishable from theoretical activities such as sociology and philosophy because their central purpose is to discover/invent truths about the world (Langford 1973). Both practical and theoretical activities are, however, composed of combinations of observations and actions. Thus, for instance, natural scientists perform experiments to test hypotheses and nurses utilise the 'truths' that they themselves or others invent/discover to inform the goals they pursue and the means to their achievement. In addition, in the normal course of events there is no temporal distinction between acting and observing but action is monitored by observation of the task situation within which a person finds herself.

Despite this, practical and theoretical activities are clearly different and their difference hinges on the purposes/intentions with which they are pursued. Nursing is a practice; it aims to bring about positive change in the health status of individual people and communities and it is distinguishable from other similar practical activities, like medicine and physiotherapy, which might also claim the same overarching purpose, by the beliefs and values about nursing which nurses possess and which issue in their practices.

Nursing exists only in nursing activities which are reflective of the beliefs and values of nursing held by the nurses undertaking such activities. In addition, it is the reflection of the beliefs and values concerning nursing and nursing work which allow nursing activities to be identified as *nursing* activities, rather than something else. Such beliefs and values are internal representations concerning nursing and nursing work and, as such, imbue it with meaning. Given this, it is imperative that critically reflective nurses understand the nature and function of, and the processes underpinning, the acquisition of such representations.

Representations and their acquisition

Representations of 'objects' of experience, including physical objects, facts, values, norms, rules, events, actions, results of actions and their concomitant subjective experiences allow people to represent to their own consciousnesses all that they experience. They allow the recognition, interpretation and (re)action to presently incoming stimulation. Representations, which are also termed concepts, constructs and construals, are constructed automatically through simple exposure (Eysenck & Keane 1990) precisely to enable people to recognise, interpret and (re)act appropriately to subsequent, similar stimulation. They thus allow people to structure experience by imposing meaning on it and, thereby, render it manageable.

Representations are acquired in two ways. They are acquired either relatively deliberately and consciously through teaching or reading, or incidentally and relatively unconsciously through mundane experience (Neisser 1976, Eysenck 1984). How they are acquired, however, determines their clarity and this, in turn, impacts (or potentially impacts) on the adequacy and accuracy with which they represent experiential phenomena.

Deliberately and consciously acquired representations are usually 'clear-cut' (Howard 1987); they are typically acquired as feature lists, represented propositionally; for example:

- this wound is inflamed...
- it is red...
- it is hot...
- it is swollen...
- and painful...

Adequate and accurate representational feature lists delimit precisely what the representation includes; to be adequate and accurate implies near exhaustion of description.

Such clear-cut representations and the propositions they reflect are often constructed and tested scientifically, that is, carefully and systematically using logic and empirical evidence. Scientists call this 'theory'. Despite this, however, it would be naive to accept uncritically such scientifically derived representations. To begin with, representations typify objects of experience; through exposure to individual instances representations are constructed which include typical members/features of a class which, in turn, allows the subsequent recognition of further individual instances of it. (It is the case that individual or unique 'objects' of experience can only be recognised as unique instances *of a kind.*) This implies that they may not account for all the aspects of currently experienced reality. In any case, 'theory' deals with general or typical representations which always require application to the parameters of the individual case. In addition, scientifically derived representations are constructed by fallible human scientists who work within deliberately tight theoretical frameworks precisely to minimise the fallibility of the truths/conclusions they invent or construct. It should be remembered, too, that as fallible human beings scientists may also be prey to questionable, implicit representations reflective of certain biases; the race and gender bias of early intelligence tests is illustrative here. Whatever else scholarship for and in practice may demand, therefore, it requires that practitioners examine the practical validity or utility (see below) of such representations against the realities they were constructed to render more meaningful and more manageable. Scholarly practitioners should be open to, but critical of, the theoretical contributions of formal science (including nursing science).

Incidentally and relatively unconsciously acquired representations are rather different. These are acquired simply through experiential exposure; they are not clear-cut but 'fuzzy' (Howard 1987) and consist, typically, in largely pictorial or imaginal exemplars which do not delimit precisely what the concept includes. Indeed, their fuzziness may be such as to render subsequent recognition/interpretation problematic; in this situation, the influence of context on appropriate interpretation is critical. An example: two men are digging holes, one in the road and one in the churchyard; how would one know that they were not doing the same thing?

There are three further and important points concerning representational acquisition to be noted. Firstly, the clarity and adequacy of representations constructed is a function of the interaction between the experiential 'object', what the cogniser already knows, the current needs and interests of the cogniser, the situation in which the cogniser is found and the uses to which the representations will be put (Roth 1986). This means that representations will only be as clear-cut and as adequate as they need to be for their possessor to get by. Importantly, therefore, if clear-cut representations are not required for, or rewarded in, everyday nursing practice nurses will not construct them. This point is particularly significant for nursing because so many of nursing's central concepts are abstract. The activities associated with 'maintaining independence', for example, are not self-evident and nursing students will require structured exposure to instances of them, in practice. 'This is an example of maintaining independence...because it is...because it does...and...'

Secondly, and related to this, a person can possess potentially several representations to represent the same experiential object for use in differing situations. Thus, for example, a nurse may have one clear-cut representation of nursing as giving individualised, holistic care for assessment and assignment purposes and another 'fuzzy' representation of nursing as getting through the workload for use in clinical practice settings (Melia 1981, Seed 1991, Moorhouse 1992, Waters 1994). The former she learns deliberately and consciously from nurse academics/educators and nursing literature; the latter, relatively unconsciously and incidentally from nurse practitioners by working with them, day-in and day-out in clinical practice situations.

The critical point concerning representational acquisition, however, is this: representations are constructed to render task situations meaningful and manageable by allowing a person to interpret subsequent similar stimulation and to plan and execute appropriate responses. This means that they are activated by the environmental cues found in such situations. For instance, assessments, assignments and nurse academics/educators seem likely to trigger a repertoire of nursing concepts that are consistent with the delivery of holistic care, whereas people and objects typically found in clinical practice situations may trigger a repertoire more consistent with getting through the workload (Greenwood 1990).

Thirdly, fuzzy representations are constitutive of 'theory', too, albeit of a fuzzy, informal type (Argyris & Schön 1977, Dickoff & James 1970). Fuzzy representations are strung together in organised hierarchies with other fuzzy and clear-cut representations to enable their possessor to describe, explain, predict and prescribe their realities and their subjective experiences of them.

Fuzzy representations are 'theories' because, irrespective of their largely exemplary, imaginal nature, they are reflective of propositions in the same way as clear-cut feature lists. Each time they are deployed to interpret experience ('...this is a...') and structure action ('...therefore I should...') the truth of their propositional content is tested. The adequacy and accuracy of these fuzzy propositions are tested day-in and day-out each time they are activated and deployed and the feedback elicited confirms or disconfirms their validity. There is no requirement, however, for such feedback to be consciously apprehended. Seed (1991) provides an account of a staff nurse working in a clinical situation which graphically illustrates this point. The registered nurse, who held the nose of a patient whilst pouring fluid into his mouth was probably not acting deliberately cruelly or, importantly, atypically. The registered nurse may well have had a range of fuzzy propositions—relating to skimping work, getting through the workload and persons—unconsciously operational at the time. Had their operationalisation elicited negative feedback when previously deployed, however, they may have been modified and/or replaced.

In terms of scholarship, this highlights an important, if rather obvious point and it is this: if a person is unaware of the construction of certain representations, she will also be unaware when she is deploying them to interpret incoming stimulation and structure (re)action. This means she will also be unable to surface them, articulate them and then challenge them for adequacy and accuracy against the realities they were constructed to represent. A further and related point is that she will also be unable to challenge them against scientifically derived representations related to the same phenomena. Their modification or replacement will, therefore, be unlikely. Given this, the surfacing and challenging of fuzzy representations is pivotal to the promotion of scholarship in practice.

'Fuzzies' can be surfaced or identified in two ways. Firstly, a nurse can be asked to talk through what she intends to do, why she intends to do it, when, to whom, with what and how she will do it before she initiates action; 'fuzzies' may become manifest during this reflection-before-action (Greenwood 1993). Secondly, because they may not become manifest until activity is underway, especially when the nurse construes her activities as part of an assessment (see above), she may well require sensitive assistance to identify and examine them. This is the task of anyone who is involved in nursing education, including clinical nurses.

There is yet more to be said about representational acquisition. To begin with, representations, clear-cut and fuzzy, are not constructed serially; they are constructed as reality is experienced, that is, holistically but following 'natural discontinuities' (Roth 1986). Thus, for instance, nurses are often 'experienced' with patients, mothers with babies, birds with trees, and so on. The world does seem full of regular configurations of 'objects' (and, therefore, subjective experiences of them). When a person learns that an object is an instance of a type she also learns how it is valued in her particular culture from the behaviour, including the verbal behaviour, of other cultural indigents (see below). She also learns how to respond appropriately to it, either through the same 'observational' mechanisms or through her own trial and error attempts which elicit feedback. Thus, she learns, for example, how certain genders, races, ages, classes and abilities are valued and disvalued in her culture, just as Seed's (1991) staff nurse did.

In addition, experience is considered to be composed of two types of 'particulars' which contribute to experiential 'wholes'; these are focal and subsidiary particulars (Polanyi 1958). Focal particulars are those to which the person is currently attending; these typically include those which are consistent with her current intentions or interests or which command attention by virtue of intensity of stimulation, e.g. loudness, brightness and novelty (Neisser 1976). Subsidiary particulars are rather different; they include world views, frames of reference and social rules (or action theories) through which objects of experience can be recognised and interpreted, that is, rendered meaningful. Subsidiary particulars are not usually apprehended consciously; they are tacit (Polanyi 1958). Nevertheless, they function as explanatory frameworks which contribute meaning and add coherence to situated experience.

In addition, they include a range of physical, social, affective and evaluative stimuli inferred from the behaviour and utterances of others which allow a person to recognise experiential objects as being objects of a kind. They provide the context of action and, as such, are of critical importance in the recognition of fuzzy representations, as noted above. The 'looks' that Melia's (1981) and Seed's (1991) student nurses elicit as feedback from qualified colleagues when they are not seen to be pulling their weight are examples of such subsidiary stimuli.

Clearly, then, in the pursuit of scholarship, it is also important to identify those frames of reference which add coherence and contribute meaning to experience. Revealing them, however, can be problematic. Practitioners need to think through what sorts of frameworks would or even could make certain experiential particulars meaningful. Thus, for instance, pouring fluid into patients' mouths while holding their noses only makes sense when nursing is construed as getting through the workload (Melia 1981, Seed 1991, Street 1993). The ability to identify such frames of reference, however, presupposes a similar ability to identify the representations of experiential particulars that are operational in a task situation and it has already been suggested that practitioners may well require assistance to do this. In the same way, and because they will be attending focally to interesting experiential particulars, they may also require sensitive assistance to identify, surface and challenge these explanatory frameworks which render situated experience meaningful.

It has already been claimed that theory construction consists of the formal generation and testing of propositions by responsible (if fallible) human scientists at differing levels of complexity and inclusiveness; it has also been suggested that cognition fulfils this function automatically in 'ordinary' human beings. Information, in the form of representations, is organised and stored hierarchically and this is a function of the 'chunking' of items of information to be stored in memory (Sloboda 1986). Thus facts are chunked with their 'appropriate' values and, where relevant, their appropriate action tendencies, and input (sensory-perceptual) processes with output (motor) processes. Nursing students observing Seed's staff nurse, for instance, will learn at least two things simultaneously simply through exposure to her behaviour. They will learn that patients/clients with certain characteristics are valued less than others by professional nurses and, consequently, that they may be treated in ways which reflect this lack of value. It is precisely because 'object', which in this instance is a certain type of patient, and 'value' are experienced together that certain patient characteristics are chunked with certain action tendencies. Chunking is a function of repetitive testing (also usefully construable as practice) in relevant task situations and it accounts for the speed, 'seamlessness' and automaticity of skilled performance. Once 'input' and 'output' representations and mechanisms have been chunked a whole sequence of complex intellectual and/or psychomotor behaviours can be run off automatically, that is, quite unconsciously. This ability to automatise much that inheres in complex skills allows people to deal (relatively) successfully with their attentional limitations. Attention, that is, human consciousness, can accommodate only nine, plus or minus two, items or chunks of information (Miller 1956).

Progressive chunking is a function of practice and feedback in task situations which both promote the construction of, and subsequently trigger, the representations which allow accurate interpretation and appropriate response. Each time representations are activated and deployed the connections between them are strengthened (Brown 1968, Rundus 1977); practice, therefore, strengthens connections between representations. Feedback has two functions. It provides further information for addition to already constructed re–presentations and, thereby, facilitates subsequent activation (Howard 1987); it also provides the means to correct or modify action through the construction and activation of more appropriate sub-routines.

The promotion of scholarship for and in practice is, therefore, a function of feedback-governed practice in relevant task situations; irrespective of the nature of the skills to be developed, be they intellectual, interpersonal or practical (manual) the same principles obtain. For scholarship in practice this means that the skills (and the action representations they reflect) should be taught as far as practicable in the clinical situations they are constructed to render meaningful and manageable and which will, eventually, trigger quite automatically their activation and deployment.

There is one further point to be made with respect to representational construction. Information, in the form of representations, is organised and stored hierarchically at what are considered to be three general levels (Roth 1986, Berlin 1972). These levels are: subordinate, where maximum specific detail is stored; basic, where the most economical amount of detail is stored for efficient human functioning; and superordinate, where only generalised information which subsumes basic representations is stored. Basic level representation is the most convenient and efficient for cognitive activities such as perception, memory and communication (Howard 1987). For instance, 'getting through the workload' (Melia 1981, Seed 1991) possesses more information than 'fitting in' to the ward team whereas 'skimping work' possesses more information than 'getting through' but this additional information may well be superfluous to requirements. In this case, 'skimping work' is subordinate to 'getting through' which is, in turn, basic to 'fitting in'. The latter is, in this representational hierarchy, the superordinate concept. Basic level representations are, therefore, the normal components of everyday discourse. What counts as 'basic', however, is problematic (Rosch et al 1976). Basic level representations may vary between individuals or between groups depending on culture or, more particularly, knowledge.

This has important implications for both nurse educators/academics and experienced clinical nurses who may, by virtue of specialist education and training, work from a set of 'basic' representations that are more sophisticated than those of the people they are observing. This, again, implies that the accuracy of the level of representation imputed to the people being observed should be checked against the level of representation actually operational in their cognitions. It also provides opportunities to furnish less expert nurses with elaborative feedback which will, in turn, promote their own more sophisticated representational construction.

The hierarchical organisation of representations is undertaken automatically by human cognitive systems; unremarkably, therefore, representations are also organised hierarchically by human scientists as they, too, attempt to render experiential particulars meaningful. This hierarchical organisation is reflected in the levels of theory they construct.

Levels of theory

A theory is a conceptual framework invented to describe, explain, predict and prescribe the phenomena experienced in reality (Dickoff & James 1968). Action theories are prescriptive, situation-producing (Dickoff & James 1968) or control theories (Argyris & Schön 1977) and they presuppose predictive theories (Naish & Hartnett 1975). Accordingly, the analysis will begin with predictive theories.

Essentially a predictive theory is a statement of relation (or proposition) between two states of affairs, of the type '...if A...then B...' Such propositions are normally tested exhaustively by quantitative scientists/methodologists to demonstrate the veracity or validity of them; verification through exhaustive testing warrants the proposition being accorded the status of causal law. Causal laws describe the necessary and sufficient antecedent conditions to 'cause' certain subsequent conditions, and to cause them always.

Causal laws thus allow the prediction of consequences which follow from the bringing about of certain antecedent conditions but prediction, in turn, requires some representation of both the existing conditions and the to-be-brought about or subsequent conditions. These latter representations presuppose further representations, that is, of the salient or significant factors and their interrelationships in both the existing and to-be-brought-about conditions or states of affairs. Both representations, that is, the representation of factors and the relationships between them are modes of theorising which necessarily presuppose predictive or causal theory. These more primitive levels of theorising are termed, respectively, factor isolating and factor relating, by Dickoff and James (1968). Prediction, as a statement of causal relation between two states of affairs, therefore, presupposes more primitive levels of representation. It is, of course, possible to conceive of relations other than the merely causal between two conditions or states of affairs and, indeed, of relations between more than two states of affairs. Such representations are theories related to the promotion or inhibition of certain causal effects; they capture the 'subtleties of causal relatedness' (Dickoff & James 1968). Thus factor isolating, factor relating and situation relating, which includes predictive, promoting and inhibiting theories are all presupposed in situation producing or prescriptive theory.

Each level of theory presupposes the existence of theories at the lower levels. Situations are described in terms of factors already isolated and predictive theories represent relationships between described situations. Similarly, situation producing theories prescribe situations (realities) in terms of available predictive theories and use factor isolating and factor relating theories in the representation of goal(s).

The purpose of situation producing theories is to bring about desired states of affairs; they are action theories which describe what an agent must do in order to bring about a desired state of affairs. They have three essential ingredients:

a a goal content which specifies the characteristics of the situation to be produced
b prescriptions for the activities required to produce such situations
c a survey list to supplement the prescriptions (Dickoff & James 1968).

Dickoff and James (1968) remind us that the survey list is a particularly significant ingredient of situation producing theory because it draws attention to two special considerations. Firstly, it aids the identification of other theories at different levels which will assist in the realisation of the intended goal. Secondly, it assists in the identification of relevant factors and aspects of activity which are inadequately represented in action directives (and, therefore, require elaboration and/or refinement).

Recognition of the survey list is, in turn, reflective of a recognition that the activity described in the prescription is not solely determined by goal and prescription. A person's judgement is central to intelligent action as judgement is required to choose and produce appropriate sub-activities in particular task situations in an attempt to realise the goal. Such judgements, however, are normally made unconsciously and they are reflective of automatic intellectual skills (Greenwood 1990) the exercise of which allows people to consult the salient features in a particular situation and make instant adjustments to routine sub-activities and actions in response to fluctuating situational demands (Benner 1984, Fitts & Posner 1967). The quality of these judgements will, therefore, reflect the relative degree of scholarship in practice operational at the time.

The function of the survey list is to enhance the effectiveness and appropriateness of activity. It is for this reason that Dickoff and James (1968) suggest that the survey list should be organised on the basis of the salient aspects of activity; these are:

- Agency—who or what performs the activity?
- Patiency—who or what is the recipient of the activity?
- Framework—in what context or in which terms is the activity performed?
- Terminus—what is the end point of the activity?
- Procedure—what is the guiding procedure, technique or protocol?
- Dynamics—what is the energy source of the activity?

It should be noted that answers to these questions will describe relationships between two or more concepts which represent two or more existent or to-be-brought-about states of affairs. In other words, they must be framed propositionally. A further if obvious point is that levels of theory or theorising are merely reflective of human reasoning or inferencing. Human reasoning is theorising; it is concerned with the manipulation of propositions at differing levels of inclusiveness and awareness.

Propositions are of two types (Scheffler 1960, 1965), namely, fact-stating (...this is a person...) and norm-stating (...she should be treated with respect...) and they are organised logically in representational hierarchies which connect those representing experiential particulars to those representing wider interpretive frameworks and 'world views'. Fact-stating propositions link factual beliefs at differing levels and norm-stating propositions link ideal beliefs or values to action directives, again at differing levels of complexity. It is precisely because norm-stating and fact-stating propositions are logically and hier-archically organised that meaning can be imposed on reality.

The manipulation of propositions is, however, non-propositional. Propositions can usefully be construed as contents of mind and their manipulation, that is inferencing or reasoning, as acts of mind. Such acts of mind, of course, include judgements.

Theoretical and practical reasoning

Human beings reason (or theorise) for two purposes; they reason to complex conclusions about the world in order to describe, explain and predict objective and subjective phenomena in it and they reason to action in order to bring about the changes they consider desirable (Langford 1973, Carr 1981). The former reasoning is termed theoretical reasoning, the latter, practical reasoning.

Theoretical reasoning proceeds logically through inductive and hypothetico-deductive manipulation of propositions at differing levels of inclusiveness and generality, which is reflected in 'levels' of theory and logically begin in basic, observational propositions of a 'this is a...' and 'it is related to...' nature, to complex truths or conclusions about the world. In contrast, practical reasoning proceeds again, logically, but only through the hypothetico-deductive manipulation of propositions of an 'if...then...' nature at progressively decreasing levels of inclusiveness and generality related to action prescriptions and survey lists which logically begin with complex human intentions or purposes (goals) to their successful execution in a (surprisingly) finite range of simple actions (Carr 1981, Sloboda 1986).

Practical reasoning, that is, reasoning which underpins situation producing or action theories, enables the identification and manipulation of the plethora of salient propositions which logically connect intention to action.

The propositions operational in practical reasoning are valid or true if they lead to the successful bringing about of the state of affairs that is desired (Carr 1981). There is, however, a complexity to be noted. Practical reasoning must be responsive to fluctuating situational demand because practice is char-acteristically ambiguous and uncertain. (This is why, of course, observation monitors action.) What this implies, therefore, is that the propositions operational in practical reasoning are valid or true if they do or would have led to the successful bringing about of the desired state of affairs, *other things being equal.*

This has important implications for scholarship in practice. Firstly, it indicates that scholarship in practice is a function of the quality of the practical reasonings of practitioners. This, in turn, is a function of both the validity of the propositional content of such reasoning and the intellectual skill with which it is manipulated. Secondly, that practical reasoning must reflect a sensitivity to the exigencies of practice. What this means is that practitioners must continually and intelligently observe their actions and sub-routines (and the propositional content they reflect) for accuracy, adequacy and appropriateness, that is, salience, in dynamic and changing practical situations. Thirdly, and in light of this ongoing monitoring, they must be able to operationalise, at differing levels of complexity and awareness, alternative more appropriate actions and sub-routines (and the propositions they reflect) as situational idiosyncrasy dictates. In short, they must skilfully *reflect-in-action* (Schön 1983).

The role of nursing research

It has already been stated that scholarship in practice is a function of the validity of the propositional content of practical reasoning schemes and that these propositions can be scientifically and/or experientially derived. On this account, it is the task of nursing research to generate and test propositions/ theories for potential inclusion in such practical reasonings. What follows concerns the role of interpretivist and action research in this; I have already alluded, albeit tangentially, to the role of 'quantitative' research in propositional validation.

It should be remembered that although practical reasoning underpins scholarship in practice, theoretical reasonings (or, at least the end products of theoretical reasonings) are subsumed within it. This seems important for interpretivist nursing research. To begin with, when an interpretivist questions another person about her beliefs she is, in an important sense, questioning her about a conclusion (albeit at differing levels of sophistication). This conclusion is the end result of a process of theoretical reasoning or inferencing, probably long forgotten and buried in some superordinate representational structure, involving propositions relating to both focal and subsidiary experiential particulars, which logically began in some simple proposition of a 'this is a...' nature.

In addition, and similarly, when an interpretivist observes action she is observing the conclusion of a process of practical reasoning or inferencing which, at some point, related propositions of an 'if...then...' nature (Sloboda 1986) to the intention(s) they attempted to execute. These propositions, too, will relate to both focal and subsidiary experiential particulars and be buried, more than likely, in superordinate representational structures.

The task of interpretivist nursing research is clearly awesome (Greenwood 1994a). It is to construct a valid mirror-image of the descriptive, explanatory, predictive and prescriptive propositions that are operational, at differing levels of complexity and awareness, in the minds of those being observed. Furthermore, this can only be accomplished through the inferencing of the prior inferencings (reasonings) of those being observed. These must then be 'played back' to the practitioners involved (and the wider nursing community) to allow their examination as both interpretive (this is a...) and action structuring (so I should...) devices, in the situation wherein they were initially identified, and more widely.

The role of action research as it is now commonly construed, or action science, (Argyris & Schön 1991) is even more daunting. For it aims to emancipate or liberate individual practitioners and groups of practitioners from maladaptive or otherwise inappropriate fuzzy representations, and the propositions they reflect, which operate, again, at differing levels of inclusiveness and awareness, and replace them with those of more validity. This involves the same sort of inferencing undertaken by interpretivist nursing research and the construction and testing of alternative propositions to achieve strategic change. Clearly, too, in order to be *action research* it has to capture and map the logic of these alternative propositions (Greenwood 1994b).

In short, the role of nursing research in the development and promotion of scholarship in practice is, firstly, to reveal the propositions that operate to sustain maladaptive practical situations and, secondly, to assist practitioners to examine and selectively replace them. This latter is, to my mind, the most critical. For it is to encourage practitioners to reason systematically and carefully from their strategically chosen intentions to their successful execution in action. In other words, it is to promote precisely the sort of practical reasoning (Greenwood 1994b) that scholarship in practice depends upon.

The role of nursing education

The development and promotion of scholarship for and in nursing practice is the raison d'être of nursing education; I take this to be necessarily true. Education is concerned to furnish nurses with the most valid fact-stating and norm-stating propositions, the intellectual skills with which to manipulate them and a deep respect for nursing and scholarship; all three are required to ensure nurses' commitment to a scholarly approach to practice.

When fact and norm-stating propositions are manipulated in schemes of theoretical reasoning they describe the logic of propositional knowledge; when manipulated in schemes of practical reasoning they describe the logic of procedural knowledge. Their cognitive manipulation enables practitioners to reason with more adequacy and accuracy to complex conclusions about aspects of practice and related phenomena and to simple actions to change aspects of their practice. The former, on this account, is an expression of scholarship *for* practice, the latter, of scholarship *in* practice. How these might be developed and promoted has already been described (see above); however, four important and related pedagogical points remain to be made. These relate, respectively, to the systematic use of feedback, the assessment of practical performance, the valid assessment of values (norm) acquisition and the importance of role models in the promotion of practical scholarship.

The systematic use of feedback

The informal and formal elicitation of feedback in representational construction through the observation or monitoring of action by a person herself or a teacher/ peer has been alluded to previously in this analysis; the provision of feedback on feedback is, however, critical to the promotion of scholarship in practice. By requiring nurses to give feedback to themselves prior to, during and following nursing activities they are being required to monitor these activities closely. Furthermore, through the provision of elaborative feedback, that is, feedback that adds to and embellishes existing knowledge, the quality of their subsequent feedback to themselves will be enhanced. Moreover, if these exercises are undertaken on a *sufficiently regular basis* nurses will learn to monitor their activities in this fashion quite automatically. Rigorous and continuous self-monitoring of practice or, *reflection-in-action* is scholarship in practice (Greenwood 1990).

The assessment of practical performance

The quality of nurses' self-monitoring that they learn to incorporate automatically into their practice is a function of the quality of the assessments (or monitoring by others) to which they are exposed. Practical performance can be assessed against two criteria; firstly, the success of the performance in terms of goal(s) achievement and, secondly, the intrinsic worth of the goal(s) in terms of some overarching values system or purpose. The first requires the revelation and examination of situationally salient propositions that are/were operational in the cognitions of the nurse, related to goal(s), prescription and survey list. In short, it requires the critical examination of the logic of the propositions which link goal(s) to actions. The second requires all this, too; however, it requires it at a more inclusive, generalised level of representation for it requires critical examination of the logic of the propositions which link sub-goals to overarching purposes and intentions and the values they reflect.

An example: a nurse is able to complete all the daily hygiene activities required by patients assigned to her care by morning coffee-break; this is an expectation in the clinical facility where she is working. She is able to accomplish this because she alone makes decisions related to patient care needs in light of what she knows of the patients. However, should her constructions of nursing include valuing patient autonomy, independence and the recognition of certain rights of patients to be included in decision-making related to their care, etc., she would be successful, somewhat paradoxically, in performing activities that should either not have been performed at all or, at least, not in the manner that they were.

Both levels of assessment describe aspects of the logic of procedural knowledge; both are necessary, therefore, in teaching nurses how to nurse. Arguably, however, it is the examination of sub-goals against overarching purposes which teaches nurses to be the sorts of deeply reflective nurses we would wish to develop.

The valid assessment of fact and norm-stating propositions

The validity of propositional knowledge, both fact and norm-stating, requires the fulfilment of three conditions, namely, a belief condition, an evidence condition and a truth condition (Scheffler 1965). Thus one could impute to a nurse knowledge that, say, the trachea lies between larynx and bronchi, if and only if, she believes it does, she has good evidence that it does and, it does. Similarly, one could impute to her knowledge that, say, she should organise care on an individual basis if, and only if, she believes she ought, she has good evidence that she ought and, she ought.

These examples are instructive in that they illuminate the problematic nature of the evidence condition. Firstly, there are concerns as to the legitimacy of claims to propositional knowledge when it is acquired vicariously, that is, when one is merely told or otherwise made aware that something is the case; this indicates that a person can possess propositional knowledge in both weak and strong senses. Propositional knowledge in the weak sense depends solely on having true belief; that is, believing that the trachea lies between larynx and bronchi and that one ought to organise care on an individual basis. Propositional knowledge in the strong sense, however, requires something further, namely, the appropriate substantive evidence.

Much of the propositional content of nursing curricula is propositional knowledge in the weak sense; much of what students learn related to fact and norm-stating propositions is accepted by them on the plausible assumption that the relevant conditions have been satisfied and this clearly has implications for the development of critical scholarship in nursing. Much of what is taught in nursing curricula is the end-product of processes of enquiry and, moreover, it is often taught didactically; 'hands on' data collection and analysis, in the broadest sense, is disappointingly uncommon and even the *critical* use of corroborated research findings in nurse teaching is less frequent than one would hope. Irrespective of the reasons for this (see for example Marquis et al 1993) it does indicate that currently nurse educators themselves do not always exhibit a real spirit of enquiry. Until they do, however, it is unlikely that nursing undergraduates will learn to appreciate its importance.

There are three further and interrelated complexities to be noted with respect to norm-stating propositions that differentiate them from fact-stating propositions. The first is that only justifications count as 'evidence' in norm-stating propositions and some of these at least will not be verifiable empirically. The second is that 'ought' statements, per se, cannot be true or false, only the hypothetical imperatives generating them may be. Thus, if a nurse wishes to...then she ought...The third is that norm statements possess both active and non-active interpretations of knowing that.

On an active interpretation of knowing that, the imputation of such knowledge to a nurse rests on the satisfaction of a further condition beyond truth, evidence and belief, namely, evidence of the incorporation of the norm in question into her actions. An example: how would we know a nurse knows that the trachea lies between the larynx and bronchus? We would be satisfied that she knew if she could state this fact, demonstrate it on an anatomical model or even draw a diagram to illustrate it. In contrast, however, in order for us to be satisfied that she had learned that honesty is the best policy we would require evidence that she was honest. Flagrant dishonesty would constitute a refutation of any claim that she knows that honesty is the best policy.

Of course, on a non-active interpretation the acquisition by a nurse of this pattern of behaviour is not required by the truth of these statements; evidence of her dishonesty due to weakness of will, behavioural inconsistency and so on, would not be incompatible with the truth of the statement. All that would be required is evidence of her ability to state that..., demonstrate ability to discriminate between examples that..., and so forth but this amounts to using evidence criteria for fact-stating propositions for determining the veracity of her claims to norm acquisition.

Thus failure to examine conduct with respect to norm acquisition as opposed to examining utterances or statements with respect to norm acquisition is fallacious (Scheffler 1960). The fallacy is, moreover, facilitated by the 'verbalism' prevalent in education, including nursing education. A similar fallacy occurs when nurse teachers promote the learning of norms in the same way as anatomical facts. Teaching someone *to be* something or other involves teaching her *to be* something or other always, in all sorts of situations; this amounts to equipping her with strong action tendencies or dispositions to act in a certain way consistently across a range of situations. This in turn requires that the student learn both *to be*...and to believe that she *ought to be*...Teaching a nurse to be..., therefore, requires both the acquisition of the norm in question and some sort of intellectual acknowledgement of its authority. It is to teach a nurse *to be*...out of conviction (Scheffler 1960).

The importance of role-modelling in the promotion of practical scholarship

Role-modelling is an exceptionally powerful teaching/learning strategy. This is because human action, that is, the purposive physical activities of people, is represented in cognitive systems both pictorially and imaginally, because they are *physical* activities, and semantically, because they are *purposive* (meaningful) activities. In contrast, human utterance is represented almost entirely semantically. What this implies is that, in a sense, action contains twice as much information as utterance. Thus when a nurse's actions and utterances are discrepant the former will be construed as more faithfully representative of her belief systems. Importantly, of course, these belief systems will include those related to the nature of nursing and nursing work. More positively, however, when action and utterance are congruent the meaning of the action will be clear; its representation will be correspondingly clear and subsequent activation and retrieval in similar task situations will be enhanced. In a nutshell: the promotion of scholarship for and in practice is critically dependent upon exposure to professional role models, clinician, academic/educator and manager, whose own professional practices clearly manifest a 'hunger for understanding' (Diers 1988).

The role of nursing management in the promotion of scholarship

The importance of role-modelling a scholarly approach to practice has already been highlighted; there are, however, additional requirements for nursing management, including educational management, if scholarship is to be systematically promoted. These concern strategy and structure and their relationship to the view of scholarship that I have been at pains to explicate.

For if scholarship for and in practice is a function of the manipulation of salient norm and fact-stating propositions, at differing levels of inclusiveness and complexity, as I have argued that it is, then what counts as scholarship in nursing practice, education, management and research should not be restricted to the traditional, university view that scholarship is the generation/invention of new knowledge or truths. The critical application of insights to practical activities, the critical integration of insights into more inclusive theoretical schemes and the appropriate presentation of these to neophyte practitioners should all be recognised as reflective of scholarship. In this, I am at one with a range of scholars in nursing (e.g. Hanson 1993, DeTournyay 1990, 1991, Tanner 1991, Rice 1990, Boyer 1990).

Management strategies in health care agencies and academic schools of nursing should reflect this view of scholarship, particularly with respect to staff development and research strategies and resources should be targeted to support such strategic plans (DeTournyay 1990). Importantly, too, management structures and processes should be implemented to facilitate this view of practical scholarship; these could usefully include the implementation of appropriate selection and promotion criteria.

Patients are currently nursed and student nurses are currently socialised in health care facilities that, in general, neither require nor reward a scholarly approach to practice (Moorhouse 1992). Clearly, therefore, systematic improvements in both nursing care and nursing education hinge on a re-orientation of fundamental clinical and educational management imperatives (Poteet et al 1987). Thoughtful, skilled, humane nursing care is a function of scholarship and this, in turn, is a function of clinical and educational management strategies and structures which foster its promotion.

Conclusion

Scholarship for nursing practice is expressed in the theoretical reasoning of nurses and scholarship in practice, in their practical reasoning. Theoretical reasoning seeks to construct 'truths' and conclusions about nursing practice and practice-related issues; it involves conscious and unconscious inductive and hypothetico-deductive manipulation of fact and norm-stating propositions at progressively increasing levels of inclusiveness and complexity. In contrast, practical reasoning seeks to construct prescriptions for practice; it involves conscious and unconscious hypothetico-deductive manipulation of fact and norm-stating propositions at progressively decreasing levels of inclusiveness and complexity. Theoretical reasoning enables nurses to render meaningful their practice-related activities and practical reasoning, to render them manageable.

The propositional content of theoretical and practical reasoning schemes is stored in memory in both clear-cut and fuzzy representations. The former, typically, are scientifically-derived and are acquired by nurses deliberately and consciously through teaching and reading; the latter, typically, are experientially-derived and are acquired incidentally and relatively unconsciously through everyday nursing activities. Representations are constructed to render situated experience meaningful and manageable; they are constructed and triggered by the environmental cues found in such situations.

The purpose of nurse education is to furnish nurses with the most valid fact and norm-stating propositions related to nursing practice and with the intellectual, interpersonal and practical skills to enable their appropriate deployment. The purpose of nursing research is similar; it is to identify maladaptive and inappropriate fact and norm-stating propositions and replace them with those that more faithfully represent the realities they seek to render meaningful and manageable. Finally, the purpose of nursing management, both clinical and educational, is to create the conditions wherein practice both requires and rewards the acquisition, deployment and continual refinement of such propositions.

REFERENCES

Argyris C, Schön D 1977 Theory in practice. Jossey Bass, San Francisco

Argyris C, Schön D 1991 Participatory action research and action science: a commentary. In: Whyte W F (ed) Participatory action research. SAGE, California

Benner P 1984 From novice to expert: excellence and power in clinical nursing practice. Addison Wesley, California

Berlin B 1972 Speculation on the growth of ethno-botanical nomenclature. Language in Society 1:51-86

Boyer E L 1990 Scholarship reconsidered: priorities of the professoriate. The Carnegie Foundation for the Advancement of Teaching, Princeton

Brown J 1968 Reciprocal facilitation and face recall. Psychonomic Science 10:41-42

Carr D 1981 Knowledge in practice. American Philosophical Quarterly 18(1):53-61

Diers D 1988 On clinical scholarship (again). IMAGE Journal of Nursing Scholarship 20(1):2

De Tournyay R 1990 Teaching as a scholarly activity. Journal of Nursing Education 29(6):101

De Tournyay R 1991 Reconsidering scholarship. Journal of Nursing Education 30(4):147-148

Dickoff J, James P 1968 Theory in a practice discipline: Part 1. Nursing Research 17(5):415-435

Dickoff J, James P 1970 Beliefs and values: bases for curriculum design. Nursing Research 19(5):415-426

Eysenck M W 1984 A handbook of cognitive psychology. Lawrence Erlbaum Associates, London

Eysenck M W, Keane M T 1990 Cognitive psychology: a student's handbook. Lawrence Erlbaum Associates, Hove

Fitts P M, Posner M I 1967 Human performance. Brooks/Cole, California

Greenwood J 1990 Learning to care: thought and action in the education of nurses. Unpublished PhD thesis. Leeds University, United Kingdom

Greenwood J 1993 Reflective practice: a critique of the work of Argyris and Schön. Journal of Advanced Nursing 18:1183-1187

Greenwood J 1994a What is it precisely that interpretive social research researches? Journal of Advanced Nursing 19:996-1002

Greenwood J 1994b Action research: a few details, a caution and something new. Journal of Advanced Nursing 20:13-18

Hanson S M H 1993 Scholarship and academia. Unpublished paper presented to the Board of the School of Nursing, Flinders University of South Australia, 14 May

Howard R W 1987 Concepts and schemata: an introduction. Cassell Education, London

Langford G 1973 The concept of education. In: Langford G, O'Connor D J (eds) New essays in the philosophy of education. Routledge & Kegan Paul, London

Marquis B, Lillibridge J, Madison J 1993 Problems and progress as Australia adopts the Bachelor's degree as the only entry to nursing practice. Nursing Outlook 41(3):135-140

Melia K M 1981 Student nurses' accounts of their work and training: a qualitative analysis. Unpublished PhD thesis . Edinburgh University, United Kingdom

Miller G A 1956 The magical number seven, plus or minus two: some limits on our capacity for processing information. Psychological Review 63:81-97

Moorhouse C 1992 Registered nurse: the first year of professional practice. La Trobe University Press, Victoria

Naish M, Hartnett A 1975 What theory cannot do for teachers. Education for Teaching 96:12-20

Neisser U 1976 Cognition and reality. W H Freeman, San Francisco

Polanyi M 1958 Personal knowledge: towards a post-critical philosophy. Routledge & Kegan Paul, London

Poteet G W, Edlund B J, Hodges L C 1987 Supporting scholarship in the health care system. Journal of Nursing Administration 17(9):4, 8

Rice R E 1990 Rethinking what it means to be a scholar. Teaching excellence: toward the best in the academy. Newsletter, Teaching Effectively Program, University of Oregon, Winter-Spring

Rosch E, Mervis C B, Gray W D, Johnson D M, Boyes-Graem P 1976 Basic objects in natural categories. Cognitive Psychology 8:382-439

Roth I 1986 Perception and representation: a cognitive approach. Open University Press, Milton Keynes

Rundus D 1977 Maintenance rehearsal and single-level processing. Journal of Verbal Learning and Verbal Behaviour 16:665-681

Sanford A J 1984 Cognition and cognitive psychology. Lawrence Erlbaum Associates, New Jersey

Scheffler I 1960 The language of education. Charles C Thomas, Illinois

Scheffler I 1965 Conditions of knowledge. The University of Chicago Press, Chicago

Schön D 1983 The reflective practitioner. Basic Books, New York

Seed A 1991 Becoming a nurse: the students' perspective. A longitudinal qualitative analysis of the emergent views of a cohort of student nurses during their three year training for general registration. Unpublished PhD thesis. Leeds Polytechnic, United Kingdom

Shorter Oxford English Dictionary 1983, 3rd edn. Book Club Associates, London

Sloboda J 1986 What is skill? In: Gelatley A (ed) The skilful mind: an introduction to cognitive psychology. Open University Press, Milton Keynes

Street A F 1993 Inside nursing: a critical ethnography of clinical nursing practice. SUNY Press, New York

Tanner C A 1991 Scholarship in nursing education. Journal of Nursing Education 30(8):339-340

Waters K R 1994 Getting dressed in the morning: styles of staff/patient interaction on rehabilitation hospital wards for elderly people. Journal of Advanced Nursing 19:239-248

8

Advanced nursing practice: different ways of knowing and seeing

FRAN SUTTON, COLLEEN SMITH

Currently within nursing there are a number of unexplored taken-for-granted ideas about the concept of advanced nursing practice. Even though this concept has been the subject of numerous debates, these debates have offered little to inform our current understanding of this type of practice. The dominant view expressed in the literature emanates from our North American colleagues. We believe these have been influential in the way that Australian nurses think about, see and experience advanced nursing practice.

Like our North American colleagues, we have recently incorporated the term 'advanced nursing practice' into our everyday language and use it synonymously with expert practice and specialist nursing practice. However, unlike our North American colleagues we have not taken the time to clarify what these terms mean and how they accommodate the needs of Australian nursing. Rather, we have accepted their interpretation of these terms. This acceptance could be problematic for Australian nursing as it assumes we share the same understanding and that there is no other possible meaning for the term. Further, it implies that nursing in Australia has features no different from that practised in North America.

Lawler (1991a) acknowledges that Australian nursing has been strongly influenced by 'culture, products, dreams and ideas' exported from North America. This, she believes, is due to the deluge of nursing literature crowding the market, the passive acceptance by Australian nurses of its superiority compared with nursing literature emanating within Australia, and the continual flow of visiting North American scholars. In discussing the notion of imported ideas, Lawler suggests 'we cannot...continue a relatively unquestioned adoption of imported ideas and not systematically explore, understand and value our own practice and its interface with the international nursing community'. Essentially she believes we need to be more critical of imported ideas and recognise there are cultural differences. Thus what is appropriate in the North

American context may be inappropriate for Australian nursing. We contend that a major issue confronting nursing as a profession and a discipline relates to the nature and notion of advanced nursing practice and how it relates to both specialist and expert practice.

The intent of this chapter is to explore the concept of advanced nursing practice and to establish some beginning relationships between advanced practice, expert practice and specialist practice. To provide a framework for this exploration we begin by describing the current and dominant perspectives of advanced nursing practice. This includes descriptions of expert and specialist nursing practice. It is followed by our beginning theorisations into the different ways in which advanced nurse practitioners think, see and experience nursing practice.

As there already exists considerable diversity about these matters, we intend this chapter to be provocative and stimulate thought but not necessarily agreement. It is our belief that these concepts have not undergone sufficient theorising or been subject to critical analysis or debate. These debates are important to the nursing profession in Australia as they provide opportunities for us to clearly distinguish important elements of nursing practice in this country. Additionally, the insights to be gained from discussion of these issues may illuminate important aspects of nursing practice with the outcomes providing clear direction for the personal and professional development of registered nurses.

Expert nursing practice

The word 'expert' has a number of meanings, each contributing to our understanding of this concept. These meanings include such elements as being especially skilled in any art or science and possessing special knowledge or experience. These meanings also suggest individuals become experts as the result of experience which enables them to develop specific skills and dexterity combined with the acquisition of discrete knowledge.

Benner (1984) offers one of the most recent and influential perspectives on expert nursing practice. In her descriptive study of nurses in practice, Benner applied the work of Dreyfus & Dreyfus and identified five varying levels of nurse expertness. She specifies a number of aspects demonstrated by practitioners functioning at the highest level, referred to as experts, which she extrapolated from exemplars collected during her study. Benner's work as a consequence is worthy of consideration as it provides useful insights into the nature of expert practice and the attributes of expert practitioners.

Benner (1984) identifies that expert nurse practitioners develop clinical expertise and that 'the hallmark of clinical expertise is an indepth knowledge of a clinical population; advanced recognitional abilities; and increased use of past whole situations or situation specific referents for understanding the clinical situation'. Inherent in this explanation of clinical expertise is that expert practitioners have an indepth knowledge of a particular clinical population; that they are able to recognise subtle changes in the patient's condition; and that this is done within the context of specific situations.

Benner (1984) believes that 'expertise develops when the clinician tests and refines propositions, hypotheses and principle-based expectations in actual practice situations'. She suggests this can only be done through experience. At the same time, Benner acknowledges the role of reflection as critical in the process of identifying the knowledge and skills held by expert practitioners. Benner suggests that 'expert nurses have a wealth of untapped knowledge...embedded in (their) practices'. She suggests that it is only through the processes of reflection that nurses can bring this knowledge into their conscious awareness and explicate the nature of expertise.

Patterson (1991) also explores the nature of expertise in the context of acute care nursing. She suggests we should not confuse expertise and excellence. Informed by the work of Peplau, Patterson states that 'expertise is an individual quality, whereas excellence is broader and relates to practice within an institution or work unit'. Essentially Patterson proposes that expertise is embedded in the individual and this is reflected in the degree of excellence exhibited through the individual's practice. Excellence is therefore the expertise made visible via the practice of experts. If we accept this notion then we are accepting that a person with expertise exhibits characteristics and dispositions that are not necessarily reflective of the expert group. A counterview suggests that while it is important to acknowledge that expertise is exhibited by the person, the characteristics which give meaning to the nature of expertise must represent those of the expert group.

Constancy in enacting a range of specific skills and in using particular knowledge or abilities enhances the opportunity for practitioners to develop expertise. Once expertise has been established the practitioner is likely to be acknowledged as an expert by colleagues. This latter point of legitimisation is important as it can only be undertaken by someone who understands the field and the knowledge and skills required. Thus, the state of being an expert is not one that an individual can claim for themselves but must be granted by the acknowledged expert group.

Thompson et al (1990) offer views on the nature of expertise and the problems inherent in defining and conceptualising this concept. They question whether the nature of expertise 'is...actual performance, ability to perform, or simply domain knowledge'. Additionally, they further question Benner's understanding of expertise as she advocates the use of situations to interpret expert practice but offers little information relevant to understanding the knowledge and thinking exhibited by experts. They elaborate further by suggesting that a better understanding of expert practitioners can be gained by disclosing the cognitive nature of their problem solving abilities. Consequently, issues requiring further exploration and debate within the profession include whether expertise derives from personal qualities of the nurse which are made evident in daily practice or whether expertise is dependent on practising within specific clinical settings.

Benner & Wrubel (1990) argue that experience is necessary for practitioners to move from one level of expertise to another. Consequently, experience means living through actual situations in such a way that it informs our perceptions and understanding of subsequent events. Factors that influence the way in which we experience the world of practice include such things as language, time and gender. The issue of gender is significant when discussing nursing as the majority of nurses are female. Thus it is likely that nurses' perceptions of experiences will differ from that held by males (Harding & Hintikka 1983). However, this factor must be understood as occurring within the context of an occupation that is strongly biased toward the masculine with respect to its structures, knowledge and emphasis (Sutton 1993).

Expertise in nursing, then, derives from familiarity with the 'doing' of nursing and requires a practitioner to be fully immersed in practice. It is clear therefore that only individuals concentrating their focus and attention on a field or aspect of nursing practice can develop and maintain expertise and therefore become nurse experts. Therefore the very notion of expert practitioner refers to the work of clinicians rather than that of the nurse academic, administrator or researcher. This has major implications for the ongoing professional development of experts. If we accept that they derive knowledge from experience and learn while doing we need to ensure such opportunities are provided. It is in this area that nurse academics, administrators and researchers can do much to assist.

Reflecting on the work of Dreyfus and Dreyfus, Patterson (1991) indicates that the expert nurse is one who practises with embodied knowledge developed from experience and mature understanding. These characteristics enable the expert practitioner to rapidly assess situations and take action appropriate to the circumstance. This does not of necessity require reflection but it may be engaged in when time or necessity require it. Therefore the expert practitioner is, according to Patterson, one who is well experienced and has a practice repertoire based, in part, on non-reflective embodied knowledge.

Benner also provides some useful information about the thinking exhibited by expert practitioners through her identification and exploration of intuition. She believes intuition to be a legitimate and fundamental component of expert performance and that capturing the behaviours, thoughts and feelings of expert performers as they encounter situations is difficult. Thus, 'the expert always knows more than he or she can tell' (Polanyi 1962 cited in Benner 1984).

A number of authors (Thomas et al 1991, Fox-Young 1992, Benner 1984) present features they perceive as held by expert practitioners. Thomas et al compare the differences between the way in which experts and novices solve clinical problems. Fox-Young (1992),citing a range of researchers in the field of teaching (Campbell 1990-91, Berliner 1986, Ropo 1987), identifies a range of characteristics held by expert teachers. Benner locates her features of expert nurses in the context of a developmental model of skill acquisition. The similarities between these groups of features are marked and suggest that many of these characteristics are generic. These features make an interesting comparison and have been detailed in Table 8.1.

Table 8.1 Comparison of expert practitioner characteristics

Fox-Young (1992)	Thomas, Wearing & Bennett (1991)	Benner (1984)
They have superior memory performance for facts	The expert is faster at solving problems than the novice The expert scores better than the novice on tests determining problem solving and critical thinking abilities	They do not rely on guide-lines or maxims to relate understanding to pertinent action
Can separate relevant from irrelevant facts	The use of irrelevant information is less obvious with the expert in that they are more selective	Have strong analytic ability
Unlikely to accept information supplied by others without question. Develop routines to deal with the routine and thereby free themselves up to deal with the unexpected		They use intuition in the clinical analysis stage of clinical decision making. They are flexible and able to adapt in a number of different situational contexts
Look for patterns and abnormalities as they engage in activities	The expert eliminates as well as confirms hypotheses or guesses	They have an understanding of the totality of a situation while having strong perceptual acuity to decipher out irrelevant data
Can use more than one source of information at a time	Experts draw from experience	Their perceptions become extensions of their experience. They have an intuitive grasp of each situation
Knowledge is tied to their field of expertise and the conditions and procedures for using it	The knowledge base of experts is better than that held by novices	Difficulty in telling all they know. Their knowledge is domain based. They have an extensive background of clinical experience
Have a strong sense of mission and determination to be the best		They incorporate a vision of 'what is possible'

Expert practitioners derive knowledge from their experience. Distilling knowledge from practice experiences requires the practitioner to assign meaning and develop understanding from such activity. Bruner (1986) suggests that individuals distinguish between 'experience' and 'an experience', the former being understood as a 'flow of happenings' and the latter being an 'intersubjective articulation of experience'. Thus practitioners identify from the broad flow of nursing situations, encountered in any single day, some which stand out. It is our contention that the situations which are noted as remarkable and attended to are those in which something different or unusual occurs. In the nursing context this is likely to be situations requiring the doing of something different, such as enacting a specific technical skill, or the use of something different, such as special procedure or equipment. It is therefore not surprising that the writers and theorists about expert nursing practice have found such practitioners in settings in which specific technical skills and abilities are required, such as in acute care settings. This is not to suggest that expertise in nursing practice cannot be found in other settings but rather it will be more readily discernible and visible in those where such technical and situational elements are frequently encountered.

It is our contention that the expert practitioner's expertness is linked to the technical and situational aspects of nursing practice. Thus this type of nurse practitioner will be evident in intensive care units, and acute care and other similar settings. It is likely, therefore, that they will not be strongly evident in settings wherein limited technologies and procedures are evident. For example, this would include areas such as mental health nursing, gerontic nursing, community nursing and midwifery. In these settings each nursing situation predominantly requires a focus on the personhood of the client. Consequently, each situation usually occurs in the private realm of the nurse-client relationship and differs markedly from others encountered. Thus the work of each practitioner is invisible and unknown to others. This invisibility makes impossible the recognition and acknowledgment of expertness.

Benner (1984) perceives experience to be not just an accumulation of time in nursing practice but rather the 'refinement of preconceived notions and theory through encounters with many practical situations that add nuances or shades of differences to theory'. Benner elaborates further by stating that experience 'involves a very active process of refining and changing preconceived theories, notions and ideas when confronted with actual situations'.

Clearly, we gain knowledge and develop expertise as a direct result of experience. However, it is important to recognise that the nature of knowledge is complex and can be described as having many facets. These facets are reflected in the way that we use the terms 'know', 'knowing' and 'knowledge' in interaction with the self, others and our social environment. We frequently speak about 'having knowledge of research methodologies' or 'knowing how to perform a procedure' or we 'know the earth is round'.

The knowledge derived from experience is a particular type of knowing. Specifically, experience gives rise to expert practitioners who develop and use theories in action, that is 'knowing how'. Essentially, knowledge derived from experience involves a process wherein the individual not only has to be in an experience but has also to hold an intent to gain from the experience. This may take the form of noting the salient points and reflecting on these at a later stage. Thus, the individual must have some preparedness to learn from the experience. As a result of the experience, ideas form in the individual's mind where they are sorted, separated and analysed. Some may be rejected while others are retained. Each subsequent experience attended to in this manner will be considered in one form or another in the context of these ideas. Through this process of consideration old and new ideas will be brought together to form models or beginning theories that are further subject to refinement or rejection according to subsequent experiences.

Exploration of expert practice is useful in that we believe it to be a necessary, but not sufficient, precursor to understanding advanced practice. Our belief is based on the view that advanced practice comprises something qualitatively more than expert practice. As we have demonstrated, expert nursing practice is premised on developing knowledge and or skills from a sustained range of experiences within a specific context. This enables the practitioner to develop particular forms of knowledge and apply this in direct client care. Specialist nursing practice, however, develops from a different set of premises and focuses on different elements associated with experience.

Specialist nursing practice

The notion of specialisation within the context of health care was first seen in medicine. It emerged during an era when thinking was influenced by the logical positivist movement and empiricism and reductionism were highly valued. Humans were seen as machines, ruled by the same laws that govern nature. All the parts that composed the whole person could be reduced to their smallest entities, studied, and rebuilt to reflect the whole person. The person comprised the psyche and the soma (Cartesian dualism) and the emphasis was on cure rather than care. The search for certainty was highly valued and predictability could be achieved as it was assumed that events followed a logical pathway from cause to effect (Leddy & Pepper 1989). This meant that medical practitioners could accurately predict human response to altered states of health as each person experiencing the same physiological disturbance would display the same pattern of signs, symptoms and response to treatment.

According to Chickadonz and Perry (1985), specialist nursing practice began to emerge in the 1890s in response to a demand for nurses with special training in obstetrics (as distinct to midwifery), surgical and operating room nursing. Hospitals developed specialist courses to prepare nurses to assume these roles and therefore satisfy an organisationally generated need to provide nursing support for clients receiving specialist medical interventions. Training was implemented according to the requirements of the doctor and medical institution. The ideological devotion to serve the doctor and not to question meant that nurses became passive receivers of specialist knowledge. In their quest for recognition, they sought the technical skills and 'the crumbs of scientific knowledge spread by the doctors' teaching' (Colliere 1986).

The knowledge and skills passed down from doctors was filtered in such a way that nurses learnt how, but not why, they undertook certain practices. This meant they learnt how to perform the technical skills but did not acquire the knowledge necessary to make independent decisions about why and when to implement such practices. Consequently, they were dependent on doctors orders to be able to implement the technical aspects of practice. This practice is still evident in that we see treatment orders written by doctors stating four hourly temperature, pulse and respirations, daily urinalysis, and four hourly blood sugar levels. Whilst these orders legitimise the implementation of technical skills, they negate the capacity and autonomy of registered nurses to make independent nursing decisions relevant to the use of such technology.

Over time, as medical practitioners increasingly developed indepth knowledge and skills and began to segregate clients on the basis of their disorder, the supportive nursing services followed. As nurses worked for lengthier periods of time with specific client groups they developed additional and 'specialised' knowledge and skills grounded in the scientific knowledge of medicine. This, combined with the increasing acceptance by the health care services of the medical ideology and the need for nurses to share knowledge with one another, resulted in their coming together within each 'special' field.

The model of nursing specialities predicated on medical ideology and specialities, is increasingly perceived by nurses as an inadequate reflection of contemporary nursing thought and practice. Bajnok (1988) states that 'speciality practice must move away from the medical model designations to a classification system that accurately describes the fields of nursing'. Bajnok acknowledges that attempts to reclassify nursing specialities has only served to replace the medical model terminology with titles which are meaningless and do very little to reflect the nature of nursing speciality. Bajnok is not arguing against the notion of speciality nursing practice, rather, she points out that nursing should disregard the medical ideological notions of specialisation that are clouding our present understanding of speciality nursing practice and begin with a new vision which is grounded in the practice of nursing. Chickadonz and Perry (1985) continue this line of thought suggesting specialist nurses fail to explicate the specialist nursing knowledge associated with each field of practice. Rather, they have only taken on aspects of knowledge and skills which were previously the province of doctors.

Lane (1985) believes that specialisation is a maturation process that occurs in almost every profession. It arises in response to an improved knowledge base and social and technological changes. As a profession becomes more complex and diverse, there is a necessity for practitioners with more specialised knowledge and skills.

What does this mean for the future practice of nursing? If we accept the argument by Bajnok (1988), and Chickadonz and Perry (1985), that nurses need to identify specialist nursing knowledge and believe Lane's (1985) notion that specialisation is a maturation process which arises from an improved knowledge base, what implications are there for the practise of nursing?

The writers believe we need to rethink the idea of specialist nursing practice. In doing this, we need to acknowledge that nursing is at an early stage of maturation in terms of knowledge development. Consequently we need to look beyond our present understanding of specialist nursing practice and develop a new vision which is grounded in the true essence of nursing. Nursing is a profession which is only beginning to articulate its true essence of being. As this essence develops further and new knowledge emerges, we will come to understand the true nature of nursing. From this we can then begin to identify specialisations which are grounded in the meaning of nursing.

We believe the historical antecedents which have shaped the current knowledge held by specialist nurse practitioners and the recurring emphasis on their role and function, coupled with the need to provide nursing services to clients in the medical specialist field, still strongly influence the present nature of specialist nursing practice. All these elements serve to distract specialist nurse practitioners from identifying whether or not they have a unique body of nursing knowledge. Consequently, the issue of what constitutes specialist nursing knowledge, and also what constitutes specialist nursing practice are interesting questions worthy of further scholarly debate. We are not arguing against the notion of specialisation, rather we are arguing that specialist knowledge as currently perceived is not specialist nursing knowledge, rather it is still 'the crumbs of scientific knowledge spread by the doctors' teaching' (Colliere 1986).

Exploring the evolution of specialist practice provides us with the guidance we need to move into the future. It allows us to delve into the work of our pioneers and discover how their thoughts have influenced present day practice. Through a historical journey we often open the doors and discover the roots of our being which influence the way we come to know and perceive areas of practice.

The advanced nurse practitioner

The previous exploration of current literature makes clear what comprises expert and specialist nursing practice and that these terms are used synonymously for advanced nursing practice. We postulate, however, that advanced nursing practice differs from expert and specialist nursing practice. All practitioners experience nursing situations and as a result some become experts and focus on a specific technical aspect of nursing practice; some become specialists by moving into discrete identifiable fields of practice and some become advanced practitioners and focus on a specific realm or aspect of nursing practice. In this section we offer our beginning conceptualisation of 'advanced nursing practice' and highlight what is different about the way in which advanced nurse practitioners think about, see and experience nursing. We further explore how this difference contributes to the development of nursing practice and scholarship within the discipline.

Our understanding of advanced nurse practitioners is derived from three primary sources of information. The first source comprises personal observations of registered nurses and clients in interaction. Secondly we have gained many insights and learnt much from the discussions and ideas of the students enrolled in the Master of Nursing (Advanced Practice). Finally, ideas and understandings gained from critiquing the literature associated with this and related concepts form the third source.

In discussing advanced nursing practice the literature offers two perspectives. Firstly, one view describes advanced nursing practice as relating to the role and function of nurse practitioners. This is depicted in the following definition of Castledine (1992), who states 'advanced nursing practice includes significant inputs of direct clinical work, research, teaching, evaluation, sophisticated case work, consultation, leadership and management across broader specialist areas of nursing care'. This view emphasises the discrete roles ascribed to the practitioner and establishes views depicting advanced nurse practitioners as either experts or specialists.

The second view focuses on characteristics and dispositions of advanced nurse practitioners. Again, this is illustrated in the following definition: 'the advanced practice nurse uses expert clinical judgement which is the result of complex reasoning and analytical intellectual processes' (Spross & Baggerley cited in Sparacino 1991). That is, this perspective focuses on internal forces that shape the practitioner. For this group of writers, advanced nursing practice is characterised by the practitioner's capacity to think and guide inquiry, to engage in reflection and display effective clinical judgement in order to create new possibilities.

Spross and Baggerly (1989) focus on internal characteristics of the advanced nurse practitioners that shape their practice. They describe the concept of clinical judgement as an essential component for an advanced nursing practice model. While they recognise that all nurses make clinical judgements, they argue that this concept needs to be described in terms of its specificity to advanced nurse practitioners.

Nursing patterns of knowing described by Carper (1986) and further developed by Chinn and Jacobs-Kramer (1991) provide a useful beginning for exploring the cognitive characteristics of the advanced nurse practitioner. That is, the way they acquire, structure and use knowledge to inform their practice. We acknowledge that advanced nurse practitioners use all ways of knowing gained from the whole of experience to inform their practice. In addition, we contend they do more than this. They come to understand through a process that Chinn and Jacobs-Kramer (1991) describe as 'bringing a critical perspective to that which is known in order to create new insights and new knowledge'. This critical perspective is informed through a process of critical thinking which requires thoughtful reflection and dialogue with others. This process brings together different perspectives and allows ideas to be challenged, rethought, and reframed to reveal new meaning and thus move beyond what is to what might be. Further, this process exposes and critically questions the social and political ideologies that impact on what is known by the practitioner.

Thus, advanced nurse practitioners use all ways of knowing gained from the whole of experience to inform practice. This assists them to understand and express what is and create new meaning. Practitioners who offer critical thinking as an added dimension to inform their practice engage in critical reflection about their practice, rather than accept theories which often constrain them from seeing things as they really are. Birx (1993) states 'the ability to imagine an alternative leads us to question the current system and move toward more humanistic health care environment and relationships'. As advanced nurse practitioners engage in clinical practice they continually question what is happening. According to Birx, this critical thinking process requires 'an attitude of openness and inquiry, knowledge and clinical experience in nursing, metacognition and metatheoretical reflection, the integration of multiple levels of theory, perspective taking and empowerment'. It is through critical questions and the social and political processes outlined by Chinn and Jacobs-Kramer (1991) that new insights and new knowledge is gained.

The Master of Nursing (Advanced Practice) program offered from the Faculty of Nursing, University of South Australia is premised on the view that advanced nursing practice can be:

> viewed in both theoretical and practical terms in that it refers to a level of nursing practice in which clinicians seek to develop and apply knowledge related to micro or mid-range theories of nursing...In this context the clinician strives to develop higher levels of excellence in nursing care through purposeful and analytic thought combined with pragmatism (Accreditation Document 1990).

This view offers a clear indication of the dimensions associated with advanced nursing practice and highlights attributes held by the advanced nurse practitioner. Firstly, the extract from this Master's program indicates that advanced nursing practice can be viewed in both theoretical and practical terms. However, we argue that it would be impossible to understand this type of practice without considering each view and how each relates to the other. We understand advanced nursing practice to be a blend of the theoretical and practical. In this sense we agree it comprises a type of practice in which such clinicians develop, from their practice, knowledge and theory that are micro to mid range in nature (Hardy 1988). That is, advanced nurse practitioners concentrate and focus their efforts on the client and situations which enhance positive outcomes for the client. As such, the practitioners' actions are purposeful, directed towards excellence (in client terms) and pragmatic.

In seeking to undertake practice, advanced nurse practitioners carefully consider and critically reflect on all aspects of care provided to the client. This level of analytic thought ensures that such practitioners remain focused and also shapes the manner in which they perceive their world of practice. For advanced nurse practitioners, the client is the centre of that world. Their skills and abilities are offered so as to ease the client's situation. They recognise that their contribution to client care makes a difference. That this difference might be minor, and/or relative to the contribution of other caregivers, is inconsequential. From the practitioners' perspective the contribution made comprises the totality of what they have to offer. Because the client is central to their efforts they are willing to 'bend' the rules. However, this, like other aspects of their work, is undertaken silently and invisibly. For this reason advanced nurse practitioners are difficult to recognise both by others and by themselves.

Advanced nurse practitioners locate themselves in the immediacy of client situations. They not only respond to the demands of the situation but do so with a recognition and acknowledgment of potential future situations and with an understanding of their own and the client's history. Given these attributes, advanced nurse practitioners are constantly 'stretching' the boundaries of nursing practice. While the care they provide resides in the heartland of nursing, its very essence, the manner in which this is undertaken acknowledges opportunities yet to be fully recognised by the profession. Advanced nurse practitioners therefore uses an 'emic' (culturally specific) perspective (Tripp-Reimer 1984) to effect 'etic' (culturally universal) changes to nursing practice. This capacity on the part of advanced nurse practitioners has its genesis in their etic understanding which in turn informs their emic perspectives and therefore their implementation of practice. In this sense, the advanced nurse practitioner develops a truly reflexive relationship between theory and practice and establishes praxis.

Advanced nurse practitioners articulate and define nursing practice by constant reference to the client and, when involved in research, make significant contributions to the discipline by generating practice-based theory. This way of thinking about practice is facilitated by their personal conceptualisation of nursing and capacity to communicate effectively with clients, other health care workers and the community generally. Because advanced nurse practitioners function at the emic level these communications are not large or public in scale and focus. But, like their interactions with clients they tend to be personal and undertaken in one-to-one or small group encounters.

Consequently, advanced nurse practitioners achieve high levels of credibility which in turn are strengthened by their continuing self-evaluation. This is undertaken via a process of critical reflection on practice and integration of the outcomes with what they know in order to further develop. This activity and its outcomes provides a sound basis for interaction with other individuals. The unification of theory and practice provide them with distinctive ways of thinking about their practice. This is evident in small infrequently seen but nonetheless taken-for-granted practices that can be observed in clinical settings. For example, when meeting a client on the first and each subsequent occasion the advanced nurse practitioner does not immediately attend to the technology attached to the client, if there is any present, but rather concentrates on the client and ascertains their state of being. Attention to technical and other matters follows this initial approach.

Advanced nurse practitioners have a clear vision for the future of nursing. It is generally one in which nurses function to serve the client and in which the role of advocate becomes a reality. This latter role however, is perceived as being undertaken on the clear understanding that it is a temporary measure enacted only until the client is able to do this for themselves. Consequently, their current practice contains an emphasis on encouraging and supporting clients to express their views enabling them to speak for themselves.

Practitioners engaging in this type of practice constantly effect change in a number of areas. Firstly, they effect changes for the client by creating a milieu in which the client can heal. Secondly, by providing alternative role models for colleagues and students of nursing they generate changes in the way other nurses practise. This latter aspect establishes them as clinically based leaders. However their capacity to lead is limited by a number of factors which include a reluctance to move away from the direct provision of care to the client. They perceive acceptance of leadership roles as creating a situation in which they will of necessity be forced to make management, rather than the client, their central concern. This is a view held even if such a leadership position is within established clinical pathways, such as clinical nurse consultant or clinical nurse specialist.

A second reason for their non-acceptance of leadership roles resides in the devaluing of those aspects in which they are skilled, that is, the personal. As in other countries, nursing in Australia values more highly expert and specialist technical skills rather than those elements demonstrated by advanced nurse practitioners, and which we believe comprise the essence of nursing.

The attributes demonstrated by advanced nurse practitioners are further enhanced by their valuing of the uncertainty generated in many practice situations. They perceive these as opportunities for growth and development in that they offer opportunities to legitimise and validate the perceptions and knowledge obtained from earlier experiences. Advanced nurse practitioners do not rely on intuition, rather they perceive the totality of situations as they impact on the client. They are clear about why they choose a particular course of action as opposed to another. That is, the action taken is in the best interest of the client. Because they relate strongly to the client's situation and continually engage in critical refection of their practice, they are able to identify the various cues to which they respond. However, these are frequently seen by others as limited and non-reliable as they are premised on a well developed under-standing of the unpredictability of human interaction and responses to health and illness.

However, we also believe that the features of expert practice, outlined by Benner (1984) and Fox-Young (1992) and other writers are also able to be identified in many advanced nurse practitioners. Thus, in our view advanced practice may incorporate expert practice. In these instances advanced nurse practitioners are expert practitioners who have developed mechanisms for extending their knowledge across practice fields. In this sense advanced nurse practitioners are emancipated from affiliation with one specific field or aspect of nursing practice.

Kitson (1987), Colliere (1986) and Lawler (1991b) offer a number of significant ideas that contribute to discussion of advanced nursing practice. The need for a practitioner of the type we have begun to describe in this chapter is reflected in the work of Kitson, who suggests that nursing must start to rely less on the scientific and objective and more on fostering a sense of the individual.

Kitson's view is based on understanding the complexity of nursing practice which has its genesis in the humanity of both the nurse and the client. She argues that nursing care requires more than establishing static protocols and rigid systems, and suggests it would be better to have stout hearts and gut reactions. Her reasoning includes the view that in searching for what is best for the client the knowledge we use as nurses is never value free. Consequently, we must recognise where our ideas and notions come from. She also suggests that nurses function on two levels each enabling them to tune in to the client. Firstly, they function at the level of clinical skills and knowledge which enables them to make observations of the client, and develop judgements based on that information. Secondly, nurses function at the personal level.

Kitson (1987) asks, if recognition of the humanity of the client is an integral part of our practice why then do we pay it so little regard and subject it to so little investigation? She suggests this is because this way of thinking is not highly regarded and is therefore dismissed or viewed with suspicion because it is seen to be unimportant, unscientific and therefore unreliable. This supports our view that the empiricist influence on nursing has led us to this point wherein little value is placed on that which cannot be measured in some way. However we also argue that the scientific components of nursing comprise only part of what nurses do, albeit the most visible parts of the care provided. Nurse practitioners, however, to be truly effective and to give the highest quality care possible need something else. 'There needs to be an emotional charge, one which discerns, synthesises, puts together that which has been dissected by the cold hand of science' (Kitson 1987).

Like Lawler (1991b), Kitson suggests that nursing's failure to address this issue has resulted in the development of a social system and process of nursing that seeks to defend the practitioner from experiencing the full affective component of nursing practice. This has included the establishment of ritualistic behaviours that serve to distance the nurse from the emotional life of the client. Similar distance from the complexity of nursing has occurred as the result of the routinisation of nursing practices and institutionalisation of personal responsibility for the delivery of care.

Kitson (1987) also suggests that 'an alternative way of denying the need for tenderness and concern is to argue that competent practice is primarily about skills and knowledge, about developing new techniques, improving treatments'. The notion that nursing is about caring is one that has been posited for a significant number of years. It cannot be emphasised enough that it is this feature which unites all nurses regardless of the field in which they practise. This of course might be to state the obvious to many nurses, but it demonstrates the need for nurses who do care. If an individual cares about their practice then they will value that practice. Like any individual that cares, nurses that care will have feelings about what they do, they will be motivated to take action and to place value on what others might perceive as the ordinary and mundane.

Lawler's work (1991b) focuses on exploring how nurses assist clients to deal with the experience of illness and dependency. In this exploration she suggests that:

> Nurses learn from experience that during illness the mind and body are emotionally, intellectually and practically inseparable...They also learn that

despite the aesthetically unpleasant and potentially nauseating things that occur during illness, the patient is also a person, and that by their manner (among other things) nurses help patients cope with the body and what ails it.

Lawler indicates that expert nurses understand this well and that the data associated with her study into the relationship between nurse and patient is derived from expert nurse interaction. She emphasises, however, that even non-expert nurses understand the patient is more than a body but frequently 'get through' a procedure by concentrating on the routine of that procedure. We postulate that Lawler uses the term 'expert nurse' synonymously with advanced nurse practitioner, and that the advanced nurse practitioner moves through a procedure by focusing on the client and assisting them to 'get through' the situation. In this sense we concur when she states that: 'Nursing care, therefore, takes place in the context of the acknowledged personhood of the other'.

During the development of our ideas a number of similar views were being developed in the United Kingdom and Canada. The emergence of these ideas is significant because it indicates that, even in those countries which have been largely responsible for shaping the way in which Australian nurses think about advanced nursing practice, this concept is being questioned and challenged. In this sense, our contribution, from Australia, to this scholarly debate is timely. It is also important to note that the emerging ideas are moving away from the structural functional perspective of advanced nursing practice to one that describes and emphasises practitioners in terms of their personal characteristics and attributes. This is exemplified by the following definition by Patterson and Haddad (1992) who describe the advanced nurse practitioner as:

> those nurses who push beyond the known boundaries of their profession; who have the vision and flexibility necessary to consider new possibilities for improvement and/or expansion; who have the urge to ask questions and seek out the answers; who are willing to take the risks and face the challenges associated with breaking new ground; and who have the ability to articulate their thoughts clearly as they move ahead such that they contribute to the understanding and development of new knowledge and skills within nursing and thus lead their profession forward to meet the needs and demands of society.

Conclusion

In concluding this chapter we challenge the profession to carefully consider whether it wishes to re-establish a focus on the client or whether it wishes to maintain its current emphasis on the technical and procedural elements of practice. We ask the questions: 'What is the specific focus of nursing?' and 'Is nursing so broad that the only way we can understand it is to fragment it or concentrate on the technical and procedural elements we have inherited from others?' This latter approach to our development can be successfully undertaken if we all envisage nursing to be a technically based profession rather than one which is grounded in the essence of the nurse-client relationship.

If it is the former direction we wish to take then we believe we should continue to explore the concept of advanced nursing practice. The different ways of thinking about, seeing and experiencing practice offered by this group of practitioners will, we believe, enable us to develop a fuller understanding of what comprises nursing. Disclosing and articulating what is unique about advanced nursing practice is important if we are to recognise the contributions made by advanced nurse practitioners to all fields of nursing practice. To do this we need to identify or develop processes that provide the data we need for interpreting and extrapolating the meaning of this complex concept.

In turn, studies of the nature suggested will result in clear direction for the development of the discipline. Scholarship in nursing will also undergo significant redirection away from the functional, and away from the positivist into exploring meaning and understanding. Once this is achieved we will, as a profession, be able to fully value what it is our practitioners do every day with clients.

REFERENCES

Bajnok I 1988 Specialization meets entry to practice. The Canadian Nurse 84(6):23-24

Benner P 1984 From novice to expert: excellence and power in clinical nursing practice. Addison-Wesley, Menlo Park

Benner P, Wrubel J 1990 The primacy of caring: stress and coping in health and illness. Addison-Wesley, Menlo Park

Birx E 1993 Critical thinking and theory-based practice. Holistic Nursing Practice 7(3):21-27

Bruner E M 1986 Experience and its expressions. In: Turner V W, Bruner E M (eds) The anthropology of experience. University of Illinois Press, Urbana

Carper B 1986 Fundamental patterns of knowing in nursing. In; Nicoll L H (ed) Perspectives on nursing theory. Scott Foresman, Illinois

Castledine G 1992 The advanced practitioner. Nursing 5(7):14-15

Chickadonz G H, Perry A M 1985 Clinical specialization versus generalization: perspectives for the future. In: McCloskey J C, Grace H K (eds) Current issues in nursing, 2nd edn. Blackwell Scientific Publishers, Boston, pp 73-90

Chinn P L, Jacobs-Kramer M K 1991 Theory and nursing: a systematic approach. Mosby, St Louis

Colliere M 1986 Invisible care and invisible women as health care providers. International Journal of Nursing Studies 23(2):95-108

Fox-Young S 1992 The assessment of experts for continuing practice; proaction/reaction? A paper delivered at the 1st National Nursing Forum, Royal College of Nursing Australia, Adelaide

Harding S, Hintikka M B (eds) 1983 Discovering reality: feminist perspectives on epistemology metaphysics methodology and philosophy of science. D. Rediel Publishers, Dordrecht Holland

Hardy L 1988 Excellence in nursing through debate: the case of nursing theory. Recent Advances in Nursing 21:1-13

Harper D 1985 The process of advanced nursing practice. Journal of Professional Nursing 1(6):323, 385

Kitson A 1987 Raising standards of clinical practice: the fundamental issue of effective nursing practice. Journal of Advanced Nursing, 12:321-329

Lane B 1985 Specialization in nursing; some Canadian issues. The Canadian Nurse 81(6):24-25

Lawler J 1991a In search of an Australian identity. In: Gray G, Pratt R (eds) Towards a discipline of nursing. Churchill Livingstone, Melbourne

Lawler J 1991b Behind the screens: nursing somology and the problem of the body. Churchill Livingstone, Melbourne

Leddy S, Pepper J 1989 Conceptual bases of professional nursing. J B Lippincott, Philadelphia, p. 103-119

Master of Nursing (Advanced Practice) course accreditation document 1990. South Australian College of Advanced Education, Salisbury, pp 11-14

Patterson B 1991 Excellence and expertise in nursing. Deakin University Press, Victoria, pp 5-7

Patterson C, Haddad B 1992 The advanced nurse practitioner: common attributes. Canadian Journal of Nursing Administration (Nov/Dec):18-22

Sparacino P 1990 Strategies for implementing advanced practice. Clinical Nurse Specialist 4(3):151-152

Sparacino P 1991 The reciprocal relationship between practice and theory. Clinical Nurse Specialist 5(3):138

Sparacino P 1992 Advanced practice: the clinical nurse specialist. Nursing Practice 5(4):2-4

Spross J A, Baggerly J 1989 Models of advanced nursing practice. In: Hamric A, Spross J (eds) The clinical nurse specialist in theory and practice, 2nd edn. W B Saunders, Philadelphia, p 19-40

Sutton F 1993 Occupational culture, feminism and nursing curriculum. A paper presented at the Critical Theory, Feminism and Nursing Conference, Melbourne

Thomas S, Wearing A, Bennett M 1991 Clinical decision making for nurses and health professionals. Harcourt Brace Jovanovich, Sydney

Thompson C G, Ryan S A, Kitzman H 1990 Expertise: the basis for expert system development. Advances in Nursing Science 13(2):1-10

Tripp-Reimer T 1984 Reconceptualizing the constructs of health: integrating emic and etic perspectives. Research in Nursing and Health 7(2):101-109

9

The handover: three modes of nursing practice knowledge

JUDITH PARKER, JOHN WILTSHIRE

Introduction

How do we conceptualise nursing practice knowledge? In this chapter we propose a way of theorising nursing practice knowledge which has been developed out of an intensive study of the nursing handover in a major metropolitan hospital. In patients' progress notes, as we have previously argued (Parker & Gardiner 1992), the nurse's voice is often silenced.

Nursing practice knowledge, whatever mode it took, was rarely visible in the formal records of nursing practice. We suggested that the silencing of the nurses' voices in written documentation could be understood in relation to powerful hegemonic forces linked to medical dominance and control. The nurse's voice, when it emerged, was a weak echo of the medical voice, saying what had already been said, voiceless on those matters that are at the heart of nursing practice.

This research led us to wonder about the extent to which the nursing handover, the oral record of nursing practice, is a site which reinforces the status quo: firstly, by legitimising the secondary role of nurses to doctors as they exchange already given medical and technical information; secondly, by providing a venue for emotional catharsis—sympathetic acknowledgment of shared situations and common crises—thus restoring emotional equilibrium. But we meditated, on the other hand, about the extent to which the nursing handover provides a site at which nurses may reclaim their own voices and attempt to challenge the structures that render them silent.

In a subsequent preliminary study (Parker et al 1992), we proposed that the handover is indeed a significant site at which nurses articulate and communicate their practice and sense of professionalism. We identified a range of functions that the handover serves. We suggested that it:

offers a forum in which nurses can demonstrate their professional competence, and at the same time seek group validation for performance decisions or at least air and share problems. Through the ritual of the handover the nurse is made to feel part of a working community. In addition, the communal or collaborative narrative (which constitutes the handover) allows the containment and support needed for the nurse to deal with what is often disturbing material. The characteristic lay language and informal exchange are important too, in the exploration of problems and aspects of nursing care which might be better not discussed in the presence of patients. Additionally, imparting information gathered in the course of their duties brings a sense of closure to the departing shift. They can hand over the sense of responsibility they have for the wellbeing of patients in their care.

Whatever the form of handover, and in this study we discerned several variants, nurses communicate to each other in a formalised setting and in largely (though not exclusively) verbal form. At handover, nurses exchange the knowledge that constitutes their practice, and exchange it in a form that is available and observable for study. But in order to identify the dimensions of this nursing knowledge, whether medically derived or authentically created as an expression of nursing voices, we need first to sift it, to separate it out, from that other knowledge which, on a superficial view, the handover seems designed to communicate.

In this chapter we first describe how we went about the current study and provide an outline of the theoretical positions that have informed our thinking about nursing practice knowledge. We then delineate three modes of nursing practice knowledge we have discerned and describe how these are brought together into an incorporative and reflective mode of nursing practice knowledge. We offer some comments on how the structuring of the handover facilitates or impedes opportunities for transmission of aspects of nursing practice knowledge.

The study

In this research project, we collected data on two forms of nursing records, the oral handover and written patient progress notes, in a major metropolitan teaching hospital. We selected two general medical wards in which to undertake the study. These were matched as closely as possible in relation to size and staffing levels, patient populations, acuity and length of stay. Each ward admitted patients under the medical care of three different general medical units. One ward also had a small geriatric assessment unit. We were able to demonstrate comparability of the nurses in the two wards through analysing sociodemographic data of education, age, sex, ethnicity and post-registration practice experience of the nurses who participated in the handover.

We observed and tape-recorded handovers at each change of shift (three per 24 hours) over three consecutive days in each ward, and interviewed key personnel to provide us with background material for our study. We also examined a selection of the progress notes of patients who were discussed in the observed handovers in order to compare written and spoken accounts of practice.

In this chapter we concentrate upon understanding the knowledge embedded in the accounts of practice given at the end of the shift handover. In theorising our study we draw particularly upon the work of Michel Foucault (1973, 1977) for the concepts of panopticism and the medical gaze, and Donna Haraway (1991) for the notion of situated knowledges. The relationship between the handover material and the patient progress notes, analysable from a variety of perspectives, remains a field for further study.

Theoretical position

Foucault, panopticism and the medical gaze

In writing about the nature of knowledge, Foucault moves away from both philosophical realism and idealism and links knowledge to the notion of discipline. He thinks of a discipline in relation to scholarship, such as in the discipline of medicine, and as an institution involving social control, such as in a hospital. For Foucault, (in Rabinov 1991) power is central in the production of knowledge. He states:

> We should admit, rather, that power produces knowledge (and not simply by encouraging it because it serves power or by applying it because it is useful); that power and knowledge directly imply one another; that there is no power relation without the correlative constitution of a field of knowledge, nor any knowledge that does not presuppose and constitute at the same time power relations...In short, it is not the activity of the subject of knowledge that produces a corpus of knowledge, useful or resistant to power, but power-knowledge, the processes and struggles that traverse it and of which it is made up, that determines the forms and possible domains of knowledge.

According to Foucault (1977) disciplinary power is exercised through techniques of social control. Drawing upon Jeremy Bentham's designs for a prison, the Panopticon, in which a single gaoler would be able to view all his prisoners at once, Foucault defined modern forms of gathering information, especially information about bodies, as surveillance. Panopticism enables disciplinary power to function through surveillance techniques aimed at bodily conformity. Hence, as Foucault (1977) argues:

> the major effect of the Panopticon: to induce in the inmate a state of conscious and permanent visibility that assures the automatic functioning of power. So to arrange things that the surveillance is permanent in its effects, even if it is discontinuous in its actions; that the perfection of power should tend to render its actual exercise unnecessary; that this architectural apparatus should be a machine for creating and sustaining a power relation independent of the person who exercises it; in short, that the inmates should be caught up in a power situation of which they are themselves the bearers.

The modern hospital is an excellent example of a panoptic site in which the disciplinary power of medicine is exercised. In medicine, the object of investigation is the human body, which is represented as a group of interacting systems of biochemical or physiological activities that, though hidden from normal sight, are finite and measurable. The history of medicine since the eighteenth century has been closely tied to anatomical investigation and to the penetration of the mysteries of the body, through increasingly sophisticated technological means. The ultrasound and the CAT scan are in a line of development following in a clear progression from the stethoscope and the X-ray (Reiser 1982). Medicine thus defines the body in terms of its interior processes and its knowledge of the body is a quantifiable knowledge of interiority. Foucault (1973) has described the mode of medical knowledge of the body as the medical gaze. As he has argued, the medical gaze simultaneously constitutes the body of the patient as an object of study, and bestows upon that study the authority and coercive power of a 'knowledge' debarred to its subject.

The metaphor of vision

As Foucault's emphasis on terms such as 'panopticism' and 'the medical gaze' suggests, knowledge in the West has been more generally conceptualised through the metaphor of vision ('I see' means 'I understand'). This mode of knowledge is based in the representational or 'spectator' theory of knowledge which as Best (1991) has pointed out, is the epistemological foundation of modernism. Such a theory of knowledge, he writes:

> involves a rigid subject-object bifurcation whereby the unbiased scientific mind confronts a neutral cosmos in a distant, analytic relation. The perceiving subject is a neutral observer and the object a neutral datum of perception. As a kind of 'mirror of nature', the mind could therefore represent the world through its objective knowledge of it and this knowledge was stable, certain and accurate in nature.

This theory of knowledge has its foundation in the Cartesian split between mind and body. In a review of a recent book by Bordo (1993), Gilligan (1994) says:

> Descartes' radical leap out of his body and into the 'I' signified an effort to transcend the limitations of perspective (because we are embodied our thought is perspectival) and to see, as it were, like God. If one had the right method, he believed, one could achieve what Thomas Nagel has called 'the view from nowhere'—a place of objectivity or unqualified truth.

Haraway (1991) draws upon Nagel's notion and refers to this mode of knowledge as constituted through the 'conquering gaze from nowhere' which 'mythically inscribes all the marked bodies, that makes the unmarked category claim the power to see and not be seen, to represent while escaping representation'. In other words, the gazer, unmarked by categorisation, is imagined to be omniscient and 'objective'. His or her own subjectivity is discountable, irrelevant, while the object of the gaze is marked through categorisation—in the case of medical science, as a disease. In this theory of knowledge, language is extricated from its enmeshment in the world of objects, becoming distinct and capable of representing the world (Foucault 1973). The meaning of the word is what it designates and the primary function of language is to inform us about objectively existing states of affairs.

Some critiques of modernism such as those offered by Best (1991), reject the dualistic separation which has resulted in the mind/body division, the split between the self and the natural world and the representational theory of knowledge. They point out that concepts that are systematised in the form of general decontextualised abstract knowledge impose uniformity upon what is a diverse and variable world. Building on the foundations laid by Foucault's critique of Enlightenment rationalism, one can envisage the emergence of multiplicity and plurality of meanings. The notion of an objective reliable universal foundation for knowledge then becomes untenable, as knowledge becomes redefined as discursive practice and the radical historical contingency of all knowledge claims is recognised.

However before one assumes that such critiques have demolished Cartesianism, it is timely to heed Bordo's (1993) warning:

> The mind/body dualism is no mere philosophical position to be defended or dispensed with by clever argument. Rather, it is a practical metaphysics that has been deployed and socially embodied in medicine, law, literary and artistic representations, the psychological construction of self, interpersonal relationships, popular culture and advertisements—a metaphysics which will be deconstructed only through concrete transformation of the institutions and practices that sustain it.

Haraway (1991) points out the dangers inherent in postmodern critiques of Cartesianism, which mean that no one perspective can claim privilege over another because 'all drawings of inside-outside boundaries in knowledge are theorized as power moves, not moves towards truth'. This relativisation, she laments, has been followed by a postmodern 'anything goes' endless play on words wherein 'all truths become warp speed effects in a hyper-real space of simulations'. The view from nowhere, 'the illusion of Modernism' becomes, as Bordo (1993) has remarked, 'the fantasy of Post-Modernism, the dream of everywhere at once.'

Haraway and situated knowledges

Haraway (1991) argues that the alternative to relativism and the postmodern 'anything goes' is 'partial locatable critical knowledges'. She supports Harding's (1986) call for a successor science which has a postmodern insistence on irreducible difference and radical multiplicity of local knowledges together with a paradoxical, 'no-nonsense commitment to faithful accounts of the "real world"'.

Haraway examines the modernist metaphor of the primacy of vision in knowledge development and explores some of its implications. She claims that 'struggles over what will count as rational accounts of the world are struggles over how to see'. She therefore argues that such an approach requires a reclaiming of vision as a metaphor in feminist discourse. She rejects the disembodied understanding of vision that has been associated with the 'spectator' theory of knowledge and argues for the 'embodied nature of all vision'. This, she claims, enables an understanding of objectivity which stems from particular and specific embodiment and which offers a necessarily partial perspective stemming from limited location and situated embodied knowledge. She declares that she is 'arguing for politics and epistemologies of location, positioning, and situating, where partiality and not universality is the condition of being heard to make rational knowledge claims'.

Modes of nursing practice knowledge

This section draws upon Foucault (1973) and Haraway (1991) and the metaphor of vision, to delineate three modes of nursing practice knowledge which are communicated by nurses during the handover. We describe these as *reconnoitre*, the nursing scan, *savoir*, the nursing gaze, and *connaissance*, the nursing look. We then describe how these aspects may be incorporated in *reconnaissance*. *Reconnoitre* is a verb meaning to inspect, observe or survey in order to gain information for military, engineering or geological purposes. It is an activity of scanning a terrain, of inspecting the topography of a place for a particular purpose. The materiality of a particular place is, if we heed Foucault, constituted through the disciplinary power embedded in the particular surveillance techniques undertaken. Thus *reconnoitre*, the nursing scan, is an activity of panoptic surveillance undertaken by nurses which produces local, situated, perspectival knowledge of the terrain in which nursing activities take place.

Savoir, the nursing gaze, is analogous to the medical gaze as described by Foucault and we argue that in its reductionist constitution it has the same type of coercive power as that invested in the medical gaze. However, we also argue that it is a fallacy of modernism to describe it as objective decontextualised representational medical knowledge to which nurses have access in a secondary and derivative way.

In defining *connaissance*, the nursing look, we use a distinction which is present in French, but not so clear in English. *Connaissance* literally means acquaintance with a person. It is familiar, concrete knowledge of persons, as distinguished from abstract knowledge, and knowledge of facts, *savoir*, which Foucault elaborated into *pouvoir/savoir*, i.e. power/knowledge—that epistemic authority which simultaneously functions as control and containment. *Reconnaissance* is nursing practice knowledge which takes account of knowledge stemming from *reconnoitre*, *savoir* and *connaissance* and which is tempered with reflective appraisal. It is located, situated, both objective and partial knowledge.

Reconnoitre, the nursing scan

From its first self-conscious texts, nursing has been concerned with the management and control of place. (We use place in preference to environment, because the latter term is now too vague and all-embracing. What we mean is a specific humanly-created site, usually a room or series of rooms, a ward.) Florence Nightingale's (1860) famous injunction: 'Windows must be open. Doors must be closed' defines in a nutshell the importance nursing has always placed on the negotiation of a place.

Within the hospital context other heath care professionals come into the ward, attend to patients, and depart. At several handovers which we monitored, the information about the patient routinely included mention of the medical unit to which they were admitted. 'Admitted on Thursday, under Medical Unit B', for example. Doctors' patients belong to these groupings which designate their speciality and disease, but patients under different units may be in adjacent beds. The medical unit, then, has not a physical but a metaphysical existence. The nursing unit, the ward, on the other hand, is a material practice, based in an actual context. This difference in the nature of the medical and nursing units can be constraining for the nurses since they are to a certain extent dependent upon doctors' visits for surveillance decisions to be made. However, their close proximity to the patients enables the nurses to feel confident about suggesting alternative measures. At a 7.00 a.m. handover the night nurse reported:

At one o'clock in the morning the doctor still hadn't come and we rang him several times 'cause he's [the patient] very rigid and shaky—when he came up he says on half hourly to hourly neuro obs. I said, if you want him on hourly neurology obs you should have seen him five hours ago—so he changed them to four hourly...so that was good, and they're fine.

The site of the nurse's work is the ward, and his or her practice is ineluctably tied to the actuality of material objects, to the spatial organisation of the physical place, and to the features of that environment which constrain or facilitate effective nursing. The nurse is concerned with the patient's ability to walk through the ward to the toilet and back, with the location of each patient in relation to the nursing station, and so forth.

A significant but taken-for-granted dimension of the routine activities of the nurse working a shift is the constant scanning of the terrain of responsibility. At a glance, a nurse may observe the sheen of the floor and the positioning of furniture, mindful of possible falls by frail patients, note whether bells, lockers and tables are in reach of bedfast patients, ascertain the location of technologies to deal with possible emergency situations, and assess the 'look' of patients and the help they may need to facilitate bodily functioning and ensure their comfort.

The institution of the handover enables the nurses going off duty to paint a verbal picture of the terrain in which the incoming nurses will work. It is a guide to the place the incoming nurses are to work in, and a map of the site. The handover functions as an opportunity for exiting nurses to verbally scan the place they are leaving, locate patients in relation to place and identify spatially related problems or issues and in so doing enable incoming nurses to have a sense of the terrain in which they will be working for the next few

157

hours. We use the term *reconnoitre* partly because one aspect of the handover is certainly reminiscent of the surveillance techniques involved in military procedures and training. The handover, in which the beds and the patients currently in the ward are listed in strict numeric order, is a process of orientation and re-orientation, by which the nurses are made familiar with the territory that they are to be traversing during the hours of their shift and the imperatives or hidden dangers of that terrain.

Much of the knowledge that is transmitted in the handover is thus devoted to practical recognition of the constraints of the physical arena for the patients:

> 'Make sure he takes his frame with him when he goes to the toilet, otherwise he won't get back.' 'If you hear a pitiful little voice near the toilet saying "Help me", that's her.'

At a 7 a.m. handover, we heard the following exchange:

> *Nurse giving handover.* Bed 5 is Mary Smith, 74 year old lady, with her pneumonia and depression um I restarted her 24 hour urine collection at 10 o'clock last night because there was hardly anything in the bottle. I watched her go to the toilet.
>
> *Nurse.* She probably needs watching.
>
> *Nurse giving handover.* Yeah, so I've got her wearing a sign around her neck to remind everyone if they see her wandering up to...
>
> *Nurse.* I think the best thing, no the best thing is put a bottle and a pan next to her and it will be...
>
> *Nurse.* She still wanders.
>
> *Nurse giving handover.* She doesn't know what...
>
> *Nurse.* She wanders off...

A specific part of the *reconnoitring* aspect of the handover is to alert the incoming nurses to the technological imperatives of the terrain, the possibilities for action and decision making inherent within the particular setting, and the need to make explicit certain expectations. For example in the terrain of the two general medical wards in which we listened to handovers, a persistent theme was the identification of patients as 'NFR' (not for resuscitation). This instruction was regularly given in regard to several of the patients following the identification of their bed number, name and age and thus highlights the expectation that the ward is a technologically sophisticated place in which a person who stops breathing would normally be resuscitated.

This aspect of the terrain was particularly apparent at one 7 a.m. handover we observed. Highlighted too, in this extract, is the taken-for-grantedness of the ward as a space in which activities of inspection and surveillance of patients' bodily functions are regarded as a normal aspect of the nurses' work.

> *Handover Nurse:* Bed 4 is Amy White, 89, not for resusc with her senility and pneumonia. Amy's the same, she's just waiting for a GAU referral. A

little bit confused and calling out overnight. Continent. Bed 5 is Bill Smith, 65, not for resusc with right cortical CVA. He's sitting out of bed for meals but you need to have the suction handy because apparently most of it goes straight down the back.

Day Nurse 1: He will be able to eat if someone stands there and feeds him by teaspoon.

Day Nurse 2: By teaspoon?

Day Nurse 1: Yes, not with a big spoon.

Handover Nurse: And he also seemed a little more confused as well. He's quite contracted. He has the air splints on during the day and he's on a fluid chart.

Bed 6 is Mr Graeme, 79, not for resusc. Haematemesis and malaena. The scopes show a 6cm CA...He was transfused, 2 units packed calls. He gets the wanders a bit, on his way to the toilet, etcetera. On a vomit chart, he had a vomit last night which is positive for occult blood. He's on a food chart and a stool chart.

It becomes clear that this *reconnoitring* aspect of the handover demonstrates the automatic functioning of techniques of panoptic surveillance described by Foucault. The ward is a site which creates and sustains power relations that are independent of the particular nurses and patients, the 'inmates' of the site. Both are part of the terrain of the ward. In our previous work on the handover (Parker et al 1992) we observed that information about all the patients in the ward was given to all the incoming nurses at the handover. It was only at the end of the handover that nurses were assigned particular patients. This was also the case in our current study. It was clear to us that the incoming nurses could not possibly absorb all the information they were given at this time and we puzzled about this process. We concluded that the collaborative narrative about the patients that was constructed at the handover provided the nurses with a sense of familiarity with the ward through the construction of stereotypical identities for patients. In this sense then the handover can be seen as a *reconnoitring* or scanning activity which gives the incoming nurses a sense of 'the lie of the land' through the construction of patients as, for example, 'good' or 'difficult' or 'needing to be watched'. To the extent that diverse individuals are constructed in stereotypical form and then related to in terms of these constructed identities, the *reconnoitring* of the handover can be seen as a technique of panoptic surveillance aimed at inducing patient conformity.

In our earlier study we also identified ways in which the collaborative narrative of the handover functions to weld the nurses into a working social group. As with soldiers risking life and limb as they scan a dangerous terrain for unexploded bombs and hidden enemies, the nurses' sense of safety and competence in managing the dangers inherent in their work is enhanced through feeling that they can rely upon the observational skills and immediate responses of one another for the duration of the shift. However the formation of this type of cohesiveness does not provide much room for individuality of responses and to this extent is an example of the disciplinary power inherent in the setting which also serves to induce docility and conformity among nurses.

Savoir—the nursing gaze

Much of the information relayed during a handover presentation deals with what we think of as objective knowledge about the patient's body, the medical history and present diagnosis, perhaps blood pressure readings or other observations, medication levels and frequency of dosages and so forth. An example from a 7 a.m. handover is as follows:

> Julie Brown, Bed 13, 51, under Medical Unit 'A'. Presented with PUO. Query atypical pneumonia. As well as unstable diabetes. She's had gestational diabetes, which she got 19 years ago. She's on oral hypo-glycaemics and a sliding scale. Um, she required 8 units of Actrapid this morning at six. Um, she's for blood cultures if her temp's greater than 37.5. She had one set of blood cultures last night. Um, her IV has been resited overnight as well, she has her intravenous in, I think it's a twelve hourly litre. Normal saline. She had a 24 hour urine collection completed this morning and her temp at six is 37.6.

What is the character of this knowledge? Much, though not all of it, is technical and medicalised, and is characterised by definiteness and cultivation of abstraction. Nurses give a recital of conditions on admission, of prescribed drugs, listing peak flows, fluid intake and output etc. each presented as a distinct, separate 'fact'. The claim to certainty of this form of knowledge is expressed in its numeric form. It is often articulated as a series of figures. ('His BM this morning for his diabetes is 11.7...It went um, it was up to 19.9 last night...down to 11.7...') This type of knowledge with its use of figures makes it appear non-personal and objective. The nurses communicate medical reports and mathematised nursing observations to each other and the knowledge communicated carries the assumption that it exists in a world of non-personal, as-if-numerical fact.

The tacit assumption is that a diagnosis has not been made by any human being making a decision (which is the case) or that any uncertainty surrounds a diagnosis (which is frequently the case), but that it has, as it were, been produced necessarily and inevitably out of the patient's condition (Hunter 1991). In the instance cited above, the diagnosis is uncertain, as the words 'query atypical' and 'unstable' inevitably suggest, but this fact, which may be the crucial one about this patient at this time, is masked by the array of indicators of certainty. The seemingly compelling and definitive reference 'PUO' is a shorthand notation of a condition wherein the patient is suffering from a fever of unknown origin, but it disguises this, in the context of interpersonal communication, by seeming to convey a precise and agreed-upon, a transpersonal, object of knowledge. The tendency of diagnoses to be expressed in such abbreviated forms, COAD for example, contributes to this air of impersonally existing information.

The Western epistemological tradition encourages one to think of this type of knowledge as decontextualised, seemingly objectively existing. We describe it as *savoir*, the nursing gaze, by analogy with the medical gaze as described by Foucault. *Savoir* is schematic and dogmatic, but it is also tremendously important. Effective nursing could not possibly be carried out without the knowledge that is communicated through medical diagnoses, readings and charts. But sometimes in the handovers we listened to, *savoir*—or something resembling it—was presented alone, the recital, as if by rote, of the 'facts' of dates, admission details, diagnostic tests, dosages and outputs. In one form of handover the dangers of this seem especially heightened. Sometimes the handover for all the patients would be given by one nurse on the previous shift, a nurse who, necessarily, had little acquaintance with some of the patients on whom he/she reported. The common characteristic of this form of handover is to deliver curt, clipped, operationalised accounts, especially of those patients that the nurse has not personally dealt with.

In these circumstances, we observed a tendency for the knowledge to be a decontextualised, processed, rather empty repetition of external facts or diagnoses, and such military-style ticking off of patients ('all present and correct') has a clear resemblance to the surveillance techniques of power/ knowledge.

In place of name and rank we hear bed number, patient's name and age, medical unit, and list of disease conditions, usually given in abbreviated and acronymic form. Whilst orientating the nurse to the domain of her practice, and facilitating the *reconnoitre*, it simultaneously designates the patient as an object, and the site of control. But that, we would argue, is to forgo, or to distort, the necessary and therapeutically enabling kinds of knowledge which the handover may more usually transmit.

Connaissance, the nursing look

The nurse also conveys, at the same time and sometimes in the same sentence, another kind of information which has two main characteristics that are quite unlike each other. The first of these characteristics is that the information is personal, in the sense that the speaker lays implicit claim to the ownership or attribution of the knowledge. The second is that the information is informal and imprecise: necessarily imprecise, we would argue. Whilst we were monitoring handovers we frequently heard nurses saying things like this: 'She's OK. She's just really tired. She looks really terrible, grey'. Or: 'The whole foot looks red and hot. Looks like he could do with antis'. Or: 'That left hand looks bad. Quite nasty.' 'She's looking very blue around the gills. She looks really blue to me.' 'She's happy.' 'His chest pain is difficult to assess. He doesn't look anxious, but I don't know...' 'Each time she goes to sleep I have to check that she's alright. Her face just caves in.'

What are the characteristics of these comments? They are certainly very different from the medicalised abstract commentaries that accompany them. Their language is largely informal, but at the same time vivid and instantly communicative. It is affective, owned language: the speakers are declaring their own responses to the patient as part of their knowledge of the patient. In fact the verb 'to look' mediates between patient and health care professional in a way not unknown, but certainly not central to, medical discourse. The patient looks, but at the same time, simultaneously as part of the same linguistic gesture, is looked at. The look of the patient (or the patient's face or body) exists only through the medium of the nurse's looking. And the nurse's looking is not the cool or scientific inspection of the nursing gaze but a process of empathic understanding or reasoning in which patient and nurse are melded for a moment into one. 'The look remains faithful, even subservient to the object's integrity, seeming to caress it, following its "natural" contours' (Sass 1992). One must not fall into the trap of calling this a 'subjective' response. The whole dichotomy of subject/object falls away when knowledge is understood in the way we are arguing—as does the separation between self and other.

This is owned language too: each time the nurses speak it, they are taking personal responsibility for their comments. It is their deposition, their testimony to the patient's condition, and they often offer it tangentially, as if registering a private, but none the less valid, response that in its very colloquiality and imprecision is an affirmation of their community with the other nurses and with the patient. 'He's not really interested in looking after himself any more, didn't put his legs on in the morning. Very apathetic. Just seems to be...' (a gesture indicating flatness, or hopelessness). But on the other hand: 'Just before I left yesterday I looked in and I thought "this lady will kick in and she'll be OK"'.

This style of nursing communication often slides seamlessly into another. In progress notes, crowded with annotations by doctors, dietitians, physiotherapists and nurses, the patient, as a speaking human subject, is only marginally documented. Sometimes, as in a case noted by Poirier and Brauner (1990), the patient's 'voice' is literally obliterated by intubation or other procedures. The patient's voice, mediated, as it must be, through the words of the nurse or physician, is rarely strongly present in progress notes. At handover, however, patients are often made present, made real, to other nurses by the recall or recitation of their own words. An example is this, given at a 7 a.m. handover: 'He slept really, really well. One of the best night's sleep he's ever had'. In the context it was clear that the first sentence referred to the nurse's observation, but this became inseparable, during her presentation, from what must have been a quotation from the patient's own mouth.

In another example, given at the 1 p.m. handover, the nurse's account of a newly admitted patient is based first on actions taken in the hospital and then moves into a description that contains within it the ring of the patient's voice:

Nurse Giving Handover: Bed 29 is Mr Grindisi. He was admitted to us this morning from casualty with chest pain, post CAGS. He's a 57 year old man and it's his first episode of chest pain from 1990 when he had the CAGS and he's been pain free until yesterday morning. He had five or six episodes of typical chest pain tightness lasting five to ten minutes over an hour. He didn't have any Anginine at home. That was yesterday and he woke last night with severe chest pain, the worst he's ever had and associated shortness of breath and nausea and that's why he came in.

Often the nurse and the patient become virtually identified and speak as if with one voice: 'She hasn't slept one wink' (the nurse makes a repeated honking noise). 'Sister, I can't go home.' 'No, Joanna', I said, 'you can't.' Another example: 'They're not changing his medication before he goes home. He's really scared'. On the other hand, sometimes the tendency for the nurse and the patient to merge can lead to the suspicion that a comment such as: 'She's fine, totally self-caring. She's fine', runs the two perspectives together in an unreflective way that may substitute convenience to the nurse for the patient's own condition.

While looking is a culturally valued and dominant mode of access to knowledge, the look, in our account of nursing knowledge, is a metaphor which stands for the range of senses. 'She looks quite good. But lifting her up the bed, she feels like a rag doll. We'd better get her out of bed and sat up on Monday.' Such comments, which are common, reflect another sense-modality of nursing knowledge. The body of the nurse is inevitably involved. This is embodied knowledge, the clearest possible illustration of Haraway's claim for the 'embodied nature of all vision'. To 'feel' that the patient is enfeebled; to smell; to 'sense' the patient's despair; to capture and reproduce the patient's difficulty in breathing by honking in imitation: all these are equally manifestations of nursing knowledge, often functioning in an interplay with each other. All these are represented, in our account, by the look.

This knowledge which nurses communicate in the handover differs then from the abstract and numeric knowledge that accompanies it. It is not formalised: it is communicated in common language idioms, without specialist terms. It is approximate, probing, to an extent impressionistic, an offering to the other of an estimate, not a presumed fact. It gravitates closely towards ordinary human communication, and does not claim an esoteric, or technically-aided knowledge of the patient's inner bodily processes. Instead it offers to read the body and the face as continuous with another version of interiority. This inner self or being of the patient, to which the look or the feel gives irrefutable access, is immediately registered as having urgent implications for practice.

But for these very reasons, nurses themselves tend to overlook, even to slight, this form of communication, to regard it as 'subjective', even as unprofessional. This form of knowledge is concrete and practice-orientated. Prestige is instead given to *savoir*, to the abstract, medicalised knowledge involved in the listing of diagnoses and drugs. The very non-formality of this other form of nursing knowledge means that it is taken-for-granted and disvalued. We argue, on the contrary that this is at the heart of nursing's professional knowledge.

We describe this form of nursing knowledge as *connaissance*, the look. We suggest that much of nursing practice knowledge is a form of *connaissance*, practised in a milieu in which prestige is attached to *savoir*, the gaze. One might describe *connaissance* in our sense as 'embodied situated caring attentiveness'. It is what is called on when a nurse, passing on a patient at handover, says, for instance, 'There's a question about this patient and his urine output. Keep an eye on him'.

It is important to distinguish 'keeping an eye on him' from panoptic surveillance in the Foucauldian sense of that term. Such a conception of looking implies the rigorous maintenance of control and power. Nurses' necessarily intermittent attention to the transient physical signs of their patients cannot be readily construed merely as mechanisms of control, though questions about management and resource allocation are clearly entailed. 'Yes, but how does he *look*?' When a nurse asks this of another at handover, she is asking for guidance on a matter which cannot in its nature be definite, and is not an instance of the objectifying and detached gaze of power/knowledge. Rather than authoritarian, looking or feeling is a kind of sampling activity. The discourse of *connaissance* is immediately tied to practice, to the immediate, non-negotiable banalities of the need to act within circumstances that, far from constraining, are themselves constrained.

Connaissance in our usage is pre-eminently an activity of involvement and situated embodied understanding. It is an activity of knowledge which is inherently communicative and transactional. *Connaissance* recognises the interdependence of this form of knowledge. It registers, too, the transience of bodily signs, and tolerates the indeterminacy of their elucidation.

Through this understanding of *connaissance*, we can begin to recognise some of the limitations of Cartesian dualism and the resultant split between mind and body, self and other. The feminist writer Brennan (1993) goes so far as to describe the idea of a separate self or autonomous ego as a 'psychotic fantasy' of omnipotence and control. She says 'To allow that my feelings physically enter you, or yours me, to think we both had the same thought at the same time because it is literally in the air, is to think in a way that really puts the subject in question'. We would argue that this is precisely the nature of *connaissance*.

Reconnaissance—incorporative reflective nursing practice knowledge

In the handover then, nurses going off duty pass on to the incoming nurses local perspectival knowledge of the specific terrain in which they have practised over the shift. They point out dangers and give warnings. This *reconnoitre* or knowledge of the nursing scan is knowledge of technological imperatives, of situational constraints and possibilities. It is a knowledge which portrays patients in stereotypical form so as to present a familiar terrain. It is a knowledge which binds nurses as a reliable and dependable unity of shared understandings.

At the handover, technical and medicalised knowledge is also presented. This is *savoir*, knowledge of the nursing gaze. We would argue, however, that this is not to be understood as objective, decontextualised, representational medical knowledge to which nurses have access in a secondary and derivative way. Such a way of understanding *savoir* is, we would suggest, a fallacy of modernism. *Savoir*, the nursing gaze, is not a gaze from 'no where' or 'everywhere'. It is a gaze from 'some where'. We would argue that so called objective decontextualised medical knowledge when incorporated by a person is embodied, partial knowledge understood from a particular point of view and situation. That is to say it is incorporated, understood and utilised according to particular situations and circumstances and in relation to specific disciplinary, ethical and political positions. A diagnosis can appear as an abstract, objective piece of information, or radiate out immediately into concerns with practice and work. Knowledge in this sense comes out of the interrelatedness, the enfolding, of thing and world. A word, a term, a diagnosis, does not always have the same referent. All medical terms, like language in general, have situated, embodied and constituted meanings, according to the situation in which they are articulated and the pressing concerns of those who use them and listen to them.

Knowledge, presented in medicalised form as *savoir*, may be effectively transmuted or recreated in its listeners into nursing *connaissance*. If medical knowledge is a labelling of pathophysiology, 'COAD' for instance, what this diagnosis in effect means will differ with the differing disciplinary positionings of its users. For a physician it refers to the interior of the body, to malign processes within the bronchial tree: for nurses it may, in effect, convey something tied to the material conditions of their practice. It may communicate, in fact, 'this patient might need a wheelchair' or 'She needs lots and lots of pillows'. But not only the disciplinary or professional positioning of the listener may alter the meaning of a diagnosis. 'COAD' will mean something different in the situation of critical care nursing from that of an aged care assessment unit. In other words, the meaning of a series of medical conditions when read out at a handover need not be inert, or a manifestation of nursing's deprivileging of its own knowledge modes.

Handovers which present *savoir*, the nursing gaze, should, we would argue, be the occasion for *reconnaissance*. By *reconnaissance* we mean the reflective integration of the three aspects of nursing knowledge, that we have identified as *reconnoitre*, *savoir* and *connaissance*. The *reconnoitre*, the scanning of the terrain, provides orientation to the potencies of the place and gives boundedness to the situated knowledge that is constituted over the shift. Medicalised knowledge must necessarily be presented to the incoming nurses at handover: but this knowledge must be re-known. It must be understood in its implications for nursing, for the immediate, as well as longer term, bodily care of the patient. *Connaissance*, as we have defined it, is a form of knowledge central to nursing care. Sometimes nurses seem to want to apologise for what is perceived as a descent into a less-than-professional mode. *Connaissance* is on these occasions felt to be an unnecessary, gauche, embarrassingly non-medical, crude, or even shameful aspect of handover discourse. But its centrality should be recognised rather than passed over or elided.

Connaissance is a form of knowledge which is increasingly validated within philosophy, an exemplary focus of cogent critiques of enlightenment configurations of human rationality. *Reconnaissance* draws upon the knowledge of the *reconnoitre* and tempers *connaissance* with reflective appraisal. It is a revalidation of *connaissance* undertaken with full recognition of the complementary mode of *savoir*. *Reconnaissance* recognises and attends to the situation- and context-bound exigencies of nursing without succumbing to the surveillance and dominance inherent in all forms of power/knowledge. *Connaissance*, as we have defined it here, complements and sometimes qualifies or redefines medicalised knowledge, but in the best handovers, *connaissance* is subject to reflective understanding, and has become *reconnaissance*, a form of embodied, situated, reflective, objective knowledge stemming from a partial perspective.

Conclusion

In this chapter we have attempted to show that the nurses' voice in the oral handover is not necessarily a weak echo of the medical voice that we identified in patient progress notes. We would argue that the handover can provide a significant site for the expression of authentic nursing practice knowledge. However, we do not claim to have seen many expressions of this form of practice knowledge in our observations of the handover. Because of the dominance of the medical voice in the hospital context, supported as it is by the disciplinary power of medical knowledge, it is not surprising that the nursing voice is somewhat muted. The Foucauldian notions of panopticism and the medical gaze help in understanding the complex terrain of disciplinary power relations within which hospital based nursing practice takes place.

Furthermore, to understand *reconnaissance* as we have formulated it requires a different understanding of the nature of knowledge from that which gives primacy to a view of knowledge as abstract, decontextualised and universal, 'the view from nowhere'. If knowledge is understood in such Cartesian terms it is difficult to identify nursing knowledge at all. Rather what can be identified is a body of abstract scientific medical knowledge which nurses draw upon from a less well informed position than doctors. They are taught this knowledge and use it in their observations of patients and in carrying out technical medically derived procedures to support the medical enterprise of diagnosis and treatment of disease. The *savoir* dimension of nursing knowledge can thus only be understood as secondary and medically derived. The knowledge of *reconnoitre* and *connaissance* become disparaged and underestimated, reduced to local 'savvy' and inappropriate personal involvement.

Bordo's (1993) warning is timely in indicating the enormity of the task of deconstructing the metaphysics of mind/ body dualism. However, Haraway's notion of situated knowledges is very helpful for nursing in describing practice knowledge as embodied and partial, incorporating a 'view from somewhere', i.e. from the situations and circumstances of specific practice locations. *Reconnaissance*, however, does not emerge when the information conveyed about a patient at handover is given by a nurse who was not involved in the direct care of the patient. It does not emerge when the information conveyed is limited to medical history, current diagnosis and medications. It seems to us that the only rationale for this information is if it facilitates effective nursing care. When priority is given to well rehearsed past conditions and nursing care is omitted, something is wrong. *Reconnaissance* does not emerge when the exchange between nurses focuses only on painting stereotypical portraits of patients or when nurses use the handover simply as a means of ensuring a sense of camaraderie. *Reconnaissance* emerges when the nurse can confidently identify salient dimensions of the terrain, can give an appropriate account of the medical parameters involved in nursing decisions and can reflectively discern the aspects of *connaissance* knowledge that need to be communicated to nurses coming on duty.

In this age of cost containment an argument has been mounted that the nursing handover is a cumbersome, unnecessary, outdated, costly and time wasting ritual. We would suggest that the oral transmission of nursing practice knowledge provides an important means of ensuring continuity of nursing practice knowledge and hence continuity of nursing care over the span of the patient's period of hospitalisation. However it is also clear to us that some current handover practices might be reviewed, and this could facilitate a milieu which enhances the likelihood of the expression of the practice knowledge of *reconnaissance*. We suggest that the nursing practice knowledge of *reconnaissance* enables nurses to make rational, objective knowledge claims stemming from their embodied, situated partial perspectives.

NOTES

Handover excerpts reported in this chapter are part of a study of the Nursing Handover and Patient Progress Notes funded by the Victorian Nursing Council and the Australian Research Council and the Australian Research Council Small Grants Scheme.

REFERENCES

Best S 1991 Chaos and entropy, metaphors in postmodern science and social theory. Silence as Culture 2(11):188-226

Bordo S 1993 Unbearable weight: feminism, Western culture and the body. University of California Press, California

Brennan T 1993 History after Lacan. Routledge, London

Foucault M 1973 The birth of the clinic, an archaeology of medical perception. Sheridan A M (trans). Tavistock, London

Foucault M 1977 Discipline and punish: the birth of the prison. Allen Lane, London

Gilligan C 1994 The dream of everywhere. Review of Books, March, London

Haraway D 1991 Simians, Cyborgs and women. The reinvention of nature. Free Association Books, London pp 183-201

Harding S 1986 The science question in feminism. Cornell University Press, Ithaca & London

Hunter K M 1991 Doctors' stories: the narrative structure of medical knowledge. Princeton University Press, Princeton

Nightingale F 1860 Notes on nursing: what it is, and what it is not, 2nd edn. Harrison & Sons, London

Parker J, Gardiner G 1992 The silence and the silencing of the nurse's voice: a reading of patient progress notes. Australian Journal of Advanced Nursing 9(2):3-9

Parker J, Gardiner G, Wiltshire J 1992 Handover: the collective narrative of nursing practice. Australian Journal of Advanced Nursing 9(3):31-37

Poirier S, Brauner D J 1990 The voices in the medical record. Theoretical Medicine 11:29-39

Rabinov P (ed) 1991 The Foucault reader. Penguin Books, London

Reiser S J 1982 Medicine and the rise of technology. Cambridge University Press, Cambridge

Sass L A 1992 Madness and modernism: schizophrenia in the light of modern art, thought and culture. Basic Books, New York

10

Scholarship in a practice discipline: the logical consequences

BARBARA A. HAYES

And heart from its prison
Cries to the spirit walking above:
'I was with you in agony.
Remember your promise of paradise',
And hammers and hammers, 'Remember me'.
'Triste, Triste' (Gwen Harwood 1972)

Introduction

The major logical outcome to scholarship in a practice-centred discipline such as nursing is naming and claiming the intellectual bases of nursing practice. Ethics is a fundamental intellectual influence on nursing practice and research. This chapter explores the consequences of being a practice discipline, i.e. both a profession and a discipline and the links which the ethical dimensions of scholarship provide. The evocative words, above, of one of Australia's prominent women poets, Gwen Harwood, are both literally and symbolically a 'cri de coeur'. In fact, if one can imagine the 'heart' as nursing practice and the 'spirit' as the intellectual aspect of nursing, this poet signals what could be the sub-title of this chapter: 'Healing the intellectual-practice split in nursing'.

Scholarship and scholarliness

In a curious twist of language the noun 'scholarliness' which bears the same attributes as 'scholarship' appears in the North American literature. Perhaps 'scholarship' is thought to be contaminated by its attendant use as a bursary or endowment of funds for the goal of learning, while 'scholarliness' betokens the possession of an extensive and profound knowledge of an academic discipline. For the purposes of discussion within this chapter, the nouns are used interchangeably.

Scholarship or 'scholarliness' became a focus of concern in nursing with the emergence of the discipline as distinct from the profession (Donaldson & Crowley 1978, Holzemer & Chambers 1986, May et al 1982) heralded by the development of doctoral programs in nursing in the United States, the United Kingdom, Europe and, more recently, in Australia and New Zealand as well as in several countries in Asia. These programs were, and are, a direct stimulus to the consciousness of scholarship as the quality of the programs is measured formally by intra-university and inter-university quality assurance assays (DEET 1994) and informally by potential students as consumers. Scholarship, as a concept in academia is a more taken-for-granted one than an explicated one and seems to resist any consensual definition. However, scholarship as a criterion for appointment, promotion and tenure is widely used in universities so that in universities there is a degree of consensus about the evidence required to meet this criterion. The following are some examples of such evidence: literature citations; review articles in books or journals of recognised international standing; invitations to address scholarly meetings and conferences; services as an editor or referee to scholarly journals or books; and/or professional awards and fellowships. It is pertinent that no one piece of this evidence alludes to practice—let alone to the centrality of practice. Thus, if scholarship is linked to nursing as a practice discipline, what are these links?

This author posits that one of the links of scholarship to practice is ethics. Given that scholarship pertains to depth of intellectual activity, this link often goes unrecognised. In nursing and other health care professions, the ethical dimensions of practice and research have been addressed and continue to be so but, to date, little has been written concerning the ethical dimensions of scholarship. Thus, one conceptualisation of the relationship of ethics to scholarship is captured in the following equation:

intellectual depth + ethics of intellectual activities = scholarship.

Taking the foregoing equation as a provisional conceptualisation of scholarship, this chapter posits that the following consequences are logical if scholarship applies to nursing as a practice discipline:

- that the ethics of practice and the ethical dimensions of scholarship are inextricably linked
- that nursing as a profession and nursing as a discipline are a continuum along the search for intellectual depth in nursing.

Each of these consequences have implications for practice, education and research which are addressed after each section.

The ethics of practice and the ethical dimensions of scholarship: an enduring connection

The primary aim of ethics is to seek to maximise the interests of all persons equally. Bioethics is focused particularly on identifying and protecting the *vulnerability* of one or more persons in a relationship or context. Vulnerability is derived from the Latin root *vulnerare* which means 'to wound'. Therefore, anyone who is vulnerable may be wounded, susceptible to injury or exposed to damage. There is a subtle difference between being vulnerable, that is, susceptible to injury, and being violated, which is to *be* injured. Being vulnerable leads to an *imbalance of power* which bioethical reasoning, based on critical reflection upon several moral principles, hopes to redress. The person or persons who are most vulnerable in the health care delivery system are those who receive its services and so become either patients or clients or consumers within the system. There is a variety of relationships between the recipient of care and health care professionals just as there is a variety of contexts in which the care is delivered.

As the reader will realise, the titles for the recipient of care vary within practice and within the literature but, in this chapter, the title of either 'patient' or 'client' is used with the respect which all these titles can engender. In addition, these titles are inclusive of the recipient's significant other/s.

Beckstrand sparked a lively debate within academic nursing circles by writing three articles (1978a, 1978b, 1980) around the notion of a practice theory for nursing. The core of the debate was that Beckstrand took issue with other writers such as Dickoff, James and Weidenbach (1968), and also Jacox (1974) who espoused the need for a practice theory in nursing. Beckstrand's arguments lacked clarity and consistency but did, at least, challenge the assumption of theory for practice as opposed to theory from, for example, science and ethics being applied to practice.

This section of the chapter traces the connection between the ethics of practice and the ethical dimensions of scholarship and suggests that a significant link between these is through the ethics of research. The notion of vulnerability is the linchpin here.

Ethics of nursing practice

In the past, teachers in education programs in nursing and health care often either conflated or confused professional etiquette with ethics. Currently, ethics, ethical principles and ethical reasoning are taught at varying depths in all undergraduate nursing curricula in Australia. Inclusion of the ethics of research is mandatory in graduate courses. It is interesting to note that the main findings of an Australia wide survey of professional ethics and honesty found that Australians rate nurses as a professional group with the highest degree of honesty and ethical standards. The survey was conducted by the Morgan Poll Australia wide in April 1994 when 1212 people aged 14 years and over were interviewed face-to-face. Australians rated 86% of nurses as maintaining 'high' or 'very high' honest and ethical standards followed by pharmacists, medical doctors, school teachers and dentists.

The moral principles, which are the basis of ethics, function by specifying that some type of action or conduct is either prohibited, required, or permitted in certain circumstances (Solomon 1990). Moral rules such as 'Never hit a patient' or 'Always tell the truth' are drawn from these principles. Practising nurses apply these principles, mostly well and sometimes badly, every day. For example, the decision about the degree of 'persuasion' or 'force' which can be justified to ensure that patients in a general medical unit maintain medication regimens that are 'for their own good' can be argued by the nurse. This justification for the exertion of force seems to be based on the judgement by the nurse that the patient's mental capability is diminished to the point that the patient cannot exercise autonomy at that particular moment. The justification by the nurse can be expressed verbally or non-verbally, e.g. by an expression of exasperation, raised eyebrow or simply a statement such as 'They don't know what's best for them'. Thus, in the application of a moral principle, practising nurses make moral judgments.

In the following extract Johnstone (1989) cites an example of the implicit obligation for the practitioner in applying the moral rule of 'Always tell the truth':

> ...if a patient asks an attending health care professional a question concerning a diagnosis and proposed treatment, the health care professional could be said to be obliged to give the information which the patient has requested. The apparent 'obligation' here finds its force not just from the moral rule of 'Always tell the truth' but also from the moral principle of autonomy which demands that rational people be respected as autonomous choosers and be given the information required to make an informed and intelligent choice.

Adherence to moral principles is not just part of the day-to-day practice of nursing but is also part of the minute-to-minute decision making. Thus the complexity of interactive nursing care demands time, energy, insight and patience.

Four of the moral principles which are commonly quoted as the basis of ethical decision-making in practice are: autonomy, non-maleficence, beneficence and justice. *Autonomy* literally means 'self-governing' and, as a concept, usually refers to a person's ability to make or to exercise choice. Inherent in applying the principle of autonomy is exhibiting a positive attitude towards the dignity of an individual and demonstrating a respect for the person's rights, beliefs and actions. In the health care professions autonomy is the principle underlying the patient or client's exercising choice over treatment. Hence there is an 'obligation' to ensure that when eliciting consent for treatment the patient is informed of available choices. The range of choices ought always to include the choice to refuse treatment even though this may seem foolish to others such as family members or health professionals (Beauchamp & Walters 1982).

Non-maleficence literally means 'above all do no harm'. Operationally, this is sometimes a difficult principle to distinguish from that of *beneficence* which demands that 'above all, do good'. The problem is particularly difficult in nursing practice when nurses are often required to inflict pain (which in another context would be seen as 'harm') in order to do 'good'. Johnstone (1989) explicates the argument from the literature and states that in the application of the principle of non-maleficence any act which unjustly injures persons or causes them to suffer an otherwise avoidable harm would be condemned. But in the application of the principle of beneficence in nursing, the obligation for the 'provision of benefits' such as pain relief, comfort and correct treatment there is also 'a balancing of benefits and harms' such as the infliction of a harm (pain) in order to achieve a good (healing), e.g. in the dressing of a patient with major burns. Clearly, the line between these two principles is a fine one. Madjar (1994) provides several examples of nurses negotiating this fine line in a chilling exposition of the embodied experiences of patients enduring pain during therapeutic experiences.

The principle of *justice* in ethics draws on the tenets of moral philosophy rather than on the sense of seeking justice before the law; for the seeking of justice before the law can have little to do with morality. Justice, as a moral principle, continues to generate widespread debate and the application of the principle generates even further debate. However, nurses often display an innate sense of the following two interpretations: that of 'justice as fairness' and 'distributive justice'. For example, the former fuelled the historic removal of the 'no strike' clause from the Victorian industrial agreement in 1984 and the latter guides the fine balancing of resources at the micro level of patient management with the guideline 'to each according to their needs (or severity of illness or level of discomfort or brevity of prognosis)' being a rough but effective 'rule of thumb'.

Because of the embodied, interactive reality of nursing practice—that is, the nurse-patient relationship involves a high level of personal care often delivered on a one-to-one basis—*intimacy* becomes an added dimension to vulnerability. Because of the nature of intimate relationships, both the patient *and* the nurse can be vulnerable.

Since Florence Nightingale's pioneering work, nurses have sought to shape and explicate an ethical framework because of this very complexity of their practice. In 1973 an international code of ethics was adopted by the national representatives attending the International Council of Nurses (ICN) meeting in Mexico City and, in 1993, a more context-specific Australian code of nursing ethics was adopted. In the raised consciousness of ethics in nursing and health care following adoption by the ICN of an international code of ethics, useful texts focusing on the application of ethics to health care emerged such as Beauchamp and Walters (1992) and Davis and Aroskar (1983). It is thus refreshing, but perhaps not surprising, that an Australian viewpoint evolved in a brief period of time. Megan-Jane Johnstone (1989), an Australian nursing academic, has contributed significantly to both the profession and the discipline of nursing through her scholarly work *Bioethics: a nursing perspective*. Johnstone's sophisticated approach to bioethics leads the reader to a deeper understanding not only of the complexity of nursing practice but also of the ethical infrastructure which underpins daily practice. The relative recency of recognition of nursing practitioners as being independent decision makers both responsible and accountable for nursing care is noted as an issue: this recognition, in and of itself, can buffer vulnerability. Johnstone threads numerous Australian nursing practice examples of embodied vulnerability—

be it that of either patient or nurse—through the work, in addition to formal examples emanating from major theories.

That patients can be ethically vulnerable is fairly obvious and has been explained earlier, but the sense of *embodied* vulnerability which nurses can experience is not as easy to recognise and arises from many sources, e.g. accountability to the patient, to the family, to the employer and to the profession for daily adherence to moral principles. These several lines of accountability can be a source of conflict. Australian scholars are making a major contribution to the literature on embodiment and its accompanying vulnerability and this has been addressed in another forum (Hayes 1992). From this discussion, it seems that the three ethical principles which impact directly on nursing practice are *autonomy*, *beneficence* and *justice* and that *both* the patient and the nurse are subject to vulnerability.

Ethics of research: the bridge between practice and scholarship

Clearly the notion of vulnerability extends also to research and this author suggests that the ethics of research can be a bridge between practice and scholarship. The rights of human subjects in research are probably now better defined and protected than the rights of patients receiving treatment within the health care delivery systems of the Western world. The history of abuses of subjects in research echo from the infamous Tuskagee experiments in the 1930s when treatment for syphilis was withheld from black male prisoners in the United States (Brandt 1978, Rothman 1982) to the withholding of treatment from women suffering from cervical cancer at Green Lane hospital in Auckland, New Zealand which began in 1958 (Coney 1988). Resulting from these tragic failures to protect vulnerable populations, vigilance is now the operative imperative of research ethics committees in universities, regional health authorities and hospitals. The pattern in Australia varies from either separate research and ethics committees to a combination of that expertise in one committee. In addition, single departments or units may have their own ethics committees.

Although most research ethics committees in Australia conform to the guidelines set down by the National Health and Medical Research Council (NHMRC), two particular problems face these committees. The first is that very few professionals, be they from health, law or theology, have a substantive grounding in philosophy/ethics which means that many of these committees simply function on precedent or rely on the previous experience of individual members. Thus, the researcher who presents a proposal that does not fit within those categories may find permission to conduct research refused.

The second problem is that the research ethics committees are fully autonomous and do not come under any formal review. The Secretary of the Australian Health Ethics Committee of the National Health and Medical Research Council, which this author believes could hold this brief, has stated that the powers of the Committee are limited to those of being an advisory body to federal government. Obviously realising this deficit, the NHMRC, through the Australian Health Ethics Committee has called for submissions from the general public on the structure, function and effectiveness of institutional ethics committees by December 1994. Crosthwaite (1994) in her recent discussion of feminism and medical ethics notes that feminist health groups were strong voices in securing 50% lay membership for institutional ethics committees in New Zealand.

However, experimentation as a means of physical and psychological torture continues to be a daily part of political reality when there are major imbalances of political power. Both nursing and medical practitioners have been implicated. Stover and Nightingale (1985) were commissioned by the American Association for the Advancement of Science to document the outcomes of their work on the Committee on Scientific Freedom and Responsibility. The title of the book reflects the chilling nature of its contents: *The breaking of bodies and minds: torture, psychiatric abuse and the health professions*. While the book documents accounts of torture in political systems in South America and in the former Soviet Union, introductory chapters explore both the experience of the breaking of bodies and minds and the ethics of involvement by health professionals which provide food for thought on a subject which most health professionals would wish to avoid. In the Foreword, Hamburg acknowledges the dilemma of the inclusion of healers in the violation of human rights and states the following:

> This is a rare, special, and sensitive book. It deals with a subject of vital worldwide importance that we would all prefer to avoid: the gross and pervasive violation of human rights. Such violations cause great suffering and, often, long-lasting mental and physical damage. There is nothing subtle nor doubtful about them. They are harmful to the victims and to the societies in which they occur. They are the ultimate abomination of the human spirit...In technologically advanced societies, there is unequivocal evidence that the capabilities of the health professions are growing, based on great advances in the sciences. Yet, here as elsewhere great power may be used both for good and for harm.

On the other hand, both nursing and medical practitioners have also been imprisoned or killed because of their willingness to protect the vulnerable either by giving treatment to those considered to be the enemy or refusing to participate in non-ethical research for those considered to be the enemy.

From this discussion it seems that the principles of *autonomy* and *non-maleficence* are the principles most applicable in research and that the subjects of research are most vulnerable.

Ethics of scholarship: what moral principles are most applicable in scholarship and who is most vulnerable?

The longstanding, post-colonial, anti-intellectual bias which prevails against any school except the school of experience creates a diffidence within nursing which results in a distance between nursing and some of the older disciplines. After several fact-finding conversations with academics from different disciplines, the following characteristics, which seem to be part of the taken-for-granted assumption about scholars and scholarship in academe, emerged. For nursing practice, however, they may appear to be incongruous or, even, pretentious:

- a person who possesses a depth and breadth of knowledge in his/her own reputed area
- a person who communicates that knowledge—primarily by teaching but also by publication
- a person who can weigh the evidence of ideas and propositions which differ or conflict with his/her own and, because she/he is a scholar, can give due weight to both sides of the argument
- a person who values learning (practice) for its own sake and is committed to the pursuit of learning (practice) for its own sake
- a person who scrupulously acknowledges the sources of his/her ideas and who, just as scrupulously, suspends belief in the face of new data prior to judgment (Bradley et al 1991).

From the foregoing characteristics, to be a scholar in a vacuum would appear to be difficult, thus a community of peers is needed not just for companionship but also for critique (Bradley & Selby 1992). In addition, a scholar is an enthusiast for, and a champion and protector of, the intellect and intellectual pursuit (Steele 1993). Whether or not these seem pretentious, these tenets of scholarship can anchor nursing both as a profession and a discipline. Finally, the intrinsic factor in scholarship is a *personal ethic of excellence*. From this discussion it seems the moral principles of *beneficence* and *autonomy* are the ones most applicable in scholarship. Scholarship opens up the often covert relationship between the scholar as person and knowledge as a dynamic entity. One must be rigorous in the pursuit of knowledge and one must respect the data: whether they be clinical data, research data or the data of knowledge, i.e. the building blocks of knowledge. There is an intimacy operating within the relationship of the person and knowledge similar to that of the nurse-patient relationship. Thus, the scholar as person is vulnerable and knowledge can suffer by being incomplete.

Implications of the ethics of scholarship for nursing practice, education and research

Rigour and respect are two identifiable threads in the ethical fabric of scholarship which form part of a personal ethic of excellence. This personal ethic of excellence can influence practice, education and research in subtle ways which allows vulnerability to be named and the vulnerable to be protected.

In practice, developing a personal ethic of excellence creates independent thinkers who respect their own skills and who are open to new career pathways in the practice not just of nursing but of health care. Often nurses view and thus describe their practice according to the context in which the care is given, for example, operating room, intensive care or out-patients. This view—that nurses employ 'context' rather than 'skill-related attributes' as the major descriptor for their practice—is restrictive in several ways and the following is just one example.

When nurses define their practice within a certain context the perception which nurses themselves have of the range of intellectual skills which are acquired through practice is limited and thus nurses' own *respect* for these skills is minimal. One result of this diminishment of 'skills-respect' is 'skills immobility' in that any career move, even within the profession of nursing itself as well as within and without the health care delivery system, is seen as a career *change* rather than a career *progression*. Thus, only small numbers of professional nurses mobilise their skills by progressing into a range of career paths in which other health professionals deem themselves well prepared: e.g. personnel or environmental management, or local, state or federal politics. In addition to respect for one's own skills—that is the death of the lie that 'Anyone with an ounce of common-sense can be a nurse', which is often the response of skilled nurses to affirmation of their skills— the other thread of the ethical fabric of scholarship in practice is that of *rigour*.

Rigour is not often employed as a descriptor for nursing practice but can be understood as a combination of the application of above-the-minimal accepted standards and thoroughness in nursing practice. Rigour is an essential ingredient for developing best practice models in nursing and health care. Thus developing a personal ethic of excellence in nursing practice which is based on respect and rigour offers nurse practitioners the following outcomes for the future of nursing practice in Australia:

- nurses taking the initiative in conducting trials for major changes in health care delivery such as prospective payment based on diagnostic related groups (DRGs) or case-mix
- nurses providing data for the grass-roots implications of major organisational changes in patient care such as mapping critical pathways or managing care.

In education, this personal ethic of excellence which creates an independent thinker is essential for the development of the discipline. All nurses simply by their being on the register for nursing hold a broad responsibility for the development of both the profession and the discipline of nursing. However, those nurses involved in education whether they be employed in a university, a hospital or other health care agency, or be working independently, are particularly responsible for the development of the body of knowledge which is referred to as the 'discipline' of nursing. In order to fulfil the brief of teaching and research, the academic needs to examine and re-examine nursing practice through the twin filters of theory and reflection.

In fact, the tradition of academe is that its members constantly attend to the task of theorising and reflection upon practice both as a prelude to and as an outcome of research.

Developing a personal ethic of excellence by weaving rigour and respect through their portfolio of skills offers nurse academics the following outcomes for the future in education:

- the opportunity for research-based scholarly practice whether or not that is the norm in a particular context
- the opportunity to break new ground in research and theory by reflecting upon the notion of *vulnerability* within nursing practice, education and research
- the opportunity for creative leadership based on a personal sense of vulnerability coupled with independent thinking.

Research seems to be the most obvious arena to apply the threads of a personal ethic of scholarship; yet, in many ways it can be the most difficult arena. 'Research is the most public of activities' is a dictum which seems obvious but the intrinsically public nature of research, signalled by this dictum, has made research committees necessary in major public institutions in Australia and in many other countries. In addition, the vulnerability of both human and animal subjects is responsible for the existence and structure of ethics committees to review proposed research. Despite these measures, many ethical questions still remain unanswered although they are often addressed. For example, the question of 'Who owns the data?' Does the funding body own the data?

The Australian federal government, through the medium of the National Health and Medical Research Council (NH&MRC), has taken the stand that, in some cases, the researched own the data. In the NHMRC Guidelines for research involving Australian Aboriginal people, no data from Aboriginal communities can be published without the permission of the Aboriginal elders of that community. Although this is a culturally sensitive decision, it does pose an exception to the public nature of research as conducted in Australia.

However, developing a personal ethic of excellence by drawing on the attributes of respect and rigour can offer nurse researchers the following outcomes for the future in research especially research conducted on human subjects:

- selection of a research design which will match the question rather than conflating method and ideology
- selection of culturally-sensitive and gender-sensitive approaches to research
- adopting respect for the data and clarifying ownership of that data prior to the collection of data
- protection of integrity of the data during analysis
- ensuring that research conducted within the discipline of nursing adds directly to that discipline either in the development of theory or in a change in practice.

Nursing as a profession and a discipline: a continuum along the search for intellectual depth

'I was with you in agony.
Remember your promise of paradise.'

The past reminds us that remembering can be painful but McCloskey and Grace (1990) believe that an awareness of one's history is a prerequisite for professional identity. In addition, awareness of one's history is also a prerequisite for knowing its knowledge—especially in depth. The view of nursing as a profession is a more familiar one than the view of nursing as a discipline. Probably the most popular, if somewhat superficial, distinction between the two is that 'the profession' is concerned with 'doing'—that is with the application of knowledge—and 'the discipline' is concerned with 'thinking'—that is, with the generation of knowledge. To a point, this does describe the difference but, in fact, both the profession and the discipline are closer than most people may think. The birth of the discipline was not only dependent upon the presence of the profession but also upon the profession being both vibrant and visible.

From the early 1960s, the discussion which preoccupied professional nursing groups—be they focused on practice, education or administration—was one centred around the distinction between nursing as an 'occupation' and nursing as a 'profession'. Clearly, the aspirations of those who carried the title 'nurse' focused on inclusion in the latter category. This distinction was fuelled by the debate which emanated from the writings of the sociologist Talcott Parsons. Parsons (1967) wrote about the structure, internal control and self-regulation of 'the professions'. Parsons' writings can assist nurses in understanding why 'professionalism' and 'professionalisation' were goals with which nurses earnestly identified in previous decades.

Parsons posited that the development and increasing strategic importance of the professions probably constituted the most important change that had occurred in the occupational system of modern societies. The growth of the professions brought to prominence a set of occupations which never figured prominently in the ideological thinking that, after having crystallised in the late 19th century, had tended to dominate public discussion in the 20th century. Professional men and women are now seen as neither 'capitalists' nor 'workers', nor are they viewed as typically governmental administrators or 'bureaucrats'. But they certainly are not independent peasant proprietors or members of the small urban proprietary groups (1967).

Further, Parsons identified the following three 'core criteria' within the general category of occupational role:

- The requirement of formal technical training accompanied by some institutionalised mode of validating both the adequacy of the training and the competence of trained individuals

179

- The training must lead to some order of mastery of generalised cultural tradition and do so in a manner giving prominence to an *intellectual* component
- A fully-fledged profession must have some institutional means of making sure that such competence will be put to socially responsible use.

Parsons' writings then indicate that an intellectual component is not only necessary but also prominent to a profession. If nursing accepted these criteria of a profession, then the question would be 'What is the intellectual component of the profession of nursing?' rather than 'Does the profession of nursing *have* an intellectual component?' But for those readers who believe that Parsons' opinions were somewhat ad hoc or who simply do not grant credence to a sociological construction of categories of social status, a short review on the rise of nursing as a profession may assist in tracing the development of the intellectual component of the profession as well as identifying the connection between the profession and the discipline.

Professional nursing in Australia developed in the post-Nightingale era (Russell 1990). For the first seventy years of the life of the European colony, nursing was managed by those who had a flair for it or by those to whom it fell by default. In 1858 the first two 'trained nurses' to arrive in Australia were two Sisters of Charity, who later helped to establish St Vincent's Hospital in Sydney, followed by Lucy Osburn and five Nightingale nurses, at the request of Henry Parkes, in 1868. Lucy Osburn, as the Lady Superintendent of the Sydney Infirmary (1868-1884), was entirely responsible for the female staff of the hospital and for the internal management of the wards. She also established and supervised a training school for general nurses which played an important role in establishing and disseminating the Nightingale system of nursing throughout New South Wales and, later, the rest of Australia. Nursing's history as a profession in Australia dates from this time and was strengthened by the struggle for registration of 'trained nurses' which lasted from 1899 to 1924 (Russell 1990).

Interestingly, the notion of the nobility of nursing as a calling, and later as a profession, is an amalgam of at least three sources which contribute to the post-Nightingale picture of a professional nurse: that of the religious sister; that of the personal servant or personal attendant for the upper classes in England and the Continent in the 18th and 19th centuries; and that of the military nurse from Nightingale's highly political and widely publicised mission to serve the injured British soldiers in the Crimea. The teaching of Christ in the Sermon on the Mount provided the mandate and the motivation for religious orders of women and men to serve the ill (both poor and rich) and thus generated one dimension of the 'nobility' of nursing as a vocation and a basis for lay people to take up this calling in a professional sense. The wealthy of all cultures and classes have always been in the position to employ personal attendants both in health and illness—that is one of the marks of privilege. This intimate caring for another for material recompense instead of for charity provided a further basis for the employment of carers in a professional sense. Then Nightingale's taking the somewhat ill-assorted group of 38 nurses to the Crimea to care for the wounded British soldiers was both a precedent for and a precipitant to the foundation of the first modern school of nursing in the Western world at St Thomas' hospital in London.

Nightingale's influence was profound and its effects were felt in many other countries in the British Empire as well as in the United States of America. Russell (1990) reminds the reader that when the Nightingale system was introduced to Australia, it was considered to be the most advanced scheme in the world. This system was so successful in improving the quality of nursing services that any attempt to change the system was strongly resisted. As a result, the Nightingale method of training remained substantially unchanged in Australia for some 100 years. The seeds of change began post-Second World War with the establishment in 1949 of the New South Wales College of Nursing and the College of Nursing, Australia (now Royal College of Nursing, Australia). Both of these colleges conducted education programs for already registered nurses in areas such as education, administration and unit (ward) management. The education programs offered already registered nurses not only the opportunity to increase their professional knowledge in specific areas but also the opportunity to complete their general education—an opportunity which had been denied many nurses for a variety of reasons not least of these being that they were, predominantly, women.

This philosophy of 'bringing the profession forward together' served nursing well but also delayed any change to the basic education system for a further twenty years. The first non-hospital, non-waged basic nursing preparation course was commenced at the headquarters of the College of Nursing, Australia in 1974. Several similar courses commenced in other States in the following year. These courses provided the blueprint for the historic transfer of nursing education from hospitals to colleges and universities—mandated by the then Prime Minister the Rt Hon Robert Hawke in August 1984. This Federal Government decision was preceded by that of the New South Wales Government in November 1983, which saw the total transfer of basic education to the tertiary sector in that State in 1985. Nationally, the transfer was completed in December 1993. The high point of professionalism reached in Australian nursing leading up to the transfer provided a rich milieu for the emergence of the discipline. The depth of knowledge in nursing practice and in nursing curricula provided the beginning for the profession/discipline continuum.

However, during the 1950s and 1960s, the discipline had been developing in the United States, the United Kingdom and in some other countries in Europe and also Asia. Many factors contributed to the emergence of the discipline in the United States of America not least of which was the development of university undergraduate degree programs in the early 1920s. These degree programs may have remained an isolated phenomenon in contributing to the development of the discipline were it not for one article which proved seminal in raising the consciousness of nursing being a discipline as well as a profession: the authors were Donaldson and Crowley. In 1978,

Donaldson and Crowley named nursing as a 'professional discipline' and anticipated both theoretical and scholarly development within that discipline by presenting some major conceptualisations and some general structure: for example, 'nursing studies the wholeness or health of humans'. This article has had a wide impact on scholarship in nursing by being a catalyst in defining the discipline.

For Australia, a national consciousness regarding the discipline emerged over a very short period. In 1989, at the inaugural meeting of what later developed into the National Nursing Research Network (NNRN), under the sponsorship of Royal College of Nursing, Australia, the 'profession' was the overall umbrella term used to embrace nursing research, nursing in academe and nursing practice. Yet in 1991, Gray and Pratt published a landmark volume in the history of nursing in Australia—*Towards a Discipline of Nursing*. This publication embraced writing at a previously undemonstrated level of theoretical sophistication in Australian nursing. Bennett (1991a) acknowledges the timeliness of the publication and the courage of the editors in the following excerpt from the Foreword:

> This book represents a significant development in the history of nursing in Australia. By bringing together a number of Australian scholars to address the issues associated with the emerging discipline of nursing, many of the shackles holding back development in this country have been broken. The editors are to be congratulated on their foresight and courage in facilitating such timely change. Australian nursing is reaching new heights in its development as a substantive discipline.

Australian scholars had reaped the harvest sown earlier in the United States of America. In the early perception of nursing as a discipline in that country, scholarship was at first narrowly defined. For example, early in the 1980s, May et al, drawing on Donaldson and Crowley (1978), found it necessary to mount the following plea, in the name of 'scholarliness', to have as much weight given to nursing theory as to nursing research in doctoral programs:

> Nursing is in dire need of true scholars who not only empirically test nursing theories but who also continue to search for new propositions. There is need for scholars to produce quality work characterized by theoretical soundness, methodological neatness, and an ability to amplify and extend nursing's theoretical propositions. Knowledge of the meaning and the goals of science is essential in enhancing the potential to produce such work (May et al 1982).

Prior to the publication of *Towards a Discipline of Nursing* in Australia, a decade of debate by international scholars generated a much broader view of scholarship. Meleis, from the University of California, San Francisco, made a major contribution to the debate through exposition and discussion in her major synthesising work devoted to the development and progress of nursing theory (1991). Meleis states the following as characteristics of the stage of scholarliness in any discipline and of nursing in particular:

1 relationships between theory, research, practice and philosophy become more apparent
2 pluralism in paradigms is encouraged
3 boundaries of the domain become more identified
4 the domain guides nursing practice, research and theory.

Bennett (1991b) believes that the debate about these criteria of nursing as an emerging scholarly discipline is well developed in Australia, and Gray and Pratt (1991) state that the discipline has moved towards the criteria of scholarship outlined by Meleis in many ways—not least of which is moving beyond the debate issuing from the spurious dichotomy between 'qualitative versus quantitative' approaches in research methodology and theory generation. Gray and Pratt suggest that the focus on exploring and promoting the relative strengths of a variety of qualitative approaches now engages nursing scholars to a greater degree than previously. Hayes (1992) believes that the deep connection of Australian nursing writers with the complexity of the body using a range of methods indicates a quality of relevance which is fundamental to scholarly endeavours in nursing as a practice discipline.

It is both interesting and exciting to reflect on why the consciousness of nursing as a discipline and the exploration of scholarship within that discipline has emerged to its current level of sophistication in such a relatively short time. The following are some of the factors which have contributed:

- Establishing the first non-hospital based and non-salaried pre-registration nursing course in 1974 at (then) College of Nursing, Australia. This built on both the experience which the College had derived since its establishment in 1949 and also the experience of the 1600 hour hospital-based curriculum in Victoria. Other States had also increased the quality of hospital based pre-registration curricula and pilot programs of college based pre-registration programs followed quickly in several States.

- Implementation of the W K Kellogg Australian Nursing Fellowship scheme. This scheme which was funded by the third wealthiest benevolent foundation in the United States provided both short term (six months) and long-term (two years) for potential nursing leaders to study in the United States of America. Seventy-eight nurses benefitted from these fellowships which were granted over five years from 1978-1983.

- Commitment by the federal government in August 1984, to move all nursing education courses from the State health sectors into the federal higher education sector over a 9 year period beginning in 1985. This political will had been the result of unified action and relentless lobbying by the profession for a decade. Although undergraduate pre-registration courses are now well established within the higher education sector, there seems to be some dilution of political will to allow some advanced nursing courses to move from the health sector in some States and Territories.

- Establishment of the Unified National System of universities in Australia seeded by the Dawkins papers (1987, 1988a, 1988b). After 1984, most nursing education courses had moved into the post-secondary system of college of advanced education. But with the amalgamation of these colleges into universities and the establishment of schools, departments and faculties of nursing in already established universities, the consciousness of the discipline, the stimulation of research and the acquisition of scholarship all expanded exponentially.

Implications of the profession/discipline continuum for nursing practice, education and research

One of the major benefits of indepth knowledge in both the profession and the discipline of nursing is the generation of reflective practice. Benner (1984) explored some pathways of bringing intellectual depth to nursing practice and demonstrated the deepening complexity of clinical nursing practice through the use of clinical narratives, which she calls paradigm cases and which others call exemplars. These clinical narratives are all of the following: micro-units of professional nursing practice; densely packed research data; transcendent moments. Benner's work proved very influential because it demonstrated what nurses had known for some time and that is, that the expert nurse demonstrates rapid decision making based on understanding at the cellular level, the systems level and the multicellular level of the body. The expert nurse moves quickly through those complex realms to assist the person to weave together the thoughts and perceptions of the experience with the *actual* experience of the body whether it is birth, death, joy, pain, achievement or loss. The process of generating clinical narratives is by retrospective reflection on a critical incident in practice—critical because it was either a situation where nursing judgment or intervention made a palpable difference or one which peeled off a layer of practice to discover a deeper level of meaning. Just as linguistic philosophers sometimes refer to a phrase as a portmanteau phrase because it is one which can be unpacked, so one could refer to the critical incidents of reflective practice as portmanteau situations. They can be unpacked to access the rich and often taken-for-granted meanings with professional nursing practice.

Garratt's (1992) exposition of reflective practice as a learning strategy outlines complementary paradigms of 'reflecting on' and 'reflecting with' and posits that both are necessary to gain a full understanding of a situation. 'Reflecting on' arises from the intellectual skills of analytic thinking derived mainly from the logical-positivist tradition, and 'reflecting with' arises from the intellectual skills inherent in adopting a phenomenological stance. Following Garratt's argument, both are necessary to unpack the dense data of a clinical narrative. The following clinical narrative is offered to the reader as an example of the interface of the following: vulnerability, intimacy, indepth knowledge and a personal ethic of excellence.

Helen was a 14-year-old patient in a major metropolitan paediatric oncology unit when I knew her. She suffered from acute lymphocytic leukaemia and had undergone several courses of chemotherapy. Throughout the course of the illness, which required frequent monitoring by blood sampling and by sampling of cerebro-spinal fluid, she faced many crises precipitated by pain and by the side-effects of treatment. After she had conquered these, in answer to the query of 'How are you today, Helen?' she often replied 'I think that it is a green pyjama day'. Helen was slightly built for her age with fine, curling red hair and pale skin, and her green pyjamas not only suited her but had become both symbol and emblem of successful transitions.

As the nurse in charge of the unit I would spend my first 30 minutes of each day with those who were acutely ill performing my own baseline assessment of their physical and psychological response both to the illness and to treatment. Helen was admitted several times as her leukaemia was not responding to treatment—thus we formed a strong bond and those quiet early morning moments spent with Helen are still a privileged memory.

Finally the decision to cease treatment was made. The team of nurses, doctors and other specialists responsible for Helen's care were well trained, dedicated and fine-tuned and the decision to tell Helen frankly of her prognosis, to tell her that there was no further treatment which could be offered was weighed carefully. The telling was done with sensitivity and in detail. This divulging of the prognosis of an illness to the patient was not common practice in paediatric oncology care in Australia at that time and was a significant decision for the team, and we all wanted to know what a difference this would make. On the following morning I went into Helen's room being alert for any reaction or response and after a few gentle probes, on my part, Helen looked at me with gentle directness and said 'I think that it's a green pyjama day'. She made no further reference at all to the news of the previous day then, or later, and died quietly some weeks later.

All of the team wondered about the efficacy of the decision. What intellectual pathways can assist in unpacking such a narrative? The tools of reflective practice (both reflecting 'on' and reflecting 'with') are invaluable but so, too, is the imagination. The imagination is the *sine qua non* of literature and it is the author's belief that it is essential for both analytic and phenomenological exploration. Garratt (1992) states the following about reflecting 'on': 'Reflecting "on" something is the way in which students can critically examine their practice and come to terms with evaluating their own learning'. This aspect of reflection leads to what Ricoeur (1976) calls 'explanation'. The reason that explanation finds its origin in the reductionist paradigm becomes clear when the association of explanation to laws, theories, hypotheses, verifications and deductions is made. Ricoeur links explanation to causation and effect to outcome. Thus reflecting 'on' assisted understanding of Helen's disease process and the suffering of her illness but did not assist in understanding her reaction to the news of her prognosis and to the cessation of treatment.

Garratt states the following about reflecting 'with':

> In teacher education the student may reflect with the coach or supervisor to a certain extent, but in nursing reflection 'with' is different. This difference lies in the relationship of the nurse with the person seeking care. The student nurse in the practice setting is learning from, and sharing in, the experience of another person who is living through an event. To enter this lived world of experience belonging to another human is a privilege that nurses are given. To grasp shared meaning from this experience is essential learning for the true art of nursing (1992).

Thus reflecting 'with' can assist in moving to an understanding of Helen's reaction to the news of her prognosis and to the cessation of treatment in the following way.

A range of interpretations could be made about Helen's choice not to engage in the conversations which would have told the team what they wanted to hear; but it seems that when Helen was told that she had a limited time to live she seemed to be hearing something she already knew. A different language was used to name the experience but her own experience of embodiment had already informed her. For, the symbol of the green pyjama day signalled to all who wished to understand that she *knew* that she was undertaking another major transition—in fact, her last transition.

The search for intellectual depth for nursing practice, education and research: implications

The immediate implication of the search for intellectual depth in nursing is the recognition that both the profession of nursing and the discipline of nursing co-exist along a continuum—both requiring intellectual skills. Both are interdependent and both serve to improve the quality of care given to the individual person who is nursed and to contribute to the expectations of quality care which the community at large can anticipate.

The following implications for nursing practice frame the challenge for the future: to disembed nursing care from the context of health care delivery; to strive towards continuity of care by the individual practitioner; to prepare practitioners who are aware of the intellectual basis of their practice; and to employ both research and theory as the basis for that practice. The struggle to disembed nursing care from the context of health care delivery has been a long one. It seems that the most tangible way to do this is by generating the cost of care. Over the last three decades the cost of various components of care have been extricated from the overall cost of care within the health care delivery budget—one of the earliest being that of specialist medical care when the fee-free 'honorary' system of specialist medical care was replaced by the 'consultant' system which consequently attracted a consultant's fee. The development of patient acuity systems based on Australian (rather than overseas) data and the

186

institution of career structures for nursing have both assisted in identifying key outcome-oriented components of nursing care and have also shaped the cost profile of care. There has been a tentative identification of intellectual skills within both of these processes by a recognition that expert nursing care is the result of experience coupled with education. Those nursing leaders who recognise and reward intellectual skills in the nurses they employ will be laying the *building blocks* for the best practice models of care.

Continuity of care is one of the performance indicators which contributes to the community's perception of quality care in many arenas and not least in health care delivery. However, provision of continuity of care by the individual practitioner has often eluded nursing practitioners. For example, the necessity for nursing care to be delivered over a 24 hour period often militates against continuity by an individual practitioner. Many creative approaches to address this perceived deficit have emerged such as 'team nursing' and 'primary nursing'. However, often the very structures established to assist nursing hamper the continuity of care by an individual practitioner. For example, the hard-won industrial awards reducing and regulating the number of hours nurses give care during any one 'shift' can now be just another inflexible constraint upon the continuity of care, such as attending to a woman throughout her birthing or staying with a child until a procedure is completed. Those nursing leaders who ensure flexibility in the delivery of nursing care and, where possible, continuity by an individual practitioner will be building the *walls* of best practice models of care.

The much-talked-about 'theory-practice' gap in the practice professions such as nursing, medicine, psychology, teaching and social work is often a puzzling phenomenon for it seems to have little to do with where the beginning practitioners receive their education. That is, this phenomenon, which is shorthand for both a gap in the application of the theory to practice and the employment of research findings, is seen also in health professions such as medicine which has been university based for several decades. It seems that there needs to be not one but many bridges built between education and practice. Those nursing leaders who can build such bridges will be placing the *roof* on best practice models of care.

The implications of the search for intellectual depth in nursing seems to be similar for both education and research so they will be addressed together. Intellectual skills and intellectual depth of skills require a 'community of scholars' (Gortner 1985) in order to thrive. The post-colonial anti-intellectual bias which has pervaded Australian culture still ensures that Australians are somewhat diffident about naming and claiming both scholars and scholarship. However, there are definite signs that this diffidence is fading. For example, the overall title of this volume—*Scholarship in the Discipline of Nursing*—signals a change. If a community of scholars is needed, how is that community built? There are several ways in which this is achieved but one of the most effective ways to achieve this is to foster the preceptor/mentor continuum. Both are in some ways an intellectual 'coach'—a notion which is extrapolated from Benner's (1984) teaching-coaching function in the continuum of novice to expert nurse. A preceptor can be a temporary connection of a few days or a few weeks but a mentor is usually someone with whom the mentee is connected over time. Both preceptors and mentors can be developed by promoting team teaching and generating collaborative research projects. For a recent discussion of the preceptor/mentor continuum the reader is directed to Watson and Knight (1994) who proffer a useful detailed analysis of the continuum and its application to nursing. Both preceptor and mentor strategies are time and person-intensive but they do create communities where the discourse of nursing becomes the mother tongue. Those nursing leaders who can foster such communities will provide *citizens* who will dwell within and who will embody the best practice models of care.

Conclusion

The sub-title of this chapter is 'Healing the intellectual-practice split in nursing'. The two approaches to this goal posited by the author are that the ethics of practice and the ethical dimensions of scholarship are inextricably linked and that nursing as a profession and nursing as a discipline are a continuum along the search for intellectual depth in nursing. The implications for nursing practice, education and research which are the outcome of exploring these two approaches are presented in the hope of supporting the concept of nursing *as* both a practice profession and a practice discipline and of stimulating debate around the logical outcomes of acknowledging the intellectual bases of both.

REFERENCES

Beauchamp T L, Walters L (eds) 1982 Contemporary issues in bioethics, 2nd edn. Wadsworth, Belmont, California

Beckstrand J 1978a The notion of a practice theory and the relationship of scientific and ethical knowledge to practice. Research in Nursing and Health 1(3):131-136

Beckstrand J 1978b The need for a practice theory as indicated by the knowledge used in the conduct of practice. Research in Nursing and Health 1(4):175-179

Beckstrand J 1980 A critique of several conceptions of practice theory in nursing. Research in Nursing and Health 3:69-79

Benner P 1984 From novice to expert: excellence and power in clinical practice. Addison Wesley, Menlo Park

Bennett M 1991a Foreword. In: Gray G, Pratt R (eds) Towards a discipline of nursing. Churchill Livingstone, Melbourne

Bennett M 1991b Teenage mutant nurse researchers. In: Gray G, Mayner L (eds) Proceedings from first international conference of the Centre for Nursing Research, Inc. Nursing research: proactive vs reactive, Adelaide, Australia

Bradley B, Selby J 1992 James Cook University, Australia. Personal communication

Bradley B, Gallagher D, Innes M, Leonard J, Selby J 1991 James Cook University, Australia. Personal communication

Brandt A M 1978 Racism and research: the case of the Tuskagee syphilis study. Hastings Center Report 8(6):21-29

Coney S 1988 The unfortunate experiment. Penguin Books, Auckland,

Crosthwaite J 1994 Feminism and medical ethics. Monash Bioethics Review 13(3):13-19

Davis A J, Aroskar M A 1983 Ethical dilemmas and nursing practice, 2nd edn. Appleton-Century-Crofts, Norwalk, Connecticut

Dawkins J 1987 Australian Department of Employment Education and Training. The challenge for higher education in Australia. AGPS, Canberra

Dawkins J 1988a Australian Department of Employment Education and Training. Higher education: policy statement overview. AGPS, Canberra

Dawkins J 1988b Australian Department of Employment Education and Training. A new commitment to higher education in Australia. AGPS, Canberra

Department of Employment Education and Training (DEET) 1994 Quality assurance report. AGPS, Canberra

Dickoff J, James P, Wiedenbach E 1968 Theory in a practice discipline: Part II—Practice orientated research. Nursing Research 17(6):545-554

Donaldson S K, Crowley D 1978 The discipline of nursing. Nursing Outlook 26(2):113-120

Garratt S 1992 Reflective practice as a learning strategy. In: Gray G, Pratt R (eds) Issues in Australian nursing 3. Churchill Livingstone, Melbourne

Gortner S 1985 University of California, San Francisco. Personal communication

Gray G, Pratt R (eds) 1991 Towards a discipline of nursing. Churchill Livingstone, Melbourne

Harwood G 1972 Triste, Triste. In: Heseltine I (ed) The Penguin book of Australian verse

Hayes B A 1992 Voices in Australian nursing: a turning point for the twenty-first century. Royal College of Nursing, Australia, Melbourne

Holzemer W L, Chambers D 1986 Healthy nursing doctoral programs: relationship between perceptions of the academic environment and productivity of faculty and alumni (research). Research in Nursing and Health 9(4):299-307

Jacox A 1974 Theory construction in nursing: an overview. Nursing Research 23(1):4-13

Johnstone M J 1989 Bioethics: a nursing perspective. Harcourt Brace Jovanovich, Sydney

McCloskey J M, Grace H K (eds) 1990 Current issues in nursing, 3rd edn. C.V. Mosby, St. Louis

Madjar I 1994 The body in health, illness and pain. Royal College of Nursing, Australia and Sigma Theta Tau International, Research Conference, Sydney

May K M, Meleis A I, Winstead-Fry P 1982 Mentorship for scholarliness: opportunities and dilemmas. Nursing Outlook 30(11):22-28

Meleis A 1991 Theoretical nursing: development and progress, 2nd edn. Lippincott, Philadelphia

Morgan R 1994 Morgan poll on honest and ethical standards. Roy Morgan Research Centre, Canberra

Parsons T 1967 Sociological theory and modern society. The Free Press, New York

Ricoeur P 1976 Interpretation theory: discourse and the surplus of meaning. Texas Christian University Press, Texas

Rothman D J 1982 Were Tuskagee and Willowbrook studies in nature? Hastings Center Report 12(2):5-7

Russell R L 1990 From Nightingale to now: nurse education in Australia. Saunders, Sydney

Solomon R C 1990 Justice and the passion for vengeance. In: Solomon R C, Murphy M C (eds) What is justice? Classic and contemporary readings. Oxford University Press, New York

Steele P D 1993 University of Melbourne. Personal communication

Stover E, Nightingale E O (eds) 1985 The breaking of bodies and minds: torture, psychiatric abuse, and the health professionals. W H Freeman, New York

Watson K, Knight B A 1994 Mentors and preceptors in the nursing profession. Contemporary Nurse 3(3):121

11

The power of one: the changer and the changed

JUDY LUMBY

This chapter is about the nature and construction of the method which emerged from my doctoral study. The study itself addressed one woman's experience of a life threatening illness and the main players were Maree the woman, and myself the primary researcher. Through the emerging method, new understandings of nursing as a therapeutic relationship transformed our personal and professional practice. As well, sharing our story with colleagues both in Australia and internationally illuminated meanings for a wider nursing audience.

The critical feminist method also enabled our stories, and in particular Maree's story, to be retold in a way which exposed the layers of inconsistencies in our lives as women, mothers and nurses. This journey through methodological, ethical and personal challenges, not only from outside but also from within ourselves, forms the substance of this chapter.

Qualifying the method as 'emerging' is purposeful, since this is exactly what happened. While the philosophical approach and methodology of the study were carefully planned, it became clear that methods which enable the study of such a personal experience have few templates to critique or to follow. Having undertaken research which left me feeling uncomfortable because of the way in which it alienated those being studied (the sample population) I now understood van Manen's (1990) stance in which he states: 'The method one chooses ought to maintain a certain harmony with the deep interest that makes one an educator (or whatever role) in the first place'. As a nurse undertaking research into an area which was intimately linked to my practice, to maintain an authenticity between myself as a researcher and myself as a nurse, I needed to find a way which bridged the two. I needed to ensure that the woman who was the 'researched' remained included in the study and was not disempowered as a result of the processes used. Indeed I hoped to find a way which would be not only a method for research but also empowering for the woman.

Introduction

'What do you mean an "n of 1?"' 'Aren't you just describing a 3-year long chat between two women?' 'Your method has no rigour!' 'How can you prove the truth of your findings?' 'Where is your hypothesis?' 'How can you generalise your findings?' And so on and so on.

Perhaps this dialogue is familiar to some of you reading this. For me the question became: how does a single researcher withstand such questioning and accusation? And when the researcher comes from a clinical background in nursing there is a further credibility gap in the world of scientific research whatever her research and clinical background. To represent my journey as one of loneliness or aloneness, however, would be to deny the very heart of the method which emerged from the research. Integral to this method was my relationship with Maree whose story had to be told: the story of one woman who faced life and death simultaneously, a story which could provide a rich map for those in the future who might care for women like Maree, a map which traces the journey, the needs and the hopes of one who is dying and in turn provides a framework for the carers involved.

Recently, when presenting this study to a group of physicians, I once more confronted the challenges outlined above. Having gained distance from the intensity of the study itself I am able to be far more reflective about the context from which such questions arise and the underlying concerns which such methods and studies engender. As Becker (cited in Roberts 1981) reminds us 'the sociologist provokes the charge of bias whenever he says something that denies the legitimacy of the hierarchy of credibility'. Within the world of medical research, the hierarchy of credibility ensures that the one way of approaching research is preserved as the true way. This approach uses the experimental method, is deductive in nature, ensures objectivity by the researcher/s, quantifies outcomes and generalises results. I was challenging a tradition as well as 'the taken-for-granted dominance of one form of knowledge over another and one set of values over another' (Perry 1987). Such challenges need careful preparation and follow up through an understanding of the context and culture of the audience. Preferably one also requires others in the audience who are sensitive to and supportive of the approach being introduced.

So what was this journey all about? It warrants many descriptions. It was about a woman who took control of her destiny through the simple 'everyday', 'the taken for granted' tasks which women (say nurses) know so well. Despite her failing health, the week prior to her liver transplant, Maree struggled from her bed to prune her hydrangea. When I asked her about this she replied: '(I did it) because it is the time of the year and they need to be pruned. Nobody else will do them'.

Maree took one week to prune one bush but this was an important accomplishment which she took for granted. An act Benner (1984) describes as 'could not have done otherwise' when speaking about the work of nurses, since this group also acts as though they have no alternative or choice. This was one of the many social constructions which Maree and I critiqued together later in the study.

Maree also worked on the Christmas Day prior to her liver transplant, another sign of taking control over her mortality. She believed that Christmas Day should be special for individuals in hospital and she liked to ensure that it was appropriately celebrated. She said that she had 'always worked on Christmas Day and the only difference this time was that at home after dinner she slept through the washing up'.

It was also about a woman who shared her courage in the face of death by her willingness to allow me, indeed she invited me, into her life as an intimate traveller for what became three years. When reflecting on the research itself, Maree says: 'The research was something I had to see through...I think that the single issue of whether I would get through the transplant, the fact that I had committed myself to the research became a binding responsibility of mine to make sure that I got through'. She also saw it as 'a promise of survival because I felt that God would not put things in my path that I couldn't finish'.

And it was also about a woman (a daughter, wife and mother) who was changed forever through the experience but was seen as the same daughter, woman and mother as before her diagnosis and was expected to continue in her previously prescribed roles. Maree speaks of her experience as 'an incredible journey...a journey that I have been blessed to go on. It's been very hard and it's changed me and it's changed my life and it's changed my thinking and my goals'. But her family and friends did not recognise that the experience in and of itself had changed her forever. As Maree says: 'It (the transplant) has had a great effect on family dynamics. The children have noticed it...my parents are concerned about it...my husband is denying it'.

The beginning

Maree's experience forms the basis of my doctoral thesis (Lumby 1992). I first met Maree many years before her diagnosis in a remote town in New South Wales where she was nursing and we had professional contact several times following that meeting. One day Maree rang me to say that she had been given a tentative diagnosis of primary biliary cirrhosis which was a terminal illness. I knew little about this woman's personal life except that she was a mother. In my effort to help her through this critical stage in her life I explained how keeping a diary had helped me to make meaning of a critical stage in my life many years before. Since she preferred to talk about her concerns we devised a mutual process which would involve her recording her daily fears, concerns, hopes and experiences and I in turn would speak to her on the telephone and respond on tape. Soon after we began this process my supervisor suggested that this appeared to be a far more appropriate and meaningful study than the one I had begun to pursue for my doctorate. Thus began the story outlined in this chapter. The processes involved in the study include reflections, story telling, listening and sharing understandings and what I have named 'critical conversation'.

The very fact that this woman's illness was the work of a research study at doctoral level normally implies that her story was sought out to answer the questions raised within the usual doctoral preparation. After all, in the early stages of such a work one traditionally narrows questions or concerns down to a feasible and credible study. When a student enrols to complete doctoral work one of the first questions asked is 'what do you want to study?' or 'what are you interested in?' or even 'what is your hypothesis?' Contrary to the traditional way of choosing and clarifying a doctoral topic, the focus of my doctorate came to me in the form of Maree's phone call one night telling me of her diagnosis and the way in which she was now viewed as a 'terminal illness'. I now wonder how many other doctoral studies have arisen out of chance rather than organised and objective working through of questions and answers about the discipline one comes from in order to identify an appropriate topic. This is one of many questions which arose for me when considering the real story of undertaking a doctorate vis a vis the organised step by step accounts we all read in texts on this topic. The other issue which became the most crucial one was that of methodology. With a strong background in traditional research methods I was aware of their inadequacies for this study. How could I join this woman through what was to be an open-ended journey in terms of time and space, and how could we make sense of her experience together in a way which would not disempower her but which would be acceptable to the wider academic and nursing community and authentic for her. The first step was to consider the issues surrounding the selection and use of methodology and method.

Debate about method

Feyerabend's text *Against method* (1991) addresses the complex issue of using method/s in a way which contributes greatly to our understanding of the nature of knowledge within the world of the scientific method. Frost and Stablein (1992) claim that 'the research act as depicted in many research texts seems to us to be somewhat idealised, abstract and mechanical'. This assumes that there is only one way of approaching problems and if the recipe is followed then the problem will be solved. As a result, any deviation from such prescribed methods often brings with it accusations of non-rigorous work. Funding for such research continues to be problematic. However as Feyerabend (1991) points out, to say 'the procedure you used is non-scientific therefore we cannot trust your results and cannot give you money for research, assumes that "science" is successful because it uses uniform procedures'. He goes on to point out that the first assertion is untrue since all science is not successful, which leads to a questioning of the second assertion concerning the importance of uniform procedures. Many stories abound of scientific discovery which has been more the result of chance than following a step by step procedure. This is not to deny those scientific breakthroughs discovered through following a prescriptive method but to highlight the alternatives.

At the same time that I was struggling with my choice of methodology and method/s, the debate about nursing research vis a vis research carried out by nurses was a current one in Australia. This highlighted the evolving struggle within the profession for pedagogies which were distinctively nursing. Pedagogy in the sense it is used here alludes to the instruction and social vision spoken of by Gore (1993) in her book *The struggle for pedagogies*. Lusted (1986, cited in Gore 1993) speaks of the concept of pedagogy in this more global sense as '(drawing) attention to the process through which knowledge is produced. Pedagogy addresses the "how" questions involved not only in the transmission or reproduction of knowledge but also in its production. Indeed it enables us to question the validity of separating these activities so easily by asking under what conditions and through what means we "come to know"'.

Speaking of pedagogies here allows a more encompassing discussion than focusing only on paradigms or methodologies since they naturally form part of the pedagogical dialogue. After all, when speaking of the production of knowledge in our society we need to move our attention to many aspects. These aspects cause us to ask the following questions. Whose interests are served by this knowledge production? Who are the producers and how do they gain their authority? What projects do such productions support and whose interests are denied? These were all questions I found pivotal before moving forward in defining what was meant by nursing research and how I might contribute to nursing knowledge through this study. For Maree this was one of the most important issues since she hoped her experience would illuminate issues for nurses and nursing about others in her position in the future. Through the study she hoped that nurses could redefine their care to best meet the needs of people facing life threatening illnesses. This was not to assume that nurses were unaware of the needs of such people but in the past there had been little opportunity to base care on research carried out by nurses.

While there had been a move in Australia to embrace nursing theories and to attempt to impose these on practice, it had become increasingly clear that certain theoretical claims about nursing's central focus had not been accepted by the 'real' nurses in practice. Nurse theorists have been, and continue to be, mainly academics who may have used their clinical nursing experience as the foundation of their theory but whose final rhetoric mystifies the clinicians struggling to care for individuals in the real world of illness and crisis. Many teachers of nursing spend time demystifying such theories in order to explain the thinking behind the models but the process which this involves, in and of itself, causes much discontent and cynicism by the 'real' clinicians who question nursing knowledge being produced outside the clinical area. Part of the answer to such questioning lies in demonstrating the authenticity of the knowledge produced by using processes involving current clinical input, and by studying experiences through methods which reflect a nursing rather than a medical (say scientific) perspective.

The other side of this debate concerning knowledge development is the need to gain legitimacy in the academic arena through the use of methods which are scientifically credible and language which is scholarly. The tension lies in the fact that such methods and language can be alienating to others in the same discipline and silencing of other view points. This is not to deny the importance of rigorous theoretical development but to remind us of both sides of this debate and the way it acts on the very practice we are attempting to illuminate.

This pedagogical struggle is an interesting one which has gone on in other professions but has been delayed for nurses in Australia. The delay has occurred because of our late arrival into institutions of higher education and therefore the lack of higher degrees in nursing. The introduction of a Bachelor of Nursing as the initial degree for entry into the profession allowed the development of graduate diplomas, masters and doctoral programs in which registered nurses could pursue nursing inquiry. Since then, nurses in Australia appear to have revelled in exploring a range of research methodologies and methods. More recently several publications (Lawler 1991, Stein-Parbury 1993, Taylor 1994) emerging from Australia demonstrate a willingness and ability to move into the international debate of nursing epistemology and ontology. The ways in which nurses have undertaken research in the United States over the last thirty years have helped us to discern what might be the most appropriate paths for nursing in Australia. Strengthened by the access to graduate studies in nursing and with an awareness of a perceived widening gap between practice and theory, researchers appear to be moving back to practice to identify and expose the knowing within the knower (Lumby 1994). This 'knowing' may be nursing or it may be the experience of crisis, illness or health, and the 'knowers' are therefore the practitioners or those undergoing the crisis, the illness or even the experience of a healthy life. Such issues as those discussed above were important as I worked through the way in which I would begin this study which had such potential to contribute to nursing epistemology and ontology. One of the issues I needed to resolve was how to study the life of another in a way which enabled her real story to be told. Little appeared to be written about working with one other person within a research study and certainly not while they were dying.

Studying the subjective experience of another

Researching the subjective experiences of individuals or groups raises a multiplicity of questions, some of which do not have clear answers but form the centre of important debates within the research community. While the human experience has been a focus for social scientists well before Weber's assertion that 'sociology is a science which attempts the interpretive understanding of social action' (cited in Parsons 1947), the methods used to understand such experiences have been similar to those used by the natural sciences. Methods employed in the natural sciences insist on distancing the researcher from the researched through designs which claim to ensure objective, unbiased, quantitative measures of outcomes which can be trusted as reliable and valid. Such claims are grounded on a belief that there is one reality which can be discovered by an outside observer who is distanced from the experience itself.

Adopted by social scientists studying subjective experience these methods rationalised subjective experience rather than exploring the feelings, and they identified experience merely from an emotional level rather than looking at all aspects of the experience. So it is that there has been a 'stalled revolution' (Hochschild 1979) in the understanding of the human experience because of the lack of methodological development. While appropriate for explaining, predicting and controlling interactions between inanimate objects in a controlled laboratory, experimental style methods have constraints when it comes to understanding and exploring the gamut of individual human expression. Human experiences do not remain controlled or controllable since they embrace the dimensions of emotion and cognition as well as the physical, political, social, cultural and historical contexts of individuals in an unpredictable society. Such uncontrollable dimensions are very concerning for scientists who are used to being able to control every step of the research process, and one of the first lessons to be learned if one moves into researching subjective experiences is to accept the messy nature of such work. This is not to say that the research itself is not able to be rigorous in its approach and scholarly in nature but that there are different ways of discussing and handling aspects such as bias, validity and reliability. In debating these aspects, different language needs to be found to more accurately illustrate the different views of the world reflected in the alternative approaches to inquiry.

Perhaps the group which has best come to grips with the issue of researching the subjective experience has been that of feminist researchers. Their focus of investigation is so often on the everyday situations which may be taken for granted by other researchers but which provide access to the complex questions about life which perplex many of us (Gunew 1990, Stanley 1990, Bowles & Klein 1989). Such research brings the personal into the public arena for debate and scrutiny. This focus often necessitates negotiations of relationships since the everyday usually involves relationships either with individuals and/or groups. But feminist research not only identifies such negotiations as important, it also highlights the processes required to raise awareness of such things and to uncover inequalities involving issues such as gender, race and ability.

When speaking of feminist research it is important to remember that there are many types of feminism and each of these has its own ideology and strategy, dependent on the philosophical position from which it emerges. However in general there are similar values underpinning studies which claim a feminist approach. These values can be explicated as characteristics which include the following: a rejection of dichotomies in order to acknowledge the blurring of home and work, of personal and professional, of practice and theory; a focus on 'the whole' vis-a-vis the specific and the relationships between the various discrete units which make up a context; a valuing of the subjective nature of life, the 'lived experience' as we know it and in particular the lives of women which have often been invisible; and an emphasis on a developing awareness and change particularly for women (Campbell & Bunting 1991). More recent feminist writers such as the philosopher Moira Gatens (1994) suggest that the way forward is to move to a transformation of both feminism and philosophy:

> This developing perspective, informed by both feminist theory and philosophy offers the means of beginning to conceptualise and live—in an intertwined way—other forms of political and ethical being. In particular a

feminist philosophy can offer an integrated , though not closed, conception of being that acknowledges the connections between being and knowing, between politics and ethics and between bodies and minds.

In contrast to the emphasis only on scientific knowledge within traditional research many forms of knowledge may be taken into account and utilised in feminist research. These various forms of knowledge include practical know-how, political knowledge and skills, and theoretical, social and critical knowledge, all of which contribute to a more total picture of the thing under scrutiny. More importantly for the researcher is the way in which such a total view uncovers the complex layers of relationships and leads to a critical awareness not possible by merely exploring one layer. The very questioning of taken for granted situations, power plays, traditions and myths begins a process of revelations not possible through traditional methods. The questioning of one side of a relationship leads to the illumination of the other side which means that when feminist researchers examine women's lives, men's lives are also revealed; in telling stories of the poor, the wealthy are also exposed; and in identifying the abused, the abusers are also uncovered. In this way the subjective experiences of individuals and groups are uncovered for public scrutiny.

Framework of the study

The other important issue to explore was the fact that the study required a nursing framework in order to theorise about the journey nurses take with people in Maree's position and to understand our growth through the study as nurses and women. Given that my years of nursing practice had left me with a strong belief that wise and sensitive nursing exists as a therapeutic force within the lives of individuals and communities, now was my chance to grapple with some of the mysteries of what I had been doing as a nurse. My years as a teacher of nursing had allowed me the advantage of space to reflect on my past practice and to watch other nurses with 'new' eyes as it were. This re-visioning which space gives can be illuminating but it does not just happen passively. John Dewey (1958) speaks of the importance of regulated reflected inquiry through the stages of 'incidental' and 'sustained' reflection. He contrasts the 'gross, macroscopic crude subject matters in primary experience' with 'the refined, derived objects of reflection since the latter are only experienced because of the intervention of systematic thinking'. He claims that both are worthwhile but that the latter is essential if one is to move to a higher level of awareness.

Over the years I was lucky enough to be involved with many advanced practitioners in specialised areas and their stories of practice had continued to fascinate as well as frustrate me. Most importantly they forced me to reflect regularly and in a sustained way on the practice we so blithely call 'nursing' but are so reluctant to describe with any clarity. Like many teachers who had been influenced by educational theorists such as Dewey (1963), Knowles (1985) and Boud (1985), I had experimented with reflective diaries and the use of critical friends in order to assist students to develop an awareness of their personal knowledge development, as well as a critical awareness of the practice they were studying.

My own tendency to reflect within my personal and professional work was perhaps part of my socialisation as a nurse and woman in which a strong sense of accountability loomed large. Certainly this tendency to be not only reflective but also reflexive in my dealings with the world led me also to assume such stances in relation to the way in which I wanted to 'do' research. The traditional research I had been involved in during my graduate studies had, however, left me feeling that such stances were impossible because they lacked rigour and therefore were not scholarly. The dissonance which existed in my life between my disciplinary and professional upbringing and my knowing and experience as a woman, nurse and mother was compounded further in my studies and readings within the feminist literature.

While my initial search seemed to point to a feminist methodology it was not until I came across later texts on alternative ways of researching that I felt authenticated in this sense (Reason & Rowan 1981) since feminist work was still viewed with scepticism. The real liberation for me would come much further into the study. First of all I needed to understand how it all worked together—that is ,the questions one has, the approaches, the methods and the journey itself for the researcher and the researched. The latter was not talked about in the acknowledged and set research texts so it was difficult to find the way without asking what appeared to be naive and even stupid questions. And as I was warned by Bordieu (1988), if one asked the questions within one's own discipline, 'it is well known that no groups love an informer especially when the transgressor or traitor can claim to share in their highest values'. More recently such questions are being not only asked but openly debated, but when I began this study in Australia they were still relatively new issues.

Later on I was to find out that the very nature of a feminist framework reflected method development as an essential and even central component of any research. This was the way in which a 'new space' (Grosz 1986) emerged in which women's knowledge and experience of the world could gain voice. This development of a 'new space' is an essential part of studies which claim to be feminist.

So my search for a framework in which to place our study began. After much reading, discussion and searching, Shulamit Reinharz's (1989) 'experiential analysis' seemed to best allow me to work in a way which was congruent with most of the values we had decided were necessary for the study. These values included valuing experience as knowledge, incoporating the reality of nurse's practice, incorporating the reality of women's experiences and knowledge, acknowledging the power relationships and the roles of the individuals in the study, empowering people involved in the study and incorporating collaborative and consultative processes in influencing nursing praxis.

Experiential analysis emphasises the concept of an iterative process rather than a linear model of research. Underpinning this process are three foci based on growth and understanding in the arena of the problem under investigation, the persons doing the investigation and the method utilised. Reinharz (1979) emphasises the critical social aspect of this method by asserting that methods should not be seen merely as techniques for exploration but used as processes for socio-historical concerns. Her concept of experiential analysis has arisen from similar frustrations to those I had encountered. She described the framework as 'my methodological resolution of the inadequacies of survey empiricism and participant observation' (Reinharz 1979). While her framework was feminist it also introduced a critical perspective which was so essential if we were to develop a critical awareness of the illness experience and of our stories as women and nurses. This critical aspect had been missing from nurses' discourse about practice although it was implicit in much of the daily dialogue. This critical aspect enabled a movement towards a wider nursing praxis described by Wheeler and Chinn (1989) as 'thoughtful reflection and action that occurs in synchrony in the direction of transforming the world'.

Feminist research

While texts on feminist research are now increasing as research within this framework is being accepted as valid, in 1989 when I was undertaking my research, while texts on feminist methodology were available, feminist methods were not discussed at any length. Indeed this lack of recipes reflects the nature of feminist research which is built on certain values and processes and insists on the congruence between the question, the context, the people involved and the outcomes desired. The values include attention to the relationships, to collaborative work, to the personal, to action and to reflective and reflexive processes. The reflexivity spoken of in feminist work is the attention to thinking critically and analytically about the research process itself (Fonow & Cook 1991). This in itself is not entirely new, since Kaplan in 1964 spoke of the informal reflection which arises during the process of inquiry as 'logic in use'. The difference for feminist inquiry is in the centrality of the notion and the way in which it is used as an essential part of the research, or as Fonow and Cook (1991) explain it, 'the acknowledgement of metaphysical commitments as part of the content of scientific understandings opens the production of knowledge to a more fruitful scrutiny'. This part of feminist methodology perhaps poses the most difficulty for traditional researchers whose stance is in direct opposition. Acknowledging oneself (the researcher) as a feeling subject who not only thinks about the research but feels intimately involved in it is an anathema. To actively seek that position through the use of a reflective diary or a critical friend feels too foreign and certainly not scientific. But the main concern expressed is that this 'subjectivity' removes the objectivity and therefore the credibility and rigour of the study. When pressed to go further with this explanation most critics are unable to explain what their objections actually mean and many texts have been written which debate the possibility of objectivity claimed by scientists (Kuhn 1970, Polanyi 1958).

So while Shulamit Reinharz certainly gave me direction she made it quite clear that methods still needed to be developed. The spiral nature of experiential analysis ensured an interactivity which would demand continual reflection, analysis and synthesis individually and collaboratively. In this way we would make meaning of Maree's experience of illness and our experience through the journey of research. So it was that we began the study with some clear parameters about our relationship, our commitments and our values as nurses and women and with some guidelines concerning method. The final method would depend on our relationship.

The method

While the method began with personal preparation as suggested by Reinharz, the phases of the method as outlined below were slowly and carefully developed as we moved through our study together, feeling our way. It required trial and error as I struggled with ensuring that the study was rigorous in its multilayering of meaning yet true to the values espoused within the framework. The multilayering was ensured through the processes of continual reflection, joint conversations, story telling, sharing of reflections and finally critical conversations. Praxis was encouraged through sharing our meanings with a wider audience of nurses and is ongoing for Maree and me. Each step of the method was discussed before we trialled it. As the method became more complex so did our relationship because of all we had experienced together. Perhaps the most difficult phase was when we began the process which I named 'critical conversation' but it was through this process that we transformed our meanings to a level of critical awareness about Maree's illness experience and about our personal and professional lives.

The phases of the method were not named until we had completed the study and were reflecting on our journey together. In this way the method was unique to us although claims of uniqueness are difficult in a world where knowledge is being created at such a rapid rate.

Phase one: searching for meaning

Personal preparation

This step was one that Reinharz introduced in her methodology and we began with this although the remaining steps are unique to this study. Reinharz talks of the need for the researcher to suspend preconceptions of the phenomena under study. Thus a literature search on the experience of illness or women's relationships was not appropriate at this stage of the study. Nevertheless philosophical, nursing and feminist texts were explored in order to ground the study. I also reflected deeply on my own stance on the areas under study in order to more closely understand my personal ontology. Maree and I also spent time talking about the study and what it would mean in terms of personal commitment. We also thought that we had explored the ethical concerns surrounding such a study, but early on into the study it became obvious to me that we had no idea of the commitment or the ethical concerns which might be raised. When the study began, Maree had just been diagnosed with primary biliary cirrhosis which is of unknown aetiology. She was told that there was no cure. We needed to find ways in which to make the experience live in a way which would allow us to make meaning of it.

Incidental reflections

This step involved taping two sets of reflections. Taping reflections have been shown to be a valuable way of making meaning of experiences (Tyson 1980, Boud 1985). Dewey (1958) talks of the difference between primary experience and regulated reflective inquiry which ensures systematic thinking. Thus it was that we layered our reflections to ensure regulated and sustained inquiry. Our primary reflections were collected on tape.

Maree's reflections

Maree recorded her feelings and activities at least weekly. This involved her personal and public experiences since at this stage she was closely involved as a patient undergoing tests and investigations. At first Maree found difficulty in committing her feelings to tape since she was amazed that 'they were important and interesting to another person'.

My reflections

At the same time that Maree was recording I was also taping my reflections on her experience and my response. We spoke on the telephone almost nightly and I taped my responses to her comments. She would often cry in desperation and my reflections at this stage very much centred on her role as a mother. We both had three daughters and I pondered on my own ability to tell my daughters that I was dying. She appeared to be so brave although there were times when she was very depressed.

Joint conversations

We also met regularly in various settings and taped what were joint conversations. I always tried to find settings which were pleasant and conducive to sharing. Thus I spent considerable time organising various venues. We often had a meal or a cup of coffee, sat in a park or went to each other's homes. We taped these conversations and thus introduced another layer of meaning. As we spent time together our relationship moved onto a different level of trust and understanding.

Shared reflections

At this stage it became important to Maree that she listen to my reflections. Originally I had planned that we would listen to all our reflections at a set time together. I realised, however, that because of the focus of our conversations I was much more aware of her reflections than she was of mine. Maree needed to be reassured that she was not being used and was asking me for reassurance of my commitment. Thus we shared out reflections. When we reviewed our relationship at the end of the study, Maree commented on the importance of this change to our relationship. After listening to my tapes she was reassured of my authenticity. This is also well documented as an important part of the nurse-patient relationship and enables the relationship to move on to another plateau of trust and reciprocity.

While this was occurring we continued our incidental reflections and joint conversations, and this added dimension of shared reflections further ensured the multilayering of the study. All these steps were occurring prior to the transplant.

Informing meanings

Since Maree did not exist in the world as an isolated being I then felt that it was important to interview those who may inform the meanings we were to make out of the study. This question of who else should be involved was not considered until after the transplant because up until this time the study centred on Maree's experience of facing death and life at the same time. Once she had successfully survived the operation and had returned home in record breaking time, the study had a new dimension. On Maree's recommendation I then went on to interview those people whom she considered to have a significant impact on her life. These included her parents and her three daughters. Consideration was given to interviewing the transplant team but we needed to be selective if we wanted to keep the depth of the study. Her daughters were a particularly important component of the feminist perspective since, as we shared stories, we realised how important our roles as mothers were to the way we existed in the world.

Interviews with daughters

These interviews were discussed with Maree at length and she decided that she would not be involved but that she would listen to the tapes after the interviews. Having daughters around similar ages I had some insight into how these daughters might be feeling about me and the whole study with their mother. I decided to take each one out to dinner and to interview them separately. The choice of context was an important part of this method in order to encourage open discussion through a relaxed setting. By this time my contact with the three daughters was considerable in both their home and the hospital when Maree was undergoing surgery.

Interview with Maree's parents

Maree's parents insisted on being interviewed together and invited me to dinner. The interview disclosed their admiration and love for their daughter in a way which Maree had not realised. Otherwise their non-disclosure on certain areas revealed more than disclosure would have.

Sharing family interviews

Despite the fact that I told each daughter that their mother would hear the tape, each one chose to disclose things to me which they had not told their mother. This placed me in a dilemma since I felt responsible for these disclosures. I soon realised that I was being used as a conduit to their mother. I was also aware of how I would feel because I was in a similar situation in terms of daughters and the complexities of mother/daughter relationships. Thus when Maree called over to collect the tapes we negotiated the next steps of the method to ensure that we listened to the tapes together over several weekends. This included discussions on what support Maree required to deal with such information. We spent a lot of time on this area and began to develop a new respect for each other as mothers and women.

Sharing our stories

As in any developing relationship we began to disclose things from our past to each other and thus this step evolved naturally. Knowing the power of one's story I asked Maree to tell her biography to me on tape and during this I shared my biography with her. This step was particularly powerful for Maree as she discovered secrets about herself that she had never uncovered. This meant that she was able to explore certain areas of her life in a new way with another person who was available and willing to be there for her as she did so.

Phase two: making meaning through critical conversations

We continued to tape until the first anniversary of Maree's transplant which we knew would be particularly significant in terms of survival and memories. Thus it was that at the end of the first year we had 16 months of individual reflections, joint conversations and interviews. Somehow we needed to find a way to make meaning out of all these rich stories. I rejected transcription or computerised analysis since this would impose a barrier between our relationship. I was also aware that the stage had come when we needed to introduce a critical component into our discussions. Thus it was that through trying out several processes we came up with something I have called Critical Conversations. This part of the study took us almost eight months of weekend meetings. Since we decided to listen to every tape in chronological order I realised that the first tapes would be those we had made when Maree was so ill and facing death. Consequently I rented a house in the mountains and we spent a week there to begin this phase.

The process of critical conversation

This evolved naturally as we explored many ways to handle the mountain of material. We played the tape on one recorder and when we wanted to comment on an aspect, we would turn off the tape and record our conversation on a new tape. This process occurred naturally between us as women having a conversation about something in our lives. It also enabled the critical component to be introduced as we challenged each other on various issues and comments. Critical here is used in the sense of artistic criticism in which those involved engage in a socio-political interaction when judging a work of art. This requires an understanding of or empathy with the artist's reality as is required of the nurse when responding to the needs of those for whom they care.

Criticism is reflective in nature and insists that one moves to a deep understanding in order to develop a critical awareness of the political, ethical, practical, social and historical aspects of an act or statement. Our various roles as nurses, mothers and daughters demanded both intuitive and aesthetic knowing as well as the other more recognised forms of knowing. This step offered the opportunity to move to another level of consciousness about our various roles in the world. It did require a trusting and supporting relationship and a commitment to the process.

We managed to edit our conversations to twelve double sided tapes which we named our 'critical tapes'. They symbolised our journey together over the last two years although in no way could they capture our future possibilities.

Phase three: transforming meaning

These tapes were the result of a multilayered spiral of meaning and they held the distilled whole of the experience. It was now the time to explicate the stories from the tapes in a way which captured the truth and acknowledged the narrator of the story. As the principle researcher I had the responsibility of telling Maree's story in a way which did not damage the whole and which ensured that it did not become my interpretation of Maree's story. To ensure this I built in several steps to the method to enable Maree to comment on and interpret the story through her own narrative.

My narrative

After immersing myself in the tapes for many weeks I made comments as I went over and over the script. My intense personal involvement in the taping mean that I not only knew the stories, I was also sensitive to every aside, every pause and every emotion on the tapes. They had become part of my life and assisted me as I struggled with the various elements of Maree's experience and our developing relationship. I also included an analysis of my own growth in this narrative which I then forwarded to Maree in hard copy.

Maree's narrative

Maree spent time reading my narrative and exploring it for congruence and authenticity. She needed to identify where my understanding of our shared experience was incongruent with her understanding. It was after all Maree's story and her experience which was to be told and she needed to own the meanings and authenticate her story. Since the development of our relationship became an increasingly important component of the study through which the method was able to emerge, Maree also reflected on this aspect and what it had meant for her. She also commented on how it informed nursing practice.

Our narrative

This step was one in which we came to shared meanings of all that had happened between us over the last two and a half years. The method had allowed the richness of our story to be told and through the use of criticism we had reached consensus as to the various interpretations. The values, judgements and ethics which arise from this active type of analysis enabled us to see the choices which posed alternatives for us in the future.

After we had shared our individual meanings, I collated understandings together to produce our narrative for public examination. This was important if the story was to have meaning outside our own relationship. Congruent with feminist values it was essential that the stories were told with clarity in order to be accessible to those involved either directly or indirectly. After all, many outside our experience may find the stories relevant professionally or privately although they would never travel our route in the same way. Only Maree and I would ever do that.

Phase four: sharing our meanings

Praxis

The final stage of this method was the sharing of meanings in a way which could be understood and useful to nurses in their practice and to others in their lives. This made it necessary to give the story explicit form through writing and sharing formally and informally. This sharing involved the transplant team and nurses both in Australia and overseas, in keeping with the intent of the critical theoretical perspective. I presented a paper at an international conference in Ohio and with graduate students studying at the University of Colorado. Where possible Maree has also been involved in the presentation. This presentation is part of the praxis component since it means that through the telling of our story we are acting on our world for change.

When I returned home from overseas I found a new Maree. Here was a woman who had emerged from her illness experience as a changed person. She had found a new job and had made long term decisions about her personal life which she had never been able to make previously. At last she had a clearer knowledge of herself as a unique person and was able to exercise some control over the rest of her life however long that might be. To celebrate that I added an epilogue to the thesis which spoke of the new Maree.

Although this phase completed the formal study, the journey continues for both of us and the sharing which joined our lives for two years will always inform the meanings we will make of our future lives. In particular, our practice as nurses will have changed in direct response to the critical consciousness developed out of our shared experience.

During the study it became clearer to me that the method was similar to the relationship which develops between a nurse and the one she/he is caring for. Maree herself named it therapeutic during our final analysis. The reciprocity, the developing trust, the collaborative aspects, the highs and the lows all mirrored aspects of the relationships I had developed with patients in the intensive care units in which I had worked. This study illuminated these relationships in a way which explained the blurred aspects of my nursing. These aspects included those where I worked in ways which I knew were therapeutic for patients but which were not necessarily within the approved traditional role of the nurse. One example is that of 'not getting close to the patient or family', (this was often explained as being professional).

The method used in the study, while time-consuming and labour-intensive, was necessary to achieve the original objective of the research: to explore a woman's experience of facing a life-threatening illness and, in doing so, to develop a critical feminist method specific to the discipline of nursing. Criticisms which inevitably arise as a result of this type of research include those challenging the practical use of such a time-consuming method and the fact that such a method requires highly specialised interpersonal skills. I believe that the method can be used within a much smaller study if the values espoused include a commitment to collaborative work where the relationship is central, the researcher and the researched work as a team, sharing is reciprocal and trust is developed and maintained through open dialogue. The everyday work of nursing and the contexts within which nurses work make them naturally suited to utilise this method and feel comfortable with it. It is by recognising their own unique knowledge developed through practice that nurses can answer van Manen's call to be in harmony with one's role when approaching research.

Through the process of this method we were able to define a pedagogy which was distinctively nursing. It drew 'attention to the process through which knowledge is produced' (Gore 1993) and answered some of the questions concerning the conditions and means by which we come to know 'nursing'. As a feminist study, it also evoked the process of transformation between bodies and minds, between being and knowing, of which Gatens (1994) speaks. It provided the 'new space' (Grosz 1986) in which women's knowledge and experience of the world can find voice. Above all, it validated the importance, indeed the absolute necessity, of approaching a prolonged study with a commitment to and a passion for the subject matter, as well as a willingness to reject traditional methods which may not be suitable for this kind of research.

In Australia nurses now have the disciplinary authority, the scholarly development and the academic mentors to further develop the unique pathways they have forged within the traditional journey of research. The questioning of methodology and methods is now becoming an integral aspect of debates within the discipline. There is an increasing willingness to celebrate rather than discourage new methodolgogies which are central to studies such as the one discussed in this chapter. New approaches to research, rather than being marginalised, are now being used to initiate debate concerning difference.

ACKNOWLEDGEMENT

This chapter is only possible because Maree (the pseudonym chosen by the woman) invited me into her life and allowed me to share her journey. I also acknowledge the assistance of my supervisor Professor Alan Pearson who encouraged me in what was at times a very difficult and confronting struggle.

REFERENCES

Benner P 1984 From novice to expert. Excellence and power in clinical nursing practice. Addison-Wesley, California

Bordieu P 1988 Homo academicus. Polity Press, Cambridge

Boud D 1985 Promoting reflection in learning. In: Boud D, Keogh R, Walker D (eds) Reflection. Turning experience into learning. Kogan Page, London

Bowles G, Klein R D (eds) 1989 Theories of women's studies. Routledge, London

Campbell J C, Bunting S 1991 Voices and paradigms: perspectives on critical and feminist theory in nursing. Advances in Nursing Science 13(3):1-5

Dewey J 1958 Experience and nature. Dover Publications, New York

Dewey J 1963 Experience and education. Collier Books, New York

Feyerabend P 1991 Against method, revised edn. Verso, London

Fonow M M, Cook J A (eds) 1991 Beyond methodology. Feminist scholarship as lived research. Indiana University Press, Bloomington

Frost P, Stablein R (eds) 1992 Doing exemplary research. Sage Publications, California

Gatens M 1994 The dangers of a woman centred philosophy. In: Polity Press (ed) The polity reader in gender studies. Blackwell, Oxford

Gore J M 1993 The struggle for pedagogies. Critical and feminist discourses of regimes of truth. Routledge, New York

Grosz E 1986 Conclusion: what is feminist theory? In: Pateman E, Grosz E (eds) Feminist challenges: social and political theory. Allen & Unwin, Sydney, pp 190-204

Gunew S (ed) 1990 Feminist knowledge. Critique and construct. Routledge, London

Hochschild A 1979 The second shift. Viking, New York

Kaplan A 1964 The conduct of inquiry: methodology for behavioural science. Chandler Publishing, San Francisco

Knowles M S 1985 Androgyny in action. Jossey Bass, San Fransisco

Kuhn T 1970 The structure of scientific revolutions, 2nd edn. University of Chicago Press, Chicago, vol. 2:2

Lawler J 1991 Behind the screens. Nursing, somology and the problems of the body. Churchill Livingstone, Melbourne

Lumby J 1992 Making meaning from a woman's experience of illness: the emergence of a feminist method for nursing. Doctoral thesis submitted for the award of Doctor of Philosophy in the Faculty of Nursing, Deakin University, Geelong, Victoria

Lumby J 1994 'Re-searching the knowing through the knower.' Keynote address at the International Nursing Research Congress, A Brave New World. The Adventure of Nursing Practice through Research sponsored by Sigma Theta Tau International and the Royal College of Nursing Australia, The University of Sydney, Australia, July 11-14

Parsons T (ed) 1947 The theory of social and economic organisation. Free Press, New York

Perry J 1987 Creating your own image. NZ Nursing Journal. February: 10-13

Polanyi M 1958 Personal knowledge: towards a post critical philosophy. Routledge & Kegan Paul, London

Reason P, Rowan J (eds) 1981 Human inquiry. A sourcebook of new paradigm research. John Wiley, Chichester

Reinharz S 1979 On becoming a social scientist: from survey research and participant observation to experiential analysis. Josey-Bass, San Fransisco

Reinharz S 1989 Experiential analysis: a contribution to feminist research. In: Bowles G, Klein R D (eds) Theories of women's studies. Routledge, London, pp 163-191

Roberts H (ed) 1981 Doing feminist research. Routledge & Kegan Paul, London

Stanley L 1990 Feminist praxis: research, theory and epistemology in feminist sociology. Routledge, London

Stein-Parbury J 1993 Patient and person. Churchill Livingstone, Melbourne

Taylor B 1994 Being human: ordinariness in nursing. Churchill Livingstone, Melbourne

Tyson R W 1980 Working notes on journals, their forms and functions for the reflective practioner. Paper from the Institute for the Arts and Humanities, West House, Chapel Hill, N.C.

van Manen R 1990 Researching lived experience. Human science for an action sensitive pedagogy. The Althouse Press, The University of Alberta

Wheeler C, Chinn P 1989 Peace and power: a handbook of feminist process, 2nd edn. National League for Nursing, New York

12

Theoretical, clinical and research scholarship: connections and distinctions

KATHRYN L. ROBERTS

Scholarship is the creative intellectual activity that advances knowledge in the discipline. It involves the generation, evaluation, synthesis and integration of knowledge based on theory, research, and practice. Scholarship in nursing takes place in the academic institution or the clinical setting and is mainly carried out by academics, clinicians, and researchers.

A person who practises scholarship is a scholar: a person who is deeply engaged in the development of knowledge in a particular discipline and who 'has a high intellectual ability, is an independent thinker and actor, has ideas that stand apart from others, is persistent in her quest for developing knowledge, is systematic, has unconditional integrity, has intellectual honesty, has some convictions and stands alone to support those convictions' (Meleis 1991). Nurse scholars may be theoreticians, researchers, clinicians or combinations of those three. Some attributes of scholarliness are creativity, critical thinking, collaboration and ability to conceptualise (Armiger 1974, Meleis 1991). Meleis (1992) also states that a scholar 'has a sense of history, a vision of the whole, a commitment to a discipline and an understanding of how scientific work is related to the discipline's mission and to humanity as a whole'. Meleis sees the scholar as having a lifelong commitment to the development of knowledge in the discipline, having a passion for excellence, being flexible with a well developed theoretical orientation, and seeking and taking part in philosophical debates within the discipline (Meleis 1992). We need to develop more scholars striving to meet these ideals in order to advance the discipline of nursing in Australia.

The conduct of research, the publication and presentation of scholarly work and the acquisition of research grants are the main activities of successful scholars (Hodges & Poteet 1992). The products and activities of scholars as shown in a study of 41 schools of nursing in the United States of America also include oral presentations, awards, consulting, teaching, and journal editing (Dienemann & Shaffer 1992). These activities, particularly publications, are now expected of nurse academics in the Australian universities.

Beginnings of nursing scholarship in Australia

Nursing as a discipline has only recently developed scholars and embraced scholarship. Nursing education was initially carried on in hospital schools of nursing where nurse educators and students were isolated from contact with academe. Nursing knowledge was based mainly on trial and error, tradition and opinion, and nurses were trained rather than educated. They were expected to be the doctors' handmaidens and not to question procedures or think for themselves. Nursing knowledge was passed down through oral methods and by set textbooks which were learned by rote. Of course, there were scholars in nursing at this stage in the development of the discipline of nursing, but they were few and they were mainly found in schools of nursing, at the colleges of nursing, or in early pilot nursing education programs in colleges of advanced education.

From the early 1970s, nurse educators and administrators began to acquire diplomas in nursing education and administration from the colleges of advanced education (CAEs) in order to acquire skills, knowledge and qualifications that would enhance their job performance. They were thus exposed to the scholarship that existed among the college academics. Some acquired more advanced qualifications such as bachelor's and master's degrees and a few embarked on doctoral studies. They were increasingly exposed to higher levels of scholarship and to the methods of scientific research. They adopted the values of the tertiary system and became the early scholars of the nursing discipline. But, as a result of this historical development, the early Australian nurse scholars necessarily developed their scholarship in other disciplines such as education, administration, behavioural science and law.

The transfer of nurse education into the tertiary education sector and the resultant birth of nursing as an academic discipline led to the emergence of nurse scholars. In the early 1970s, the nursing leaders began an organised political effort which culminated in the transfer of nursing education into the tertiary education sector in the mid-1980s. Higher education at that time operated under a binary system which comprised both CAEs and universities. The CAEs had an emphasis on vocational education and were considered to be less scholarly and research-oriented than the universities. They were developing a focus on research as a means of emulating universities, but teaching remained their main mission. When nursing education transferred into the tertiary education system, the new nurse academics were suddenly expected to operate at the level of scholarship in the CAEs, and many were unprepared and underqualified for it owing to the suddenness with which the transfer took place. Most were struggling to upgrade their qualifications to bachelor's or master's degrees while at the same time developing the new diploma courses for basic nurse education. Their scholarship was developed within the context of an extra-ordinary workload and an expectation that they would do research (Roberts 1991).

The nurse academics were just starting to settle into the CAEs when the CAEs and universities were amalgamated to form the Unified National System of universities. Nurse education thus became a part of the universities in

Australia within a decade after leaving the hospital schools of nursing, a swiftness that exceeded even the most optimistic estimates. Nurse academics were consequently plunged into the university culture within less than a decade after leaving the hospital schools. They were now expected to be scholars and researchers at the level of the university academic when they had not even had time to develop the levels of scholarship expected of CAE academics. There was new pressure to upgrade the basic diplomas to bachelor degrees which increased the workload, and the nurse academics were still underqualified. They were now under pressure to acquire master's and doctoral degrees. So, underqualified and overworked and with very few fully fledged scholars in their midst, nurse academics clung precariously to the bottom rung of the university scholarship ladder. Australian nurse academics were going through the same transition that had taken place in the United States 25 years earlier.

With the consolidation of nursing as a discipline in the universities, Australian nurse scholars are emerging from their developmental stage. The growth of the nursing professoriate has undoubtedly contributed to the emergence of Australian nurse scholarship. The normal university pattern of developing research and scholarship in the discipline in which one is teaching is slowly being adopted by nurse academics. This trend has been enhanced by the opportunity for them to do postgraduate work in nursing which has only been possible in recent times.

In order to achieve the status of a respected academic discipline in the universities, nursing must make research and scholarship a very high priority and therefore must develop its researchers and scholars. Nursing cannot afford to be less rigorous in terms of scholarship than other disciplines in the university and therefore its professors must meet the same expectations for scholarly productivity as professors in other disciplines (Armiger 1974, Fitzpatrick & Abraham 1987). Over time, with the establishment of true scholarliness, the place of nursing education in the universities in Australia will become secure.

The domain of scholarship

The domain of scholarship in nursing can be divided into three areas: theoretical scholarship, clinical scholarship, and research scholarship. The distinction pertains to the thrust and intention of the discourse, the primary focus of the scholarship. Theoretical scholarship mainly focuses on the theoretical aspects of the topic, clinical scholarship concerns applications to practice and research scholarship reports research projects. The boundary between these types of scholarship is arbitrary since clinical or research scholarship will require consideration of theoretical aspects and theoretical scholarship will consider clinical practice and research findings. While theoretical, research and clinical scholarship overlap considerably, they are not necessarily the same thing. There is a large overlap between research and scholarship but there are areas which are different. There are areas of clinical practice, theoretical scholarship and clinical scholarship that lie outside research and areas of research that lie outside scholarship. In the following sections, the connections and distinctions between these areas will be explored.

Theoretical scholarship

Theoretical scholarship deals with the theoretical aspects of knowledge in the discipline without concern for its application. The main feature of theoretical scholarship is that it develops new knowledge through the integration and synthesis of knowledge, which advances the knowledge of the discipline of nursing. It is the 'scholarship of integration' which is interdisciplinary, interpretive and integrative (Boyer 1990). It is usually, but not exclusively, carried out by the nurse academics in the tertiary education institutions. Theoretical scholarship at this point in the development of the nursing profession includes the discussion of nursing theory, administration, education, professional issues, research methodology, law, ethics, philosophy, health care system, and politics. Supporting concepts from other disciplines may be used. However, it is the contention of the author that scholarship that discourses upon knowledge of other disciplines without at least applying that knowledge to nursing is not nursing scholarship. It is scholarship in the other discipline even if it is scholarship by nurses and about nurses.

Theoretical scholarship is the predominant form of non-research scholarship in Australia (McConnell & Paech 1993). Theoretical scholarship has been important for the development of knowledge in nursing. It will continue to be important as nursing develops a more scholarly approach to the construction of its knowledge base. It will continue to thrive for some time because most of the first generation of nursing professors honed their scholarly skills in the disciplines of education or administration. Much of their scholarly work is still produced in these areas although some are now producing clinical research and clinical scholarship.

A person may be a theoretical scholar without carrying out empirical research. The theoretical scholar may find and synthesise facts, concepts, research findings and insights developed by others without ever doing empirical research. Some nurse theorists, for example, developed their nursing theories by considering what nursing ought to be rather than by researching what nursing is. In a practice discipline such as nursing, it is necessary to see that the balance does not swing too far towards theoretical scholarship lest theory and research be divorced.

Theoretical scholars are also not necessarily practitioners. Most nurse academics, who make up the bulk of theoretical scholars, do not practise nursing beyond what is involved in teaching students. While some universities require their nurse academics teaching nursing to do clinical updates, this practice is not universal. Even in the clinical update, the nurse academic may not carry the total responsibility for decision making concerning the nursing care of the client. Without this responsibility, full clinical practice is not achieved. It is, however, unlikely that anyone could be a theoretician without being a scholar. In order to develop theory, the person must have a mastery of understanding of the theoretical area being developed in order to achieve the necessary synthesis of knowledge.

Clinical scholarship

Clinical scholarship is a very important link in the development of scholarship in Australia. It interacts with theoretical and research scholarship through the application of scholars' ideas to practice. Not only is it important in terms of scholarship but also it can lead to the improvement and documentation of nursing practice which will be part of the growth of nursing as a discipline in Australia.

Clinical scholarship has only recently been accepted by the nursing academic world although it had been recognised for a longer time in Medicine, as evidenced by the existence of clinical chairs, for example a chair in tropical medicine. Clinical scholarship in Nursing grew after Wald and Leonard (1964) advocated the development of theory about the practice of nursing. It is 'the study of the nature and effect of nursing. It depends on the people who do that, who are engaged in the clinical work. It helps us know what nursing is and does'. (Diers 1988). Clinical scholarship is a type of 'scholarship of application' which is carried out by professional schools and which asks how knowledge can be applied to solve problems (Boyer 1990). Nursing has a great deal to learn from expert clinical nurses who discuss, describe and document their practice. A well known North American nurse-scholar states that 'a wealth of untapped knowledge is embedded in the practices and the "know-how" of expert nurse clinicians' (Benner 1984). Clinicians increase their expertise and validate nursing knowledge when they test out theories and nursing interventions in actual practice situations (Patterson 1991).

Clinical scholarship must be based on a body of nursing and relevant scientific knowledge. Clinical events are observed by the experienced clinician, and analysed to make new connections between things or ideas, thus producing a synthesised whole. As does any scholar, the clinical scholar seeks truths, explanations, and ever more increasing information about the phenomena of the discipline (Diers 1988). The scholarliness of the clinical work is produced by the constant analysis of the work and the interpretation of the events to others. Clinical scholarship has its basis in the application of theory and research to practice. Nurses who are true clinical scholars are able to enhance the well being of their clients through improvement of nursing practice.

To be effective, the clinical scholar must communicate knowledge to fellow clinicians and other scholars. The clinical scholar can transmit knowledge in the clinical setting by means of such activities as informal teaching at the bedside, case presentations, or more formal grand nursing rounds, inservice education and conference presentations. Dolan (1984) describes clinical judgment seminars in which senior clinical nurses meet to discuss their practice; these seminars have been successful in uncovering the knowledge embedded in practice. Clinical scholarship can also take place in the university by teaching students at lectures and seminars. These are, however, mainly oral methods of transmission of knowledge. Street (1992) and Parker and Gardner (1991) have shown that the culture of the clinical practice of nursing is mainly oral rather than written. The heavy use of the oral method may well be attributable

215

to the fact that nursing is overwhelmingly female and that women rely on oral communication more than written communication. We need to find ways of acknowledging, documenting and transmitting the richness of clinical nursing scholarship that is presently communicated in oral form. One way might be to introduce, at appropriate times, computers that convert voice into transcript.

If oral methods are used to the exclusion of written methods, our clinical scholarship will not be transmitted to others and nursing will remain undervalued because it is undocumented in a system that is dominated by males who place more value on written communication than on oral communication. Until we develop ways of validating orally transmitted knowledge to augment the conventional written methods, the clinical scholar must rely on a body of written material such as papers in conference proceedings and papers in clinical nursing journals. Electronic media may well be the way of the future for disseminating clinical scholarship through electronic journals such as the new Online Journal of Knowledge Synthesis for Nursing developed by Sigma Theta Tau in the United States of America. However, these journals will need to establish that they are as rigorous as the conventional journals in terms of selection for publication if they are to be taken seriously by academe.

Who are our clinical scholars? Nurse academics have the skills to execute the written part of clinical scholarship but unless they are engaged in clinical practice they are not 'working at the cutting edge of innovative nursing practice' where the clinical scholars belong (Fawcett & Carino 1989). In Australia, clinical scholarship is in its infancy. As Australian nurse clinicians are increasingly produced by the tertiary education system, there will be more practitioners who have not only a theory-based education but also the skills to transmit their knowledge. In the short term, it may be that nurse academics who are engaged in joint appointments are the clinical scholars. They are well placed to see the important issues from the clinical side and also have skills of scholarship. Nurse academics who are employed by the university but commit a portion of their time to faculty practice are also in a position to see the clinical issues and write about them in a scholarly way. A clinical professoriate has already begun to be developed with the establishment of clinical chairs at University of Technology, Sydney and University of Sydney. While these are university chairs of nursing, partial or full funding is provided by the health sector and thus the university must be responsive to its needs concerning research and leadership of nursing practice. A professoriate with expertise in clinical practice will concentrate on the development of clinical nursing knowledge and thus will foster the development of nursing scholarship. In the next generation, these chairs will be held by scholars with doctoral degrees based on nursing practice research. In the health care sector, clinical nurse consultants are well placed to be clinical scholars as they have the depth of clinical expertise necessary as well as a tertiary education which emphasises theoretical knowledge and the skills of scholarship. Nurse clinicians in North America have demonstrated clinical scholarship at an advanced level (Fawcett & Carino 1989).

The emergence of clinical scholarship in the United States has seen the recognition of clinical scholars through the American Academy of Nursing, the Sigma Theta Tau Awards, and the establishment of a Clinical Scholars Program (Fawcett & Carino 1989). Some professional body in Australia such as Royal College of Nursing, Australia, or the New South Wales College of Nursing should take up the challenge to reward clinical scholarship as it develops in this country by establishing an Australian system of honours for clinical nursing excellence. Nurses who have consistently contributed to the scholarly development of clinical practice could be nominated for recognition. We have for too long rewarded academic and education excellence without recognising clinical excellence. It is time that this was changed and clinical scholarship was promoted to its rightful place in nursing.

Not all clinicians are clinical scholars. The clinician who is too inexpert through lack of depth of experience, or who merely does a job without thinking about the meaning of the clinical practice is not a scholar. In order to be a clinical scholar, the clinician must develop new insights into clinical practice through the integration and synthesis of knowledge derived from theory, research and observation.

Similarly, not all clinical scholars are interested in research, or are capable of doing it. The clinical scholar, like the theoretical scholar, can synthesise theoretical knowledge and research findings and apply those findings to clinical practice without doing scientific research. In a lament about the plight of the 'pragmatic practitioner', Masson (1991) suggests that a clinician may think about practice, may look up research findings and may have plenty to say about clinical practice but not have the inclination to do research. This may be clinical scholarship but it is not research scholarship.

Research scholarship

Research scholarship has traditionally been regarded as the most illustrious form of scholarship in academe since it contributes not only to the stock of human knowledge but also to the intellectual climate of the university (Boyer 1990). Research, a well-understood concept, is 'a careful search or enquiry, a course of critical investigation' (Concise Oxford English Dictionary). Scientific research is the systematic collection and analysis of empirical data in order to find new facts and relationships. Nursing has been defined by the American Nurses' Association as 'the diagnosis and treatment of human responses to actual or potential health problems' (Woods & Catanzaro 1988). Nursing research can be defined, therefore, as research that deals with the diagnosis and treatment of human responses to actual or potential health problems. It is generally applied research that focuses both on how nurses diagnose and treat health problems and on the client's response to these problems and their treatment. It is normally conducted in the clinical setting or laboratory.

The research process involves conceptualising and planning the research, finding funding, implementing the research project, analysing the results, writing up the report, and communicating the results to the profession. The researcher will first find a question to answer which may arise from other work previously done or may be a new question. The approach taken from then on depends on the nature of the question and the research paradigm to be used to answer it. It is not the purpose of this chapter to enter into the qualitative versus quantitative research debate, but the definition of scholarly research given above is meant to embrace both paradigms. Nursing research has developed more in the quantitative paradigm than the qualitative paradigm and this has influenced the scholarship of the nursing discipline.

The research process is not unlike the nursing process: both have assessment, planning, implementation and evaluation phases. In the assessment phase, the researcher assesses the question, its relevance, value and possible contribution to the discipline. In the planning phase, the researcher designs the project in such a way that it will be most likely to answer the question that is posed. In the implementation phase, the data are collected, and in the evaluation phase, the project is evaluated by the researcher and others in terms of its contribution to the field.

In the quantitative paradigm, a research question will frequently arise from theory and then the research is conceptualised so that it fits into the theoretical framework. The body of relevant literature is reviewed, a concise, researchable problem is stated, and the project is then developed using an appropriate research design such as an experiment. The research proposal is written and funding and institutional approvals are sought. The data are collected and then analysed using appropriate statistical or other techniques, and the results are extracted and conclusions drawn. The results are evaluated in terms of the validity of the study, its shortcomings, its relationship to the other work in the field and its contribution to the knowledge of the discipline.

In the qualitative paradigm, there is much less emphasis on measurement and much more on meaning. The process differs from the quantitative paradigm in that there may be no theoretical framework since the idea is to develop theory rather than be driven by it. Some approaches to qualitative research are phenomenology, ethnography, grounded theory and historical research. The researcher does not go in blinkered by an indepth review of a lot of previous literature in the field although some knowledge is beneficial. The grounded theorist ethnographer, for example, will live in the culture and collect data from it using observation and interviews as the main data collection processes. The data are analysed and theoretical insights are drawn from them. As for quantitative research, the project is then written up and evaluated. In both research paradigms, scholarship is involved in the stages of conceptualising the research project and synthesising the research findings with the knowledge in the discipline. It is therefore most important in designing, analysing, writing up and disseminating the findings.

Research scholars are mainly but not exclusively found in the universities. It is possible for clinical researchers working in the clinical setting outside the universities to be scholars. They too, however, would be likely to be receiving research training through the mechanism of acquiring formal academic qualifications. Research scholars will be produced by the universities in increasing numbers as the trend towards higher qualifications continues. If promotion in academe continues to be primarily based on research publications and research-based higher degrees, this trend will be reinforced. A PhD is the ultimate research qualification and the doctoral dissertation is the highest training in scholarly research. Not all nursing research is scholarship. Some nursing research is of a nature that does not lead to fundamental development of scholarly knowledge in the discipline. For example, replicatory research is not research scholarship. If a study is simply being done with no new methods and no fresh insights, it is not scholarship. This is not to say that the results are not used in scholarship because other scholars may derive knowledge from the cumulative body of research including replicatory research.

It is also necessary to distinguish between the different uses of the word research in order to exclude research that is not scientific. Research may mean the searching for and retrieving of information, the kind that one does in the construction of a piece of writing. It may involve long hours in the library, finding lists of papers and books to read, finding the material to read in preparation for a scholarly piece of work, and digging out the relevant bits of information. This is research that might best be called library research. It is one of the techniques used by both the scholar and the scientific researcher. Although library research is used during the process of scientific research it is not the same thing because it does not embody scientific inquiry. It is only the first step towards scientific enquiry.

Nursing research has traditionally focused on education and administration research. Although this type of research may be scientific, it is mainly research about the practitioners of nursing. It may be useful to nursing because it indirectly improves practice, but this type of research builds up knowledge in the other disciplines rather than contributing to knowledge about nursing.

New researchers may lack the mastery of knowledge necessary to produce scholarship in research. Students who do required research without mastering the area of the discipline under investigation are not scholars. It takes a considerable time before a researcher achieves such a level of mastery over the area that the research is deemed scholarly. Scholarliness is frequently not achieved until the doctoral level because it is at that level that the researcher is required to demonstrate complete mastery of a subject area. The higher levels of scholarship are not attained at the master's level because the research is less indepth and there is no requirement for the contribution of new knowledge to the discipline.

Nurses who take part in research as a member of a team and only participate in the mechanical parts of the process are not scholars. A hierarchy of ways in which nurses can participate in the research process is: reading and critiquing research reports; implementing research in practice; using a single step in the research process; combining several steps in the research process; replicating a published study; designing and conducting a small research study; preparing a grant proposal; co-ordinating a large research project and reporting the results; and consulting with other professionals about the research process (Sweeney 1985 cited in Schutzenhofer 1991). Scholarship would most likely not be involved below the steps of designing and conducting a small research study. A nurse 'data manager' is a case in point. This person designs forms, monitors protocol accrual, enters data, abstracts data, assures the quality and integrity of data and provides investigators with data reports (Cassidy 1993). The characteristics needed for a nurse data manager are an understanding of research methodology, being detail oriented, and being well organized. This is not the stuff of scholarship in research. The nurse researcher-scholar must be able to rise above the minutiae of research, see the broader picture, and contribute to its development.

The compleat scholar?

In an ideal world of nursing scholarship, the scholar would be a practitioner, researcher, and teacher. The teacher/researcher/practitioner could function at the highest level of scholarship because these components would all reinforce each other. Armiger (1974), in an early paper on scholarship in nursing, speaks of the need to combine teaching, research and application to practice. Nursing knowledge would be generated by scholars who would observe nursing problems, solve those problems through research, generate nursing theory through research, and apply theory and research findings to practice.

The model of integrated scholarship has been in place in North American universities for at least 15 years, and the concept was introduced to Australia over a decade ago at the first national nursing conference by Dr Loretta Ford, one of its key exponents in the United States of America. It is implemented by means of such devices as joint appointments in which the nurse is expected to practise in the area of expertise, do research, teach at the university and the clinical facility, and produce scholarly writing. In the present state of the profession in Australia, however, the functions of scholarship, research and practice are not generally integrated. Scholars may be distanced from clinical practice and research, sitting back in their armchairs in their ivory towers contemplating the mysteries of the nursing universe. The scholar may be involved in either clinical practice or research, but not usually both. Although the integrated model has not been recognised widely yet in Australia, some attempts have been made to implement it, notably at Deakin University. The nursing branch of the academic union (Union of Australian College Academics, an amalgamating partner of the National Tertiary Education Union) has a policy opposing joint appointments because they are seen as exploiting the workers. In the author's opinion, the union should direct its efforts toward improving the implementation of joint appointments, instead of trying to prevent a mechanism that would help to heal the breach between education and practice.

This lack of integration has primarily occurred because of the traditional separation of education (where most scholarship and research originated) and practice, where most clinical development is conceived. Another cause is the education of nurse academics in other disciplines which has led to the scholarship of the current generation of nurse scholars being developed in disciplines other than nursing which may be relevant to but not central to nursing.

In a professional discipline such as nursing, scholarship, it is argued, should aim for a high degree of integration of practice, theory, and research which can inform practice. The model of the all-in-one scholar is a wonderful ideal but requires a considerable amount of resources to support the person. Secretarial support, teaching assistance and research assistance are essential to allow the scholar to concentrate on the high level intellectual aspects of each area. Without adequate support the nurse may be unable to carry out any of the roles well. Sheer lack of time may prohibit the development of expertise in research, clinical practice, and teaching. Indeed, listening to a paper given by a joint appointee it seemed to the author that the person was carrying an impossible workload. It might be more realistic at this time to set up a model of collaboration in which the links between research, theory, clinical practice and scholarship are all present but each person does not carry out all functions. Indeed, Boyer (1990) cautions that it is unrealistic to expect all faculty to do research, and suggests that academics can remain scholarly by reading the literature in their field, keeping well informed about trends and patterns in their field and writing about these.

A community of scholars?

If nursing is to mature as a discipline, it must create a community of scholars. At present, the discipline of nursing in Australia is in the embryonic stages of this process. There are limited opportunities in Australia for publishing nursing scholarship with the result that dialogue is limited. The large size of the country combined with a geographical dispersion of the population leads to lack of communication between scholars outside their own institutions and at the national level. Conversations between nurse academics within institutions focus on industrial and parochial issues rather than scholarly discourse. Further opportunities for networking between scholars with similar interests and for building up focus groups with similar research interests within institutions need to be created. There should be more links between universities and clinical practice sites. The development of a professorial interest group, setting up of nursing research centres, and expansion of conjoint academic/clinical appointments will help to achieve this aim. While it is undeniable that nursing has made significant progress towards scholarship in the last decade, there is much more to be done. It is to be hoped that the next generation of scholars who get to positions of prominence in the 21st century will not have to inquire about the connections between theoretical, clinical and research scholarship.

REFERENCES

Armiger Sr B 1974 Scholarship in nursing. Nursing Outlook 22(3):160-164

Benner P 1984 From novice to expert. Addison-Wesley, Menlo Park California, ch 1

Boyer E 1990 Scholarship reconsidered: the priorities of the professoriate. The Carnegie Foundation for the Advancement of Teaching, Princeton New Jersey, ch 2

Cassidy J 1993 The role of the data manager in clinical cancer research: an opportunity for nurses. Cancer Nursing 16(2):131-138

Concise Oxford English dictionary, 6th edn. Sykes J (ed) University Press, Oxford, p 954

Dienemann J, Shaffer C 1992 Faculty performance appraisal systems: procedures and criteria. Journal of Professional Nursing 8(3):148-154

Diers D 1988 On clinical scholarship (again). IMAGE: Journal of Nursing Scholarship 20(1):2

Dolan K 1984 Bridges between education and practice. In: Benner P 1984 From novice to expert. Addison-Wesley, Menlo Park California, Epilogue

Fawcett J, Carino C 1989 Hallmarks of success in nursing practice. Advances in Nursing Science 11(4):1-8

Fitzpatrick J, Abraham I 1987 Toward the socialization of scholars and scientists. Nurse Educator 12(3):23-25

Hodges L, Poteet G 1992 The first 5 years after the dissertation. Journal of Professional Nursing 8(3):143-147

Masson V 1991 Clinical scholarship and the pragmatic practitioner. Nursing Outlook 37(4):160

Meleis A 1991 Theoretical nursing: development and progress, 2nd edn. J B Lippincott, Philadelphia, ch 7

Meleis A 1992 On the way to scholarship: from master's to doctorate. Journal of Professional Nursing 8(6):328-334

Parker J, Gardner G 1991 The silence and silencing of the nurse's voice: a reading of the patient's progress notes. The Australian Journal of Advanced Nursing 9(2):3-9

Patterson D 1991 Achieving excellence in nursing. Journal of Pediatric Nursing 6(6):391-395

Roberts K 1991 Institutional influences on nurse-academics' instructional planning decisions in the implementation of basic nursing curricula in colleges of advanced education in New South Wales. Royal College of Nursing, Australia, Melbourne

Schutzenhofer K 1991 Scholarly pursuit in the clinical setting: an obligation of professional nursing. Journal of Professional Nursing 7(1):10-15

Street A 1992 Inside nursing: a critical ethnography of nursing practice. SUNY Press, Albany, New York, ch 12

Sweeney M 1985 Clinical nursing research: exposing the myths. In: McCloskey J, Grace H (eds) Current issues in nursing, 2nd edn. Blackwell, New York, pp 161-170

Wald F, Leonard R 1964 Towards development of nursing practice theory. Nursing Research 13(4):309-313

Woods N, Catanzaro M 1988 Nursing research: theory and practice. Mosby, St Louis, ch 1

13

Humanities, scholarly wisdom and nursing practice

GRAEME CURRY

The humanities may be regarded as those disciplines which are primarily intent on exploring what it means to be human. Nursing practice is primarily about people (both individuals and groups) in clinical interaction in many different contexts. The goals appropriate to and congruent with the practice of nursing include the facilitation of clinical relationships (Gray 1984). Central to these relationships are such characteristics as healing, nurture, support, comfort, care, encouragement, awareness, wholeness, acceptance, dignity, integration, education, enabling, protection and liberation.

Nursing may be justly regarded as one of the humanities inasmuch as it pursues these goals within clinical interaction as appropriate to its discipline and profession. These relationships will be humane inasmuch as they are practised with patience, rigour, gentleness, alertness, attentiveness, observance, creativity, generosity, compassion, responsibility, integrity, trustworthiness, astuteness, balanced judgement, humility and simplicity. These characteristics are in fact also some of the features of what might be described as scholarly wisdom.

It is possible for nursing to degrade the clinical interaction through preoccupations with rapid outcomes or reductionist analyses; by attitudes of slovenly disinterest or obsessional inflexibility; with tendencies to regard detail in ad hoc or superficial ways; in jumping to unsubstantiated conclusions; when theories are embraced and research methodologies chosen that are unnecessarily complicated and obfuscatory rather than clarifying; by the use of inappropriate jargon or irrelevant models; and through blatant ethnocentrism, sexism and historically insensitive tunnel vision.

Such neglect of the larger human vision for nursing entails its being regarded as no longer one of the humanities. When nursing loses sight of its goals and embraces instead thoughtless and heartless mechanical techn('hand')ologies it becomes an instrument of wounding, diminishment, suffocation, inappropriate control, rigidity, superficiality, positivism, unhealthy pragmatism, undermining, neglect, abuse, disintegration, cynicism, disempowering dependencies, disabililty, enslavement and the fulfilment of selfish/egocentric purposes (compare Curry 1993). This constitutes a reversal of the goals of nursing itself. In such circumstances scholarly wisdom and humane practice would be minimally if at all present. These features may also become present in the areas of education, research and management which are intended to serve practice rather than self-interest.

Human disciplines

Systems proposing to identify, classify and arrange the fields of human activity, knowledge and interest have been many and varied. Systems developed by or implicit in, for example, the works of Plato, Aristotle, Hugh of Saint Victor, Bacon (1605), Comte, Dilthey (1923) and Collingwood (1924) are usefully and critically summarised by Bird (1976). He also includes consideration 'of the various maps of learning, the most widely used today' as 'embodied in the encyclopedia on the one hand and in the university on the other', suggesting that the latter may be 'based often only on principles of administrative, if not of personal, convenience' rather than representing 'a well-articulated division of the world of knowledge' (Bird 1976).

The location of nursing whether within or separate from medicine, health sciences/studies, biological sciences, social/behavioural sciences or humanities/arts in university structures tells us little about what fundamentally constitutes nursing knowledge and practice. Rather it says much more about the historical, political, social, economic and personal circumstances and conditions surrounding nursing's relatively naive entry into the tertiary education sector (Curry 1977), and the pragmatics of its attempts to carve out territory and achieve degrees of control in a sometimes antagonistic environment

In many of the systems proposed for the organisation of human knowledge and of the humanities in particular (yet certainly with different hier-archisations) philosophy, literature and history are often regarded as the three fundamental human disciplines. Just as nursing is about people so these fundamental human disciplines focus on the thought, expression and action of people exploring structures, purposes, motivations, implications and outcomes. Human and other 'scientific' disciplines provide ways for describing human experience of objects, ideas, relationships, connections and other persons. All forms of human description have limitations in terms of their field of inquiry and explanation, and the applicability of particular methods to particular kinds of activities and events. Thus we should talk of the limits of all intellectual activity including philosophy and even theology (Newman 1852). The present work confines its attention to the discipline of philosophy and the notion of scholarly wisdom. This should not be understood, however, to imply any lack of acknowledgment of the significance of history, literature, language, theology and philosophical anthropology for nursing practice.

Philosophy and nursing practice

Philosophy is sometimes identified as the central and foundational discipline not only of the humanities but also of all the various arts and sciences and possibly as underpinning all human activity itself. Packard and Polifroni (1992) emphasise that 'addressing the philosophical basis of knowledge development is an essential component of nursing scholarship' and it should be added that such scholarship has the intrinsic intention of contributing to the development of quality nursing practice.

The word 'philosophy' is derived from the Greek words for 'loving' or 'befriending' (*philos*) and 'wisdom' (*sophia*) (Liddell & Scott 1940). The Oxford English Dictionary (OED) notes that it refers originally and broadly to the 'love, study, or pursuit of wisdom, or of knowledge of things and their causes, whether theoretical or practical'. The ways in which 'philosophy' and related terms have been used in the Western world, let alone in Eastern systems of thought and amongst other peoples such as the Australian Aboriginal and Torres Strait Islander, Ameroindian and African peoples, have been historically many and varied. Western philosophies have often been divided into natural, moral and metaphysical philosophy and there are analogues to these divisions in other cultural systems.

'Natural philosophy' may be defined as the 'knowledge or study of nature or of natural objects and phenomena; "natural knowledge": now usually called *science*' (OED). Essential to nursing scholarship and practice is an awareness that those so-called sciences such as biology, physiology, physics, chemistry and psychology, that are often given such prominence in nursing curricula, are in their origins derived from natural philosophy and are dependent for the particular forms they now take on the social dominance of certain philosophical presuppositions often naively accepted with little critical thinking.

Such an awareness of the historical and philosophical dimensions of the natural sciences places them in their human context. The natural sciences are products of human activity within the limits of space and time. They are a fundamental component of human culture and social change. The primary sources of scientific writing (such as the works of Aristotle, Hippocrates, Kepler, Darwin, Einstein and Bernard) should be read. This could replace the rather slavish adherence to set texts in anatomy and physiology and become the norm for students of nursing. Such 'reading of primary sources' has been successfully used with school children (Matthews 1988) and nursing has much to benefit from such an innovation.

'Moral philosophy' is 'the knowledge or study of the principles of human action or conduct; ethics' (OED). This particular branch of philosophy has sometimes been over-emphasised in nursing and medicine without sufficient reference to the other branches of philosophy. Ethics or moral philosophy certainly provides an immediately relevant way of access to philosophical thinking for nurses, but it needs to be closely aligned as early as possible with broader fields of philosophical inquiry such as those of epistemology, the philosophy of language, logic, social and political philosophy, philosophical theology, philosophical psychology and philosophical anthropology to avoid narrow, superficial and muddled thinking.

'Central to any moral understanding is the concept of person' (Cassell 1991) and nurses in their clinical interaction are primarily involved with people, not with cases or diseases or syndromes or diagnoses. Nursing as a 'science' is unable to address issues or practices related to the unique individuality of each patient in the particularities of context and relationships. Such issues are sometimes relegated to nursing as an 'art' or to judgments that are perceived primarily as subjective (Cassell 1991). Such recognition points to the centrality of philosophical anthropology in the development of a moral philosophy relevant to nursing practice and such an anthropology requires a generous interaction with the other central human disciplines. Medicine has begun to recognise this in the recent moves in Australia for such study to be provided only at graduate level. One report stated that: 'We're hoping there'll be students with humanities degrees from music, philosophies, arts, whatever, as well as students with science backgrounds' (Robbins 1994).

Fundamental to nursing's moral concerns is the significance of the question of what it means to be a person and how this relates to changes in science and technology. Such questions are relevant in all areas of higher education that are intended to serve human interest and draw heavily on new technologies. There is an urgent need to increase 'the rigour and sensitivity of moral reasoning without foreclosing on fundamental questions;...produce graduates instilled with qualities of character and virtue;...require engagement with moral questions, and at the same time enhance the student's capacity to deal with them' (Leech 1993).

The exploration of such questions at a depth consistent with their complexity will enable nurses to begin to deal with 'the central dilemma facing nursing today' as referred to by Kurtz and Wang (1991). This dilemma is identified as 'the order to care by a society that refuses to value caring' where nurses 'are expected to act as if altruism (the basis for caring) and autonomy (the basis for rights) are separate ways of existing'. In referring to this dilemma they note that it is to be coupled with 'a growing concern that today's economic, bureaucratic, and technological environment is limiting nurses' caring abilities'.

If nurses are to avoid becoming mere passive cogs in the new 'in-corporations' where 'The flux and energy of human life become increasingly reduced to finite quantities of force and sensation, allowing it to be evermore efficiently subsumed and deployed in schools, factories, hospitals and households by the productivist and rationalising imperatives of a capitalist megamachine' (Crary & Kwinter 1992), then the questions fundamental to philosophical anthropologies require thorough exploration in their historical and transcultural contexts. The value of moral philosophy for nurses is certainly not confined to a 'preoccupation with *etiquette* (viz 'good manners')' nor should it be confined to the particulars of '*bona fide* professional ethics' (Johnstone 1993). A much larger vision is demanded that embraces the social, the economic, the political and the spiritual.

'Metaphysical philosophy' is 'that department of knowledge or study which deals with ultimate reality, or with the most general causes and principles of things' (OED). Metaphysical philosophy deals with the fundamental questions that underlie all branches of human scholarly inquiry and as such needs to be approached with a rigour congruent with its complexity and significance. Vague and inappropriate usage of such terms as 'ontology' which from time to time achieve popularity in nursing academe in no way serve the interests of scholarship or practice.

The rich variety of usage of the word 'philosophy' bears significant relationships to practice and scholarly wisdom. Nurses are keenly interested in issues concerning the relationship of knowledge to their practice. Clinical judgement requires a wise consideration of the relative significance of what is observed and astute discrimination regarding the results of investigations that are made. An interest in the causes of physiological and behavioural changes motivates much nursing inquiry. Systematic investigation of 'foundations' and 'principles' is regarded as essential to the development of any nursing theory that will have relevance to practice. The influence of 'attitudes' to practice and clinical outcomes is regarded as significant. The concept of 'vocation' in the history of nursing is well recognised. The relationship of nursing to 'traditional' or 'alternative' healing arts is beginning to be explored historically and transculturally. The appreciation of the aesthetic dimensions of body-image and self-concept as a result of burns, cancer or other disability are being more fully acknowledged. The perception of statistics, number and language as human constructs and the notions of reliability, variance and relevance have potentially radical implications for any hint of arrogance in the application of quantitative research methodologies. An understanding of the influence of social and political philosophies on the development of health services, models of delivery and institutional practices has the potential to illuminate the bankruptcy of 'economic rationalisms' and reductionist 'competencies'. The ability to think clearly, to argue cogently and to communicate wisely are three skills essential to excellence in nursing scholarship and practice.

The diversity of human traditions has embraced an overwhelming array of methods to explore these and the many other philosophic questions of nature, morals and metaphysics. These have included models, structures and techniques that may be variously described as logical, analytic, critical, intuitive, introspective, observational, 'common-sense', reflective, interpretative, evaluative, explanatory and synthetic. Approaches to philosophic issues have been variously referred to with such descriptors as sceptical, paradoxical, analogical, allegorical, empiricist, atomist, sophist, stoic, monist, dualist, pluralist, materialist, realist, rationalist, idealist, scholastic, analytic/linguistic, positivist (social, critical or logical), psychoanalytic, evolutionary, developmental, nihilist, anarchic, chaotic, cosmogonic, socialist, capitalist, 'oikonomic', phenomenological, existentialist, utilitarian, pragmatist, feminist, transgender, structuralist, functionalist, deconstructionist, postmodern and eclectic.

These approaches to varying extents are included in, overlap or are besides those related to particular individuals. More than 140 major Western philosophers spanning the 26 centuries from c624 BCE to the present day could be listed. Useful surveys of some of the philosophic traditions, personalities and associated schools are to be found in such reference sources as Bales (1987), Copleston (1946), Edwards (1967) and Passmore (1957).

The examples of philosophical approaches referred to above are purposefully selective, as would be any listing of major philosophers across the centuries. The intention is to psychologically 'flood' the would-be nursing theorist, philosopher, researcher, scholar, academic, student, manager and practitioner with the reality of their task of serving clinical interaction. It is this task that is so often studiously avoided by nurses because of the immensity and complexity for any individual or community not only in confronting and exploring the human condition in the supposed abstract but also in actually applying those understandings to the real world of practice.

The nurse is to be 'clever' but in the sense of true wisdom, not in the forms of superficial smartness, trickery, charade, pretence or deceit. Many of the writings of nurses moving into the previously often unchartered regions of philosophy, conceptual frameworks, theories and paradigms have been neglectful of the necessity of the admission that we know very little. This is true even of authors with an apparent breadth of understanding and impressive presentation such as Meleis (1991) who refers very rarely to the exact words of classical primary philosophical texts and as a result impoverishes her work. For example, in her chapters where she refers to Kant and Spinoza in the chapter titles neither Kant nor Spinoza make an appearance in her list of references.

Certainly what nurses do know (and this is often very significant) they often know not how to articulate clearly in words, although sometimes highly able nurses are able to communicate this knowledge to the limited audience that may be privy to their example. It is also important for nurses to discover and acknowledge that the more we come to know the less we realise we know, and that the most dangerous nurses in practice, academe and management are the ones who think they know it all!

Analogous and equally overwhelming and demanding would be a listing of a selection of the major cultural and linguistic groupings of people over historical time and geographical space. It would be the height of naivety to believe that we could ever come to grips with more than a very small number of philosophical systems, cultural mores or human languages. Yet the willingness to be acutely aware of, recognise, acknowledge and accept this lack in the face of constant diversity, change and variability is itself an ambitious task. The central significance of such cognitive and emotional 'deluging' lies in the development of a humble appreciation of our own littleness in all of this, despite the daily demand upon us as nurses to provide care and support for a myriad of unique individuals and communities in an unending variety of clinical relationships. Further, such constant openness to new possibilities enables a certain childlike or youthful excitement and attentiveness to be gently and patiently maintained and developed. This novel expectancy can act as a very significant corrective to the pervasive cynicism, obsessionality and reductionism that sometimes characterise the culture of nursing.

Wittgenstein (1958) states that 'in psychology there are experimental methods and *conceptual confusion*....The existence of the experimental method makes us think we have the means of solving the problems which trouble us; though problem and method pass one another by'. A basic acquaintance with such an overview of this richness of philosophical understandings is necessary if nursing knowledge and practice are to be developed on firm foundations. Similarly, a selective listing of major groupings of Hindu, Buddhist and Chinese philosophical schools would not exhaust the limits of the impressive variety of human philosophic traditions which have hardly been hinted at. These could include the Egyptian, Akkadian, Sumerian, Persian, Byzantine, Islamic, Jewish, Zoroastrian, Jain, Sikh, Shinto, Zen, traditional 'gipsy', African, Southeast Asian, Ameroindian and Oceanic schools and methods including, for example, the highly sophisticated traditions of the Aboriginal and Torres Strait Islander peoples of Australia and the Maori and Polynesian peoples of New Zealand. These traditions often have strong associations with theological ideas and religious practices along with developed oral, literary, musical and other artistic products arising from deeply respected historical and transcendental dimensions.

Despite much criticism and in spite of the ways in which their work might be evaluated, Rogers (along with Krieger and Orem in more limited ways) are examples of nursing writers who have attempted to demonstrate a broader vision of philosophical understandings. Rogers has developed 'an evolutionary conceptual system that has inspired tremendous creativity, research activity, and intellectual growth in the profession. Because of her knowledge of many scientific fields and her own broad education and extensive readings, she brought to nursing a questioning stance about previously accepted foundations, such as the biomedical model and logical empiricism' (Garon 1992).

Hanchett (1992) refers to analogies between Rogers' outlook and 'concepts used in Tibetan Buddhist philosophy' and quotes Sarter's statement 'that serious attention be paid to the formal systems of thought of the East, both ancient and modern, so that accurate interpretation and application, rather than vague references, can be made'. It is certainly very difficult to come to grips with the thought forms and expressions of other traditions when we have a minimal grasp of our own cultural heritage. This can be one of the weaknesses involved in recent trends to focus on Asia in its great diversity without adequate awareness of Australia's diverse range of cultural (including Asian) heritage (Ryckmans 1993). There is a definite need for historical and cultural contextualisations for philosophical understanding and an awareness of the complex enmeshment of the human disciplines of philosophy, history, literature and language. This needs to be coupled with an awareness of the necessity for these to be explored together with the study of theology and religion in the multiplicity of traditions.

Even limited exposure to the range of understandings of the nature and role of philosophical activity and endeavour in human inquiry may assist nurses in laying to rest once and for all an apparent preoccupation with '*the* critical-reflective paradigm' and with 'femin*ism*'. There are a myriad of critical and/or reflective paradigms in the diversity of the philosophical traditions relevant to the exploration of nursing knowledges and practices. Feminisms, like Marxisms and most other -isms, are also many and varied. A radical lesbian separatist feminism, for example, may certainly be regarded as intellectually respectable but its contribution to nursing knowledges and practices may be quite different to a traditional Marxist feminism or to a socialist or a more liberal feminism (Kleffel 1991). 'There is not *a* philosophical method, though there are indeed methods, like different therapies.' (Wittgenstein 1958). The philosophical inexactitude prevalent among nurses especially in academe is of grave concern for the development of future practice. Professional maturity in philosophical understanding and understanding of its limitations and ours will help guard against nurses taking for granted all kinds of implicit assumptions about various practices, activities and beliefs so often naively embraced. Issues, for example, of cultural differences, relativism, freedom, causation, scepticism, uncertainty, doubts, beliefs, rituals, *episteme*, ontology, perception, experience, intuition, memory and imagination require critical study of the history of philosophy to illuminate their relevance to the clinical setting and to avoid ethnocentrism and gender bias.

How can nurses, for example, claim to seriously understand and care for the person with supposed memory loss, hallucination, delusion or 'non-compliance', or assure quality practice, or reliably develop nursing diagnoses without coming to grips with philosophical, historical and transcultural issues related to orientation, judgement, memory and selectivity; sensation, perception, attention and alertness; cognition, intelligence, learning, belief and knowledge; volition, choice, habit formation, impulse, control and freedom; value, expectation, responsibility, dignity and integrity; order, classification, meaning, fragmentation and 'wholism'; let alone begin to construct a phenomenology or taxonomy of nursing interests and practices?

If 'the philosopher's treatment of a question is like the treatment of an illness' (Wittgenstein 1958) and if philosophy, according to Cicero, 'imparts wisdom which the statesman needs to combine with eloquence...' and 'offers training in argument' (Boardman et al 1991) and if 'the triumph' of Socrates' 'art of midwifery' is 'in thoroughly examining whether the thought which the mind of the young man (sic!) brings forth is a false idol or a noble and true birth' (in Plato's *Theaetetus* in Jowett 1892) then nursing practice and philosophy have much mutually beneficial work to perform together.

Scholarship, wisdom and nursing practice

The Oxford English Dictionary provides definitions for the words 'scholar', 'scholarly', 'scholarship' and 'scholastic' in a number of ways. 'Scholar' is sometimes used to refer to a person taught in or belonging to a school or who is associated in training, instruction or discipline with a particular master or teacher. From this notion is derived the idea of a 'disciple'. Reference is also made to those associated with the 'schools' of a university and those who have gained their learning in such institutions. A scholar as 'a learned or erudite person' is sometimes regarded as a person who is especially skilled in classical languages and literature, particularly Greek and Latin. 'Scholarship' both in its individual and collective senses is connected with scholarly achievements. Besides its particular medieval senses 'scholastic' refers to being studious or learned with a fundamental sense of being 'at leisure'; of devoting such leisure to learning; of 'having the characteristics of the scholar or student, as distinguished from the man of affairs'; or a 'man of learning...as opposed to a man of the world' (OED).

From the cluster of meanings related to the word 'schola' it might be useful to choose that of 'one who is taught in a school'. Such a school would be one of disciplined (!) 'leisure', desirous of divine wisdom, ever open, constant and ongoing—characterised by a transcendent aspect. The idea of 'e-duc-ation' is one of always going beyond and of 'leading out-of-self'. Such an idea of scholarship implies an active alertness within tranquillity recognising the necessity for time and spaciousness to explore. This is reflected in the idea of a dissertation or thesis. There is no room for rush or an anxious desire to fulfil inappropriate 'deadlines'. There are time frames and structures but these are designed to provide time to discover clarity of purpose and achieve clarity of expression. Monastic leisure (as typified by the rhythms of silence, prayer and reading) was matched by monastic productivity (as reflected in manual labour and hospital-ity) and productivity in nursing scholarship will be only matched by the permission for and conscious encouragement of leisure in nursing practice and scholarship. Leisure is the fundamental condition for attentiveness and attentiveness is integral to the heart of nursing. The work of leisure and the leisure of work and their embrace in university, hospital and hospice are essential to human dignity. To be learned in at least one particular great tradition would seem to be an essential component of scholarship and to be thus learned needs to be a fundamental intention of those nurses in both academe and practice who would purport to become nursing scholars.

Palmer (1986) defines clinical scholarship as 'knowledge and learning derived from analytic observations of clients and patients' and states that such scholarship '(1) is rooted in *observations* of the health-sickness phenomena of people, (2) mandates *extensive knowledge* in those sciences used in the practice of nursing as well as knowledge of nursing itself, (3) requires significant extensive *experiences* in the clinical practice of nursing, and (4) demands *intellectual activity*: thinking, analysis and synthesis' and notes that 'Diers includes writing as an essential activity'. The discipline associated with the study of one or more great human traditions in its philosophical, historical, literary, linguistic and theological dimensions provides a firm foundation for the development of sophisticated skills in clinical observations; facilitates the acquisition of extensive knowledge in those human sciences fundamental to the practice of nursing; enriches and enlivens the quality of experiences in clinical practice; develops rigour and balance in intellectual activity; and requires excellence in the abilities not only of writing but also of reading, listening/attending, reflection, understanding, questioning and speaking.

Nightingale is one example of a nurse who was truly a clinical scholar according to these criteria. As Widerquist (1992) points out 'under her father's tutelage, Nightingale developed as a classical rather than a scientific scholar' and her 'keen intellect combined with a classical education...fostered critical thinking and scepticism'. She also refers to the work of Nightingale in collaboration with the eminent Oxford scholar named Jowett for whom she wrote 'on religion and philosophy and assisted...in translating Plato's *Republic*'.

This scholarly sophistication of Nightingale may be compared with that of a nurse named Paula who lived from 347 to 404 CE. She also was a learned woman (Cross 1958, Donahue 1985) and her linguistic ability in Latin, Greek and Hebrew and her involvement in the work of biblical translation, places her alongside Jerome in the production of the Latin Vulgate which is usually ascribed alone to the male partner in the scholarly enterprise. Paula's practicality was not confined to linguistic and literary activity. She was also involved in the design and management of hospices and hospitals in the Holy Land, developed a sophisticated system of nurse education and herself continued to 'personally nurse' the sick.

It is clear that the so-called 'ideas' person may be at the same time a person of great practicality and efficiency. As stated in a classical Indian description of the characteristics of 'the attending nurse', besides the need for 'knowledge of the manner in which drugs should be prepared or compounded for administration, ...devotedness to the patient waited upon, and purity (both of mind and body)' is included the 'qualification' of 'cleverness' (in the Kaviratna as quoted in translation in Donahue 1985).

This scholarly 'cleverness' which is characterised by and intimately connected with practicality closely relates to those rich understandings associated with the word 'wisdom'. In classical Hebrew the verb 'hakam' has the meaning of to 'be wise', to 'make firm, sound, free from defect (by the exercise of skill)'. The noun form 'hokmah' ('wisdom') is always feminine and the adjectival form is 'hakam' ('wise'). These terms have a rich variety of referents as does the English usage of these words. According to the Oxford English Dictionary, this usage includes the characteristics associated with right judgment in issues related to everyday life and conduct; the ability to make sound judgements as regards choosing appropriate means and ends; and practical wisdom. Wisdom is usually personified as feminine and is also used as a referent to Jesus Christ as 'the Wisdom of the Father'. It is also used in reference to knowledge especially when it is regarded as particularly significant or obscure and in relation to this has a sense of enlightenment, learning and/or erudition. Early use posits a close relationship with philosophy and science. The emphasis on practical knowledge and understanding is coupled with the idea of 'expertness in an art'. Further emphases include the presence of sound, right and fitting judgement; the ability of discernment; the disposition of acting according to such judgment and discernment; perceptiveness and discrimination in choosing 'the best means for accomplishing an end'; good sense and prudence.

Wisdom may be 'distinguished from the reasoned, systematic view of the world and man which is the conscious aim of philosophy' by its characteristic 'direct, practical insight into the meaning and purpose of things that comes to "shrewd, penetrating, and observant minds, from their own experience of life, and their daily commerce with the world."' The Encyclopaedia of Religion and Ethics suggests that philosophy may seem to be more 'intellectual' whilst wisdom has a much wider appeal 'to all who are interested in life and have understanding enough to appreciate a word of truth well spoken'. Yet wisdom and philosophy may be regarded as intimately connected in the sense that 'knowledge of life reached intuitively by wisdom is the raw material out of which philosophical systems are evolved'. Such movement of definition and usage clearly indicate the constant flow between the philosophical and practical senses of wisdom—they are intimately intertwined together (Hastings 1967).

Reading and reflecting upon the great scholarly output of the classical authors is interlocked with that experience gained in 'the university of life' (Holland 1993). It is the 'lectio' ('reading') of everyday nursing practice which creates the 'practical wisdom' of the experienced nurse. 'The continuity of the wisdom tradition' and the continuity of scholarly wisdom in nursing practice is in the 'constant enlargement and enrichment of this faculty of applied intelligence' (Roth 1972).

Seneca (1928) states that 'The truest form of wisdom is to make a wide and long inspection, to put self in subjection, and then to move forward slowly and in a set direction'. This is certainly wise advice for the nurse setting out on a systematic program of scholarly reading in the humanities as well as in the day-to-day activity of clinical judgement. Too often institutions that teach nursing (and other disciplines) 'throw away the opportunity really to *educate*, for the sake of a flimsy and unpractical "training" that for the most part does not even *train*' (Flexner 1930), resulting in a 'civilisation and education' which 'while...sharpen(ing) the mind, often blunt the tongue; while...brighten(ing) the intelligence, often tarnish the imagination...(making) (p)rimitive language seem(s) often a kind of magic...(and) intellectual language, a kind of algebra' (Lucas 1955). Nursing needs intellects characterised by a practicality able to communicate scholarship with clarity and wisdom. Such intellects are not created overnight. They require a long and disciplined training comparable to that of any athlete in the gymnasium. It is only such a scholarly training in the ways of practical wisdom that will form the foundations and context for excellence in nursing teaching and research. Such teaching and research sometimes seem to be confused with the essence of scholarship itself.

The humanity of nursing

If nursing is to affirm itself as one of the humanities both in academe and in practice it is essential that each nursing scholar and practitioner immerse themselves in depth in the primary sources and experiences of at least one of the major human traditions. This will include an acknowledgment of the cultural relativism and ethnocentrism of any such immersion. Nevertheless, this will require a rigorous and systematic program of reading and reflection in key philosophical, historical, literary and theological 'masterpieces' and at least a fundamental acquaintance with the linguistic commonalities and peculiarities of that particular tradition. For some, such reading and reflection will be enriched by opportunity for interaction with those who continue to belong to that tradition. A few will be able to express in writing the relationship of their experience of this tradition to their experience of nursing practice. It is not expected that the majority of nurses (even in academe) will become expert philosophers, historians, *literati*, linguists or theologians. If nursing scholarship, however, is to develop with any degree of credibility nurses need to be more fully aware of the immensity of human understandings and traditions and of the fragmentary and minimal nature of our present knowledge.

Scholarly wisdom in nursing is not served 'by vague reading and a few scattered writings' but rather 'requires penetration and continuity and methodical effort, so as to attain a fullness of development' (Sertillanges 1946). Nursing scholarship needs to find its location in the network of human scholarship and this includes the exploration, identification and appreciation of the contribution of and presence of women's work in what is often brought forward as men's work. Such scholarship will bring a feminine eye to the maleness of the 'canons' of the classical traditions.

For example, if nurses are to take seriously the formative influences of the classical Western philosophical tradition it is essential that they develop a comfortable, yet humble familiarity with the *ipsissima verba* ('the exact words') of, for example, Plato, Aristotle, Augustine, Aquinas, Descartes, Locke, Kant and Hegel. Certainly, for many nurses, the approach to these primary sources will be through good translations rather than in the original languages of the writers. The rich experience of nurses as nurses (and, for many, as women) will bring to the wealth of such an intellectual tradition new insights and understandings often neglected by those who may claim some hegemony with such traditions.

Nursing as a humanity and the humanisation of nursing practice will not, however, be fully developed by mere intellectual activity as it also cannot be by mere technology. The 'head' and 'hands' of nursing need to be accompanied by a 'heart' that gives full respect to the dignity and unique individuality of each person and community with which nurses are involved.

ACKNOWLEDGEMENTS

I wish to acknowledge the support, encouragement, criticism and other contributions of patients, students, colleagues, acquaintances, friends and family in the preparation of this chapter, in particular John Cochrane, Sheryl Delacour, Neil Frazer, Anne Gray, Rhonda Holland, Bernadette Keane, Ophelia Lobo, Anne McKenzie, Geoffrey Parker, Wayne Stamp and Eli Statulevicius.

REFERENCES

Bacon F 1605, 1973 The advancement of learning. J M Dent, London

Bales E F 1987 A ready reference to philosophy East and West. University Press of America, Lanham, MD

Bird O A 1976 Cultures in conflict: an essay in the philosophy of the humanities. University of Notre Dame Press, Notre Dame

Boardman J, Griffin J, Murray O (eds) 1991 The Oxford history of the classical world. University Press, Oxford

Cassell E J 1991 The nature of suffering and the goals of medicine. Oxford University Press, New York

Collingwood R G 1924 Speculum mentis. Clarendon Press, Oxford

Copleston F C 1946-1985 A history of philosophy. Image Books, New York (six volumes)

Crary J, Kwinter S (eds) 1992 Incorporations. Zone, New York (Zone 6)

Cross F L (ed) 1958, 1966 The Oxford dictionary of the Christian church. Oxford University Press, London

Curry G 1977 Educating for nursing professionalism: status or competence. The Lamp October:5-7

Curry G 1993 Royal commissions, committees of inquiry and psychiatric nursing. Australian nursing...the story. First national nursing history conference. Royal College of Nursing, Australia, Melbourne 55-62

Dilthey W 1923, 1988 (transl) Introduction to the human sciences. An attempt to lay a foundation for the study of society and history. Harvester Wheatsheaf, London

Donahue M P 1985 Nursing the finest art. An illustrated history. Mosby, St Louis

Edwards P (ed) 1967 The encyclopedia of philosophy. Macmillan, New York (eight volumes)

Flexner A 1930 Universities American English German. Oxford Univerity Press, London

Garon M 1992 Contributions of Martha Rogers to the development of nursing knowledge. Nursing Outlook March/April:67-72

Gray A 1984 Proposal of diploma of applied science (nursing). Kuring-gai College of Advanced Education, Sydney (two volumes)

Hanchett E S 1992 Concepts from Eastern philosophy and Rogers' science of unitary human beings. Nursing Science Quarterly 5(4):164-170

Hastings J (ed) 1967 Encyclopaedia of religion and ethics. Clark, Edinburgh

Holland R 1993 Personal communication

Johnstone M-J 1993 The development of nursing ethics in Australia: an historical overview. Australian nursing...the story. First national nursing history conference. Royal College of Nursing, Australia, Melbourne 33-51

Jowett B [1892]1937 (transl) The dialogues of Plato. Random House, New York (two volumes)

Kleffel D 1991 An ecofeminist analysis of nursing knowledge. Nursing Forum 26(4):5-18

Kurtz R J, Wang J 1991 The caring ethic: more than kindness, the core of nursing science. Nursing Forum 26(1):4-8

Leech G 1993 Call for virtue to be on syllabus. The Australian Higher Education December 1:25

Liddell H G, Scott R (eds) 1940 A Greek-English lexicon. Clarendon Press, Oxford (two volumes)

Lucas F L 1955, 1974 Style. Cassell, London

Matthews M R 1988 A role for history and philosophy in science teaching. Educational Philosophy and Theory 20(2):67-81

Meleis A I 1991 Theoretical nursing. Development and progress. Lippincott, Philadelphia

Newman J H 1852, 1959 The idea of a university. Image, New York

Packard S A, Polifroni E C 1992 The nature of scientific truth. Nursing Science Quarterly 5(4):158-163

Palmer I S 1986 The emergence of clinical scholarship as a professional imperative. Journal of Professional Nursing Sept/Oct:318-325

Passmore J 1957, 1968 A hundred years of philosophy. Penguin, Harmondsworth

Robbins M 1994 Medicine becomes postgrad course. The Australian Higher Education 16 (February):13

Roth C (ed) 1972 Encyclopaedia Judaica. Macmillan, Jerusalem (sixteen volumes)

Ryckmans P 1993 For better universities, first abolish degrees. The Australian Higher Education 24 (November):19

Seneca 1928 (transl) Moral essays. Harvard University Press, Cambridge, Massacusetts (three volumes)

Sertillanges A D 1946 (transl) The intellectual life. Its spirit conditions methods. Mercier Press, Cork

The Oxford English dictionary 1989, 2nd edn. Clarendon Press, Oxford (twenty volumes) (OED)

Widerquist J G 1992 The spirituality of Florence Nightingale. Nursing Research 41(1):49-55

Wittgenstein L 1958, 1963 (transl) Philosophical investigation, 2nd edn. Blackwell, Oxford

FURTHER READING

Arberry A J 1955, 1964 (transl) The Koran. University Press, Oxford

Aristotle 1986 (transl) De anima (On the soul). Penguin, Harmondsworth

Barnes H E 1937, 1962 A history of historical writing, 2nd revised edn. Dover, New York

Benedict Saint 1952 (transl) The rule. Burns Oates, London

Birt L M et al 1993 Bridging the gap. The social sciences, humanities, science and technology in economic development. Commonwealth Government Printer, Canberra

Blazek R, Aversa E 1988 The humanities. A selective guide to information sources, 3rd edn. Libraries Unlimited, Englewood, Colorado

Brown F, Driver S R, Briggs C A 1907, 1966 A Hebrew and English lexicon of the Old Testament. Clarendon Press, Oxford

Bunting S, Campbell J C 1990 Feminism and nursing: historical perspectives. Advances in Nursing Science 12(4):11-24

Callahan D, Caplan A L, Jennings B (eds) 1985 Applying the humanities. Plenum Press, New York

Cassell E J 1984 The place of the humanities in medicine. Hastings Center, New York

Cassirer E 1944 An essay on man. An introduction to a philosophy of human culture. Yale University Press, New Haven

Christian J L 1990 Philosophy. An introduction to the art of wondering. Holt, Rinehart & Winston, Fort Worth

Cicero 1949 (transl) De inventione De optimo genere oratorum Topica. Harvard University Press, Cambridge, Massachusetts

Collingwood R G 1938, 1963 The principles of art. Clarendon Press, Oxford

Collingwood R G 1946, 1961 The idea of history. University Press, Oxford

Confucius 1979 (transl) The Analects. Penguin, Harmondsworth

Constantelos D J 1968 Byzantine philanthropy and social welfare. Rutgers University Press, New Brunswick, New Jersey

Conze E 1959 (selected and compiled) Buddhist scriptures. Penguin, Harmondsworth

Curry G 1987 Transcendence, theology and nursing education. Unpublished manuscript of paper presented to the Australian and New Zealand Society for Theological Studies Conference, Melbourne

Curry G 1992 Retrospective prospects: memory, re-enactment of the past and nursing practice. Australian Nursing Memorabilia and History Society, Melbourne (audio-casette and unpublished typescript)

Curry G 1993 'Self-actualisation' or self-destruction: an historical perspective on psychiatric nursing. The Australian Journal of Mental Health Nursing 2(5):234-242

Daly M 1984 Pure lust Elemental feminist philosophy. Women's Press, London

Davis S K 1992 Nursing and the humanities: health assessment in the art gallery. Journal of Nursing Education 31(2):93-94

Dechanet J-M 1972 William of St Thierry. The man and his work. Cistercian Publications, Spencer, Massachusetts (Cistercian Studies Series No 10)

Dennis W (ed) 1948 Readings in the history of psychology. Appleton-Century-Crofts, New York

Dorsch T S (transl) 1965 Classical literary criticism Aristotle/Horace/Longinus. Penguin, Harmondsworth

Dunlop M 1992 Shaping nursing knowledge: an interpretive analysis of curriculum documents from NSW Australia. Monograph Series, Royal College of Nursing, Australia, Melbourne

Eliade M (ed) 1987 The encyclopedia of religion. Macmillan, New York

Feher M (ed) 1989 Fragments for a history of the human body. Zone, New York (Zone 3-5) (three parts)

Feinberg L 1992 Transgender liberation. A movement whose time has come. World View Forum, New York

Gardiner P (ed) 1959 Theories of history. Free Press, New York

Godden J, Curry G, Delacour S 1993 The decline of myths and myopia? Recent trends in nursing historiography. The Australian Journal of Advanced Nursing 10(2):27-34

Harakas S S 1990 Health and medicine in the Eastern Orthodox tradition. Faith, liturgy, and wholeness. Crossroad, New York

Herodotus 1954, 1972 (transl) The histories. Penguin, Harmondsworth

Highet G 1949, 1985 The classical tradition Greek and Roman inluences on Western literature. Oxford University Press, New York

Horace 1964, 1967 (transl) The Odes. Penguin, Harmondsworth

Hugh of Saint Victor 1956 (transl) The divine love. Mowbrays, London

Hutchins R M (ed) 1952 Great books of the Western world. Britannica, Chicago (fifty-four volumes)

John Chrysostom Saint 1977 (transl) Six books on the priesthood. St Vladimir's Seminary Press, New York

Jonas C M 1992 The meaning of being an elder in Nepal. Nursing Science Quarterly 5(4):171-175

Josephus 1927, 1976 (transl) The Jewish war. Harvard University Press, Cambridge, Massachusetts

Kant I 1960 (transl) Education. University of Michigan Press, Ann Arbor

Klein D B 1970 A history of scientific psychology. Its origins and philosophical backgrounds. Routledge and Kegan Paul, London

Leclercq J 1974, 1978 (transl) The love of learning and the desire for God. A study of monastic culture, 2nd revised edn. SPCK, London

Lehmann J 1957 The craft of letters in England. Greenwood Press, Westport, Connecticut

Lewis C T, Short C 1879 A Latin dictionary. Clarendon Press, Oxford

McAdoo H R 1965 The spirit of Anglicanism. A survey of Anglican theological method in the seventeenth century. Black, London

MacGinty G 1986 *Lectio divina*: fount and guide of the spiritual life. Cistercian Studies 21(1):64-71

Macquarie J 1982 In search of humanity. A theological and philosophical approach. SCM Press, London

Magnusson M (ed) 1990 Chambers biographical dictionary, 5th edn. Chambers, Edinburgh

Mascaro J 1962 (transl) The Bhagavad Gita. Penguin, Harmondsworth

Mascaro J 1973 The Dhammapada. The path of perfection. Penguin, Harmondsworth

Moore A R 1978 The missing medical text. Humane patient care. University Press, Melbourne

Muller F M 1879, 1884, 1962 (transl) The Upanisads. Dover, New York (two parts) (originally volumes I and XV of The sacred books of the East)

O'Flaherty W D 1981 (transl) The Rig Veda. An anthology. Penguin, Harmondworth

Palmer G E H, Sherrard P, Ware K 1979-1981 (transl) The Philokalia. The complete text compiled by St Nikodimos of the holy mountain and St Makarios of Corinth. Faber, London (volumes one and two)

Peschel E R (ed) 1980 Medicine and literature. Neale Watson, New York

Rahman F 1989 Health and medicine in the Islamic tradition. Change and identity. Crossroad, New York

Revised Standard Version 1973 The Holy Bible with the Apocrypha/Deuterocanonical books. Collins, New York

Rieu E V 1952 The four gospels. Penguin, Harmondsworth

Rowse A L 1946 The use of history. English Universities Press, London

Scarry E 1985 The body in pain. The making and unmaking of the world. Oxford University Press, New York

Scholes P A, Ward J O 1970, 1991 The Oxford companion to music, 10th edn. University Press, Oxford

Sheikh A A, Sheikh K S 1989 Eastern and Western approaches to healing Ancient wisdom and modern knowledge. Wiley, New York

Slade J W, Lee J Y 1990 Beyond the two cultures. Essays on science, technology, and literature. State University Press, Iowa

Smith D H 1986 Health and medicine in the Anglican tradition. Conscience, community and compromise. Crossroad, New York

Spinoza B 1949, 1967 (transl) Ethics. Hafner, New York

Thomas L 1978 Notes of a biology-watcher. How to fix the premedical curriculum. The New England Journal of Medicine May 25:1180-1181

Topolski J 1976 (transl) Methodology of history. Warsaw

Traherne T 1958 Centuries, poems and thanksgivings. Clarendon Press, Oxford (volume 1)

Underhill E 1911 Mysticism. A study in the nature and development of man's spiritual consciouness. Methuen, London

Virgil 1956 (transl) The Aeneid. Penguin, Harmondsworth

Waddell H 1936 (transl) The desert fathers. University of Michigan Press, Ann Arbor

William of St Thierry 1956 (transl) On the nature and dignity of love. Mowbray, London

Wurzbach M E 1991 Judgment under conditions of uncertainty. Nursing Forum 26(3):27-34

14

Victorian influences on the development of nursing

JUDITH GODDEN

Introduction

One impact of the Nightingale revolution in nursing was a re-definition of nursing to a practice discipline that required dedication and commitment from its adherents. This ideological base was a source of short term strength but of long term weakness for nursing. The stress on dedication, on nursing as a vocation rather than occupation, resulted in an occupational status that was uniquely high for Victorian working women. A question for nursing scholarship is why nursing, especially in comparison with other predominantly female, caring occupations, came to be identified with such high levels of dedication. Are the values of the vocational concept an integral part of nursing professionalisation or simply an aspect of a strategy which is now historical baggage?

This question is particularly pertinent as the identification of nursing with vocational idealism has been both a source of occupational identity and occupational exploitation. A commitment to nursing as a vocation led, in the middle decades of this century, to a distaste for nursing unionism and the reluctance of many nurses to support efforts to improve conditions of work and pay (see for example Strachan 1991, Godden 1990). The consequences of the split between what has been termed the professional and trade union strategies has been the subject of a lively debate (for example McCoppin 1989). Numerous explanations have been given for nurses' reliance on a public recognition of their professionalism and dedication; a reliance which has led to the persistent undervaluing of nursing. One explanation is that nurses were ordered to care in a society which devalued caring (Reverby 1987). The focus in this chapter is on the Victorian ideals of womanhood which influenced the development of a professional identity within nursing. As the legitimacy of these values declined in the wider society their utility to nursing also declined. The question that such historical scholarship leaves for current nurses is to what extent is nursing professionalism still hindered by Victorian notions of womanhood.

Florence Nightingale revisited

A major influence on the development of modern nursing was the ideal of womanhood held by Florence Nightingale and her contemporaries in the Victorian age (1837-1901). Nightingale dominated general nursing from 1854-56, when she was in charge of nurses during the Crimean War. She left an enduring legacy of nursing ideology and philosophy. This legacy is shrouded in myth and, like the personality of Nightingale herself, characterised by contradictions and ambiguities. In modern terms, she was a radical conservative, someone who accepted the basic structures of society while advocating drastic changes in the manifestations of those structures. Nightingale, in Strachey's (1948) analogy, was not an ugly duckling who found her identity among the swans, but an eagle born to a family of swans. Rejecting her decorative destiny as a swan, she became instead an eagle, soaring high, dominating, inspiring awe and, inter alia, resolutely redefining nursing.

Nightingale's redefinition of nursing quickly spread to the British colonies, including Australia. At least one nurse, partly trained under the Nightingale system at St. Thomas' Hospital, joined the gold rushes of the 1850s and migrated to Australia. Margaret Clarke (nee Wilkie) nursed the poor on the goldfields and later founded a Home and Training School for Nurses in Sydney (Godden 1983). It was not until 1868, however, that organised Nightingale nursing came to Australia. This occurred with the appointment of a 'Nightingale' trainee, Lucy Osburn, as Lady Superintendent to Sydney Infirmary (later Sydney Hospital). Lucy Osburn attracted enthusiastic recruits from the colonial middle class. One recruit was Nora Barton, daughter of graziers Robert and Emily Barton, and later aunt of poet 'Banjo' Paterson. Osburn and her enthusiastic trainees were responsible for the gradual spread of Nightingale ideals throughout the colony. When Lucy Osburn resigned in 1884, general nursing in Australia was firmly based on Nightingale principles.

The timing of the introduction of the Nightingale system to Britain and Australia was crucial. The 1860s to 1880s were decades when 'the woman question' was being earnestly and publicly debated. Both sides to the debate, however, shared many assumptions about the nature of women. These assumptions were the basis of Nightingale's vision of the reformed nurse. In revolutionising nursing, Nightingale used and epitomised Victorian ideology about women while simultaneously offering a radically new role for middle class women.

Three central tenets of Victorian ideology

At the very core of Victorian beliefs about women lay three tenets and the highest accolades were bestowed on women who, inter alia, conformed to these. The first tenet was the ideal of womanhood summarised in the concept of the lady; the second was that women should do only unpaid work for the welfare of her family, church or the poor; and the third was that women and men operated in separate spheres.

In transforming nursing, Nightingale could not avoid being influenced by these ideals. To have any social legitimacy for middle class women, reformed nursing needed, at the very least, to appear consistent with these ideals. It is important to note that, to the Victorians, appearances could be as important as reality. What we may call hypocrisy was often a deep conviction that ideals should be upheld even if they were not consistently practised. In effect, this meant that the image of nursing assumed as much importance as the reality of nursing. Certainly, as Baly (1987) has demonstrated, Nightingale was able to effect radical changes on the image while the reality was less altered.

None of these Victorian assumptions and ideals about women could be met by working class women. Working class women did not have the leisure to display the lifestyle and appearance of a 'lady'. They also transgressed the second tenet completely—not only did they work, but they did manual labour which had low status for both men and women. To compound matters, they undertook waged work. Volunteer work was acceptable under Victorian ideology; that same work when paid was unacceptable. When the paid work was outside the confines of a home and family, such as factory work, it transgressed the dominant mores even more.

The ideal for middle and upper class women then was that they would not do manual work; they would not accept payment for any work; and that any such activity would be discreetly undertaken within a home, preferably their own. As Blake (1990) has noted, 'What was not acceptable was a middle-class woman earning a salary in a professional job and achieving a level of independence from men and from family'. 'Ladies', that term denoting the highest status women, generally did not work for a living: such middle class women who did do so were re-cast as 'gentlewomen', having lost status. It is a measure of Nightingale's radicalism and achievement that some of her lady superintendents and matrons were among the few exceptions to this rule.

The third assumption by Victorians was that men and women were basically different. This is the opposite to the currently prevailing view in Western society that men and women are fundamentally alike, with relatively superficial differences. The Victorian belief was that men and women were—physically, spiritually, sexually and psychologically—fundamentally different. This ideology led to a homosocial world where it was believed that only women could really understand and be friends with another woman; only a man could understand another man. These assumptions were articulated in the doctrine of the 'separate spheres'.

The doctrine of the separate spheres meant, in essence, that Victorian men and women were viewed as moving in separate world spheres and each sex was legitimately accorded power over their own sphere. Men claimed the largely 'public' sphere of politics, finance and employment while women claimed the largely 'private' sphere of home and children. It was seen as natural and proper for women to defer to men in this largely public sphere; and just as natural for men to defer to women in matters especially relating to child-raising and house-keeping. In practice, the distinction between appropriate male/public and female/private spheres was blurred and was being constantly negotiated. This was particularly so as women's supremacy over matters relating to the home and to the understanding of children and other women was not restricted to the private sphere. The distinct nature of women was claimed as a reason for public rights including their philanthropic and social reforming activities, and such diverse issues as entry to medical school and the need for women's suffrage. This fluidity in gender roles and the claims of women, especially at times of economic uncertainty, was a source of considerable anxiety. Insomuch as the women's sphere was perceived as expanding and/or threatening the male sphere (or vice versa), conflict was generated.

Conflict also arose over attempts to reject, to various degrees, the notion of female dependency. Victorian women were legally dependants but support for women escaping from this dependency grew during the Victorian era. In some cases, female dependency did not suit the interests of all men. The Married Women's Property Acts, for example, had long been pre-empted by marriage settlements arranged by the fathers of rich women to protect their daughters' property. Furthermore, male power was contested. The domestic tyrant of Victorian literature was not an admired figure. Similarly, the father who willed the guardianship of his children away from that of a 'deserving' mother was seen as abusing his rights. Women were seen as vulnerable and in need of protection and control yet that dependency was mitigated by individual circumstance. It was also mitigated by women having appropriate power over activities that properly belonged to the woman's sphere.

These were key values concerning women in Nightingale's era: they were values which she took for granted and herself epitomised. Nightingale, that egotistical, achieving, towering, radical eagle, was also a product of her class and time. During her long life, she was never an employed worker: even her brief stint as Lady Superintendent of the Invalid Gentlewoman's Institute was a voluntary position (Smith 1982). It was this work which she left to supervise nurses in Crimea. When she returned to England, to immerse herself in government reports and statistics, her name was irrevocably linked with that of nursing. As money poured into the coffers of the Nightingale Fund, she was expected to transform nursing. Nursing was to shed its disreputable aura of lower domestic service and to be opened as a profession for middle class women. These women, like Nightingale, were clamouring for 'moral activity', a worthwhile purpose in life (Nightingale 1978 [1859]). Most, unlike Nightingale, also needed to earn their living.

Redefining nursing

The enormity of the task of redefining nursing as a suitable job for middle class women is easily—almost inevitably—underestimated. Middle class women, in terms of the Victorian ideal outlined above, did not 'work'. The only exception was the profession of governess and they worked within private homes. Even so, governesses were in a vastly over-crowded occupation, socially lonely as they were caught between the upper servants and the employing family, and frequently exploited. As most were lowly-paid, they frequently faced a destitute retirement. The plight of governesses was well documented in the Victorian press and could serve only as a model to avoid for any pioneer of women's employment.

There was a successful model for women's unpaid work which had won public esteem and through which Nightingale herself had achieved international acclaim. Philanthropy, whether of the strictly charitable or broader social reforming model, was the one, and only one, high status public activity open to women in the mid-Victorian era. No other public work by lay women carried as high a status. An analogy is the current situation of females of the British royal family; as Princesses Anne and Diana have demonstrated, philanthropic activity is the surest public activity that results in high public acceptance and approval. Last century, such philanthropic activity by women was generally religiously motivated and carried out under the auspices of a church or sectarian organisation. It was an activity endorsed by Queen Victoria and had many public role models, including such household names as Quaker Elizabeth Fry and Catholic Caroline Chisholm. Women's philanthropy also had part of its roots in the 'lady bountiful' role espoused by centuries of gentry women towards their tenants and poorer villagers. Such individual efforts, however, were increasingly discredited as ineffective and inefficient. Nightingale was one of the many who disparaged and sneered at such individual and unregulated efforts (Nightingale [1859] 1978). High status Victorian philanthropy, in keeping with general trends, became increasingly institutionalised and organised.

Organised sectarian philanthropy by upper and middle class Victorian women was widespread both in England and in Australia (Prochaska 1980, Godden 1983). At a time of minimal social welfare, the philanthropic activities of women were both highly valued and public. To the destitute, such women were frequently the only alternative to other means of survival—severe malnutrition, crime, prostitution and/or the dreaded, brutal, last resort of the workhouse. To the wealthy, philanthropists were equally valued and less resented. By dividing the poor into the 'deserving' and 'undeserving', and giving relief only to the former, philanthropists were able to exercise immense power of social control. Philanthropists demanded gratitude, conservatism and the values of good employees from those they helped. Women philanthropists worked with those they understood best—children, other women and the sick. While male philanthropists were more encompassing, women philanthropists rarely succoured healthy men and both men and women increasingly challenged the appropriateness of men offering philanthropic relief to women.

When Nightingale and Osburn were re-shaping nursing in their respective countries, therefore, philanthropy was the only work whereby women gained status and esteem by working in the public sphere. Furthermore, after the Crimean War Nightingale was the centre of what we now call the cult of the personality. At St. Thomas' Hospital, where the Nightingale system of nurse training began, nurses were and are proud to be called 'Nightingales'. Other nurses also modelled themselves on the perceived virtues of Nightingale and her public work of war-time philanthropy.

The catch was that this highly visible, publicly esteemed work of philanthropy by Victorian ladies such as Nightingale was unpaid, voluntary work. Nightingale's task was to create nursing as an occupation with similar legitimacy and esteem so that it would also attract middle class women. In doing so, she transgressed a number of mores; that 'ladies' did not work; that paid work coarsened and demeaned women; and that women should not work outside the home. Nightingale achieved her goals by disguising the essential nature of nursing as public work by women. She did this by emphasising nursing as work on behalf of others; as women's work under the control of high status women but with a sub-stratum doing the manual work; and as being controlled by women but subordinate to male power. She also stressed the creation of a substitute home for the nursing staff under the control of the Matron. It was a radical act built on a conservative acceptance of assumptions about women and the legitimacy of power.

The expression of nursing as a philanthropic activity with religious overtones was summarised in the concept of the nursing vocation. The stress on the nursing vocation served an important function in attracting women who were genuinely motivated by the ideal to help those in need. The imagery of the nursing vocation was important as a beacon of idealism and sharply contrasted with the frequent drudgery and poverty that characterised women's employment. Public hospitals in the Victorian age were charitable institutions for the destitute and constituted a harsh world where patients were controlled, coerced and frequently discharged for misbehaviour; this world was transformed by the image of womanly caring. Ironically children's hospitals, where patients suffered the most from being forcibly isolated from family and friends, had the gentlest, most appealing image.

The ideal Nightingale nurse was a lady, doing work that was within the woman's sphere and, within the public hospitals at least, with religiously inspired, philanthropic intent. These ideals of 19th century nursing were strongly grounded in Victorian ideology and are examined more fully in the following sections.

Nurses as ladies

A number of authors have suggested that the Victorian concept of the 'lady' was crucial in the development of nursing. One historian, (Kingston 1975) argued that Florence Nightingale 'both created nursing as a profession for women, and lumbered it with some of the most repressive notions of ladylike behaviour ever to emerge from nineteenth-century drawing-rooms...nurses, whatever else they were, were ladies first, and for that doubtful privilege they paid very heavily indeed'.

That Nightingale was able to create nursing as a profession for women, however, was partly because she incorporated it with repressive notions of ladylike behaviour. Nightingale was able to create nursing as a suitable occupation for middle class woman because she identified it with the concept of the lady; because there were very real privileges associated with being 'ladies'.

The problem for nursing, as Kingston (1975) went on to argue, was that the 'notion of "lady" was eroded...[and] the safeguards and privileges that the notion implied also diminished'. An essential part of those 'safeguards and privileges' was the very right of middle class women to participate actively in the public sphere.

Other writers have also argued for the importance of the concept of the lady but have misunderstood the historical meaning of the term. The Victorian concept of 'lady' was one which conferred rights and privileges on high status women. It was a specific and purposeful ideal, and in nursing it was based on the model of Florence Nightingale herself. Victorian ladies were, in practice, generally a far cry from the languishing prisoners of the drawing room that appear in fiction and in the medical literature of the time. The assumption that they were 'relatively passive and subordinate' draws more on current concepts about ladies than Victorian reality (Short & Sharman 1989).

The extent to which Nightingale modelled her ideal of the nurse on the ideal of the lady can be seen by a comparison of descriptions of an ideal 'lady' with that of an ideal 'nurse'. A typical definition of the innate qualities of a lady occurs in one of the many books on Victorian etiquette (anon 1980 [1885]): 'From a lady there exhales a subtle magnetism...Within her influence the diffident grows self-possessed, the impudent are checked, the inconsiderate are admonished; even the rude are constrained to be mannerly, and the refined are perfected'.

Compare that description to Nightingale's equally lyrical description of the ideal nurse (quoted in Seymer 1954): 'A really good nurse must needs be of the highest class of character. It needs hardly be said that she must be: (1) Chaste, in the sense of the Sermon in the Mount; a good nurse should be the Sermon on the Mount in herself. It should naturally seem impossible to the most unchaste to utter even an immodest jest in her presence'.

The tone and expectations of the two articles are similar. The assumption was that control of self led to perfection in manner and character which resulted in the control of others, including the most rude and unchaste. Implicit in this concept is the assumption that both ladies and nurses were responsible for, and could control, the behaviour of others. As Dean and Bolton (1980) have outlined, public hospitals in Britain were seen as unruly places where the lower classes exhibited disorder: the concern of the Victorian nurse was to control that potential disorder. The stress on control of patients was equally clear in New South Wales. When Lucy Osburn testified before the Royal Commission into Public Charities about the discharge of patients, for example, she frequently cited the reason as being disobedience or 'transgression of the rules' rather than cure. On Osburn's and others' evidence, enforcing the wearing of hospital clothes and a ban on smoking was a major issue for nurses at Sydney Hospital.

Putting ladies in charge of the behaviour of both patients and nurses was seen as a solution to potential disorder. Nightingale stressed that nursing was the 'only case, queens not excepted, where a woman is really in charge of men' (quoted in Seymer 1954). The common solution to this uncommon case was to obtain 'ladies capable, by their intellectual attainments and moral power, of maintaining discipline and exercising the administrative authority of a ward sister' (Royal Commission report 1874). Under the Nightingale system, as introduced by Lucy Osburn into Sydney Hospital, there was a clear demarcation between nurses and the supervisory sisters. This demarcation was in accord with Nightingale's assumption that ladies would superintend while others did the 'coarse, thankless, uphill work' of nursing (quoted in Holton 1984).

Working class women were recruited and retained as nurses with no promotion into supervisory positions. Lucy Osburn, in keeping with Nightingale, believed that a woman 'may be an excellent nurse, and yet not suited for a sister' (Royal Commission evidence 1873). The reason for this lack of suitability was connected with the nurse's class, or in the Victorian code, a lack of 'sufficient education' combined with a lack of 'moral power' (Royal Commission evidence 1873). Being ladylike was vital. In Osburn's words, sisters needed to be 'as quiet, steady people as we can get' for it was expected that they would lead 'a dull, lonely life'. Nurses, on the other hand were 'a merry set, and like music and dancing, and that sort of thing' (Royal Commission evidence 1873). It was clear 'that sort of thing' were not ladylike pursuits.

Paralleling these attitudes to working class nurses, the Royal Commissioners accepted in their Report on Sydney Hospital (1874) that 'there is part of the hospital nursing service which should be undertaken by ladies, and which ladies alone are fitted to undertake—the supervision'. 'Ladies' were recruited to be supervisory sisters although, ironically, it was claimed that at Sydney Hospital they were sometimes trained by their subordinates, the nurses (Royal Commission evidence 1873). The title 'sister' was seen as essential in defining and defending the occupant's ladylike status. When the title was temporarily replaced with that of 'Head Nurse', Lucy Osburn considered that the position was 'scarcely that of a lady' as 'nurses disliked being controlled by a nurse' of similar status to themselves (Royal Commission evidence 1873).

There was little dispute within nursing that supervisory positions belonged ideally to women with the class and status of ladies. There was, after all, little other way of making such appointments as training was so brief. Lucy Osburn's qualifications were described as 'a very complete training' (Royal Commission report 1874). This training comprised visits to continental hospitals, one year at St. Thomas' and three months work (Royal Commission evidence 1873-74). A training to be a sister within the Nightingale system generally meant rapid promotion. This applied even to nurses such as Frances Gillam Holden. An Australian nurse, she was dismissed as an 'incompetent' probationer by Lucy Osburn, who considered her 'dreadfully disagreeable' (Briggs 1983, Osburn 1875). Despite this, Holden was appointed Lady Superintendent to the Hospital for Sick Children (now Royal Alexandra Hospital for Children) just five years later.

There was an additional reason for the desire for nursing to be associated with ladies. Nurses, especially in the Victorian age, were breaking strong taboos regarding viewing nudity and understanding the body in its physical and sexual dimensions (Lawler 1991). As supervisors, 'Sisters' were only partly removed from the sanctions of breaking such strong taboos. This reality of nursing work reinforced the need for nurses to be identified with, and senior nurses to be, ladies because ladies were 'pure'. Only the maverick nurse was able to challenge the taboo itself. One such was Frances Gillam Holden. When Lady Superintendent of the Children's Hospital in Sydney, Holden wrote a spirited attack on the idea that knowledge of the body, 'this pure, wise, noble knowledge...' was 'improper' (Holden 1887). Few nurses, if any, followed her lead. More commonly nurses developed work practices that helped defend them against the stigma of supposedly improper knowledge. These defences included the ritual covering of a patient's body when it was being washed. During the 20th century, the adoption by nurses of 'task' nursing (where a patient was viewed as a series of nursing tasks to be undertaken separately rather than on a holistic basis) was necessitated by the skill levels of student nurses. That it was adopted so enthusiastically is an indication that it also served as a defence against the stigma and taboos of acknowledging the body in its totality.

An important qualification to the above argument is that most nurses and sisters appear to have been, in Australia as well as Britain, 'ordinary women who needed to earn their living' rather than ladies (Dingwall et al 1988). The hope that supervisory nurses would always be ladies, rather than 'ordinary women', did not long survive the reality of insufficient numbers of 'ladies' being recruited to, and remaining in, nursing. A few hospitals in Australia (for example, Children's in Sydney) tried to set up the system where selected nursing students entered as 'lady probationers' with special privileges (Hipsley 1952). The system of unpaid lady volunteers, disliked by Nightingale, was also mooted (Royal Commission report 1873-74). Even Sydney Hospital's separate recruitment of sisters did not long survive.

Despite the realities of women's employment, the assumption remained that a senior nurse needed the authority that, outside the hospital, only flowed to women with the class and status of a lady. To boost this authority, a system of rigid hospital etiquette developed within nursing which eventually rested on the basis of seniority. The hierarchy within nursing meant that the senior nurses were treated as supervising ladies, regardless of their status outside the hospital. Even this century, most admiring descriptions by nurses of Matrons stress the qualities of an ideal Victorian lady, including unruffled claim, poise and aloofness (Godden 1990-3). The similarity of the ideal nurse and the ideal Victorian lady was also evident in nursing magazines (for example Australasian Nurses' Journal 1923).

Under this later modification of the Nightingale system, senior nurses were accorded the respect and deference due to ladies by the public, junior nurses and patients. Their status was considered to have a direct impact on imparting order and calm in 'their' wards and obtaining the confidence of the patients. This status was reinforced by symbols and in particular, by the symbolism of nursing uniforms. The caps and uniforms worn by junior nurses indicated that they did the domestic work associated with nursing such as cleaning the wards and patients. In contrast, the white uniforms, and particularly the long veils, of sisters and matrons publicly proclaimed that their work was supervisory rather than menial: a crucial distinction when determining occupational status.

The influence of 19th century ideology, however, also meant that even ladies had to work within the woman's sphere, that is, undertake activities seen as uniquely appropriate to women. It was therefore crucial to the success of Nightingale's reforms that nursing was defined as within the woman's sphere.

Work within the woman's sphere

The concept of a separate sphere of activity for women meant that ladies had power and status over their own sphere of activity and over their own sex. Ambition was directed at controlling their own sphere rather than challenging the power of their male counterparts. Nightingale and other nursing leaders aimed to define nursing so that it would be accepted as part of the woman's sphere and not a challenge to male authority. It is consistent with this belief in separate spheres that Nightingale would insist that women control nursing and not enter medicine, an occupation which was (and largely remains) a male domain.

Ensuring that nurses were females was the first requirement in identifying nursing as being within the woman's sphere. General hospital nursing in Australia, prior to 1868, appears to have been predominantly a male occupation as males predominated amongst charity inmates and patients were nursed by their own sex. At Sydney Infirmary before Osburn's arrival, for example, there were five nurses and twelve 'wardsmen' (Royal Commission evidence 1873-74). Although it can be debated whether the term 'wardsman' can be equated with 'nurse', it is clear that the displacement of such men from wards was achieved consistently as part of the Nightingale reforms. Nowhere was this more explicit than when The Alfred Hospital in Melbourne opened its Nightingale nursing school in 1880. It stressed that nursing was a woman's occupation by adopting the motto which translated as 'Where there is not a woman, there the sick man groans' (Mitchell 1977).

For nursing to be accepted as being within the woman's sphere it also had to assume a hierarchical structure. The woman's sphere was never a democratic ideal of 'sisterhood' as that would potentially challenge the structures of male society. Given the gender inequalities of the society, women could not (and perhaps, cannot), gain control over an occupation that employed both men and women. Therefore, their only hope was to limit that occupation to women and gain control over members of their own sex. A strictly gender-segregated, class-based hierarchal work force was, at this stage, a logical way to establish an occupation that could be controlled by middle class ladies.

Nightingale argued explicitly for such a hierarchical work force segregated by gender. In Australia, her views were publicised by the propagandising efforts of the New South Wales Royal Commission into Public Charities in 1873-74. The Royal Commissioners consistently attributed all the ills in social welfare provision to the intrusion of men in the woman's sphere, and evoked Nightingale to support the claim that women had to be in charge of women because 'in disciplinary matters a woman only can understand a woman' (Royal Commission report 1873-4). Nightingale actually wrote the more militant 'A man can never govern a woman' in a private letter to Sir William Windeyer, the Commission's chairman (Nightingale 1874). Such a view is consistent with Nightingale's call for a 'clear and recorded definition of the limits of these two [male medical and female nursing] classes of jurisdiction' (Royal Commission evidence 1873). It is also consistent with Nightingale's summation of her work in changing nursing: 'The whole reform in Nursing both at home and abroad has consisted in this: to take all power over the Nursing out of the hands of the men and put it into the hands of *one female trained head*, and make her responsible for everything regarding internal management and discipline being carried out' (quoted in Vicinus 1985. Emphasis in the original). With such statements, Nightingale firmly claimed general nursing as being wholly within the woman's sphere.

Nightingale also insisted on nurses' obedience to (predominantly male) doctors with such phrases as 'it is unquestionably the duty of the Nurses to obey [medical orders]...' (Nightingale quoted in Brodsky 1968). This insistence, along with a ritualised deference, was echoed in the first chapters of nursing textbooks (with titles such as 'Ethics and Hospital Etiquette') for at least a hundred years (for example Doherty et al 1963). Although nurses also had an obligation to refuse to participate in unethical procedures, the stress was on loyalty and obedience. This stress was indicative of female subordination and paved the way for crippling medical domination.

In its initial form, however, the stress on nursing obedience can also be interpreted as a shrewd understanding of the problems of women exercising authority in a male dominated society. Looked at in this light, nurses' obedience to doctors can be seen as a trade-off: Nightingale was equally insistent on nurses' control over nursing as she was on obedience to doctors. Nurses would obey doctors' medical orders but those doctors had no rights to direct nursing work or to discipline an individual nurse. Nursing was under the control of the most senior nurse and all complaints had to go through her. Osburn quoted a Nightingale pamphlet to stress both these points: 'Vest the whole responsibility for nursing, internal management, for discipline, and training...of nurses in one female head of the nursing staff...she [the head] must be responsible that their [doctors'] orders about the treatment of the sick are strictly carried out' (Royal Commission evidence 1873-74). This 'trade-off' was a way of preserving the authority of those women in charge of the woman's sphere of nursing. As long as the medical orders of doctors were obeyed, senior nurses could exercise authority in their own right, over what they called 'their' nurses, with little fear of challenge from that potentially rival source of power, the doctors.

As hospitals became larger, segregation of junior nurses from doctors was also used to preserve authority. Olson has noted the rarity of references to physicians by nurses in the American hospital he studied (Olson 1993). These segregated worlds of nurses and doctors, paralleling the women's and men's spheres, also were manifested in Australia. By the 20th century, senior nurses ensured that doctors could not over-ride their control of junior nurses by the simple expedient of segregation: junior nurses were not allowed to talk to doctors and after-hours socialisation was discouraged. One nurse recalled a typical incident during her training at Balmain Hospital (Sydney) in the 1930s in which she 'delivered the message directly to the doctor'. As she soon discovered, 'that was the worst crime I could have committed nursing etiquette wise' (Mary C 1990). It was the worst crime because it potentially challenged, however unwittingly, the concept of the separate spheres and therefore undermined nursing authority.

The Victorian world view, however, demanded more than a hierarchical woman's sphere controlled by ladies. To be accorded legitimacy, women's work within the public sphere had to be demonstratively philanthropic, that is, offer assistance to the poor and less fortunate. As mentioned above, this philanthropy generally had strong religious overtones. Nursing had traditionally been identified with charity because training took place within charitable institutions. For more complex reasons, including the influence of the nursing nuns, nursing charity had strong religious overtones.

Philanthropy and religion

Nineteenth century public hospitals were charitable institutions for the sick poor. The transition of hospitals to institutions for the use of the general public varied greatly, although within New South Wales it had generally been achieved by the first world war. During Nightingale's lifetime, however, all Nightingale nurses were trained within those charitable institutions, public hospitals. Nurses in hospitals such as Royal Prince Alfred (Sydney) were constantly reminded that their nursing was an act of charity to the sick poor (Forsyth 1994). Nightingale's own brief periods of nursing training all took place in charitable religious institutions, most notably the hospital run by deaconesses at Kaiserwerth, Germany. Within these institutions, nursing was literally an act of religion as well as charity.

Nightingale also attempted training with nursing nuns in Paris and appears to have contemplated becoming a nun. The example of nursing nuns was an important influence on the ideal of the lady nurse working within her separate women's sphere. In Australia, the influence both of Protestant and Catholic nuns was strongly felt. Nominally a secular institution, Sydney Hospital was a Protestant bastion and an alternative to the Catholic St Vincent's Hospital. Lucy Osburn faced constant criticism because of her high church Anglicanism and her brief adoption of the title Lady Superior. This did not stop her friends amongst the senior nurses referring to her as 'our beloved Lady', and one of her favourite head nurses at Sydney Hospital left to join an Anglican order (Moule 1875). Catholic nuns were also highly influential, particularly the Sisters of Charity, the first nursing nuns in Australia. The ideal of service in fiercely autonomous orders was a characteristic feature of nursing nuns and leading nuns in Australia were explicitly and consistently conceptualised as 'ladies' (for example, Godden 1983). Catholic nursing nuns were ladies also with a tradition of defending their autonomy against the encroachment of archbishops and doctors alike (Godden 1983).

Whether from a Catholic or Protestant source, religious imagery and exhortations to be 'other-worldly' permeated nursing. One example is an article about the nurses at the (public) Children's Hospital in the *Illustrated Sydney News* (7 March 1889) headed 'Working for Good'. The author of this article described the Matron as 'our Hospital Madonna of the grave, sweet face and rich, sad voice'. Also very clear in its religious, altruistic overtones, was the so-called Nightingale pledge (written by an American nurse in 1893 and repeated by generations of hospital trained nursing students throughout the western world):

> I solemnly pledge myself before God and in the presence of this assembly to pass my life in purity and to practise my profession faithfully. I will do all in my power to elevate the standard of my profession... [and ended] With loyalty will I endeavour to aid the physician in his work and to devote myself to the welfare of those committed to my care.

Similarly explicit in its religious overtones was the message to the lay nursing students at the Catholic St Vincent's Hospital in Sydney who were publicly exhorted to: 'remember that no sordid love of gain, no low selfish aims should urge them onward in the path of duty...they must be/Consecrated, set apart/ Unto a life of sympathy/These must be their aims; these their lofty ideals...thus only will the art of nursing be transformed into the highest Christian virtue...' (St Vincent's Hospital Annual Report 1910).

Even in 1949, the Minister for Health in NSW described the ideal nurse as one 'who [would] feel a spiritual urge for the work' (Kelly 1949). The sentiment was put in more secular terms by the eminent nurse tutors, Doherty, Sirl and Ring (1963), 'Service to mankind is the primary function of nurses and the reason for the existence of the nursing profession'. One can be justifiably cynical about employers who encouraged nurses to eschew material for spiritual rewards. However, such an ideal was central to the Victorian ideal of womanhood, and justified the special status and professional identity of nursing.

Impact of Victorian ideals upon nursing

One impact of the Nightingale revolution in nursing was that the concept of the nursing 'vocation' became fundamental to nursing ideology. This identification with dedication and caring drew on a number of sources, including the legacy of nursing monks and nuns and the deaconesses at Kaiserwerth. However, the centrality of the nursing vocation was not an inevitable continuation of earlier trends but part of a deliberate choice by Florence Nightingale. In particular, Nightingale chose to locate reformed nursing training in the context of Victorian public hospitals. Such places allowed student nurses access to patients on which to practise. However, they also were charities catering for the destitute poor, were only partly within the female sphere, and were disreputable. The major problem then confronting Nightingale, so I have argued, is that Nightingale had to preserve the status of women working in such a disreputable, public sphere. Nursing pioneers like

Nightingale and Osburn attempted to both legitimise, and give high status to, middle class women working as nurses in the public sphere. As progressive as these ideas were, they were still grounded in the contemporary Victorian ideology and did not challenge common assumptions about the nature of women. The most successful model of women working in the public sphere and maintaining status as ladies were the voluntary, religiously motivated, charitable ladies. In addition, Nightingale herself had the class and status of a lady and won renown through charitable action. The 'new' nurse was to be created in the image of Nightingale and other charitable ladies; an image which would share (albeit to a lesser extent) Nightingale's own purposefulness and high status. In practice, however, the contradictions between the ideal lady and the nursing reality could only partly be resolved. As the 19th century ideal of the lady faded, nursing ideology became increasingly out of step with the needs of its practitioners.

The Victorian ideological basis of nursing was a source of occupational status and was designed to justify women working, and working within the public sphere. Part of that justification was that the work was not 'work' as defined by males. Nursing was instead caring activity sited in a charitable context and insulated from male interference. On the basis of this, nursing demanded professional status from a world which should value altruistic ladies. The extent of the contradictions and ambiguities within nursing was later evident in disputes over nurses' working conditions. These disputes centred around conflict between the strategies of unionism and professionalism. The unionist strategy saw nursing primarily as work and identified nurses as workers in the public sphere. Those holding to the professional strategy partly put their faith in the special status of nurses—nurses by their high personal and professional standards winning respect, status and commensurate monetary rewards (Godden 1993).

Conclusion

The Victorian ideal of womanhood was central in the development of the ideological basis of general nursing. This identification of nurses with ideal images of Victorian womanhood conferred status and prestige upon the fledgeling profession. Such identification also gave an ideological focus to nursing work and a justification for women working in the public sphere. Now, however, the identification of nursing with Victorian values is no longer a source of strength. The ideal of the lady has faded and the right of women to work in the public sphere is rarely contested. It was with this legacy of Victorian ideology that leading nurses in the 20th century attempted to develop a professional identity for nursing. Their compromises, achievements and failures are reflected in the discipline and practice of nursing today. The challenge for nurses today is to distinguish between those values which are the essence of nursing and those that need to be jettisoned along with the accompanying Victorian ideology.

ACKNOWLEDGEMENTS

This chapter is partly based on my paper 'We are professional women' presented at Nursing, Women's History and the Politics of Welfare Conference, University of Nottingham (UK), July 1993. My thanks to Patricia Clark for her generous sharing of letters by and about Lucy Osburn in the National Library, Canberra.

REFERENCES

Anon 1980 Australian etiquette [1885]. J M Dent, Melbourne
Australasian Nurses' Journal, 15 September 1923, pp 452,454
Baly M 1987 The Nightingale nurses: the myth and the reality. In: Maggs C (ed) Nursing history: the state of the art. Croom Helm, Beckenham, pp 33-59
Blake C 1990 The charge of the parasols. Women's Press, London
Briggs B 1983 Holden, Frances Gillam. In: Nairn B, Serle G (eds) The Australian dictionary of biography, vol. 9. Melbourne University Press, pp 328-329
Brodsky I 1968 Sydney's nurse crusaders. Old Sydney Free Press, Sydney
C, Mary Interview with author, 9 November 1990. Transcript held by author
Dean M, Bolton G 1980 The administration of poverty and the development of nursing practice in nineteenth century England. In: Davies C (ed) Rewriting nursing history. Croom Helm, London, ch 4
Dingwall R, Rafferty A M, Webster C 1988 An introduction to the social history of nursing. Routledge, London
Doherty M, Sirl M, Ring O 1963 Modern practical nursing procedures, 10th edn. Dymocks, Sydney
Forsyth S 1994 Professionalisation and nursing: an historical perspective. Master of Arts thesis, Sydney University
Godden J 1983 Philanthropy and the woman's sphere. PhD thesis, Macquarie University
Godden J 1990 The unionisation of nurses. In: Radi H (ed) Jessie Street. Documents and essays. Women's Redress Press, Sydney
Godden J 1990-93 Interviews of nurses. Transcripts held by author
Godden J 1993 We are professional women: nursing as philanthropic work within the woman's sphere, Australia 1880-1930. Paper at Nursing, Women's History and the Politics of Welfare Conference, University of Nottingham (UK), July
Hipsley P 1952 The early history of the Royal Alexandra Hospital for Children, Sydney. Angus & Robertson, Sydney
Holden F G 1887 The gospel of physical salvation. The Sydney Quarterly Magazine IV(3):203-210
Holton S 1984 Feminine authority and social order: Florence Nightingale's conception of nursing and health care. Social Analysis 15(August):59-101
Illustrated Sydney News, 7 March 1889:10
Kelly C 1949 letter to United Associations for Women. December, MLMSS 2/60 ADD-On 1317 Box 1(2)
Kingston B 1975 My wife, my daughter and poor Mary Ann. Nelson, Melbourne
Lawler J 1991 Behind the screens. Nursing, somology and the problem of the body. Churchill Livingstone, Melbourne
McCoppin B 1989 The use and abuse of industrial power, the professional dilemma. In: Gray G, Pratt R (eds) Issues in Australian nursing 2. Churchill Livingstone, Melbourne
Mitchell A 1977 The hospital south of the Yarra. Alfred Hospital, Melbourne

Moule G 1875 letter to Nora Murray-Prior, 29 July. Murray-Prior papers, NLA MS7801, 16/110 Box 4, folder 22

Nightingale F 1874 letter to Sir William Windeyer, 22 March. Windeyer Papers, MSSPI, series 22/1-2, Sydney University archives

Nightingale F 1978 Cassandra [1859]. In: Strachey R (ed) The cause. A short history of the women's movement in Great Britain. Virago, London, appendix I

Olson T 1993 Laying claim to caring: professionalization, gender and the language of training, 1915-1937. Paper presented at Nursing, Women's History and the Politics of Welfare Conference, University of Nottingham (UK), July, pp. 1-20

Osburn L 1875 letter to Nora Murray-Prior, 15 October. Murray-Prior papers, NLA MS7801, 23/4

Prochaska F K 1980 Women and philanthropy in 19th century England. Oxford University Press, Oxford

Reverby S 1987 Ordered to care. The dilemma of American nursing. Cambridge University Press, Cambridge

Royal Commission into Public Charities 1873-74 Report and evidence. Votes and proceedings of the New South Wales Legislative Assembly, vol. VI, Sydney, pp 78-262

St Vincent's Hospital 1910 Annual report. St. Vincent's Hospital, Sydney

Seymer L 1954 (ed) Selected writings of Florence Nightingale. Macmillan, New York

Short S, Sharman E 1989 Dissecting the current nursing struggle in Australia. In: Lupton G, Najman J (eds) Sociology of health and illness. Australian readings. Macmillan, Melbourne, pp 225-235

Smith F B 1982 Florence Nightingale. Reputation and power. Croom Helm, London

Strachan G 1991 Sacred office, trade or profession? The dilemma of nurses' industrial activities in Queensland, 1900 to 1950. Labour History, 61(November):147-163

Strachey L 1948 Eminent Victorians [1918]. Penguin, Harmondsworth, ch. 2

Vicinus M 1985 Independent women. Virago, London, ch. 3

15

The discursive formation of caring

LIZA HESLOP, JENNIFER OATES

Introduction

This chapter identifies and maps the discursive formation of caring in nursing knowledge, as revealed by the history of nursing in Australia. It describes caring discourses from one epoch to another and focuses on nurses' struggle for meaning as they have acquired the knowledge and practices of a particular era. Extant caring scholarship tends to emphasise a natural and certain reality and focuses on human experiences and values, which, we contend, leaves hidden other possible descriptions (e.g. a socially constructed reality). One consequence of this legacy is to insufficiently address the conception and operation of power and its influence on caring knowledge and practices. We attempt a political examination of the multiple, pregnant and contradictory meanings that have shaped nursing and given it identity. A genealogical method, derived from Foucault's poststructuralism, shows how different understandings and practices of caring have come into being and have governed nursing practices and scholarship in different historical epochs. Commencing in the 18th century, five successive historical epochs are identified, each producing different understandings of nurse caring.

Extant literature on caring

Florence Nightingale is acclaimed for her role in defining nurse caring, differentiating it from medical therapeutics and curing—the realm of doctors. She is cited frequently for laying the foundation of modern nursing. Caring, seen as a particular province of nursing, is specified as denoting the separation of the discipline and practice of nursing from that of medicine. Contemporary caring literature, largely informed by the humanist position of Western thought, has generated renewed interest in caring as a formative domain of nursing and a large amount of literature has emerged. This interest has been largely North American. An important albeit smaller scholarship has developed in Australia.

Morse et al (1990) have provided a typology of caring based on an examination of the North American nursing literature. They identified five concepts of caring: an innate trait; a moral imperative and ideal; an affect; a nurse-patient interrelationship; and a therapeutic intervention. They found that the breadth of the concepts of caring were confusing for practising nurses, and favoured caring being developed as a measure of practice outcomes, promoting the professionalism of the nurse. Caring has been favoured by Chinn (1991) as a framework for developing nursing knowledge. Specifically there are three nursing theories (not all scholars agree on their theoretical status) which use caring as a central organising concept: Watson's 'Human Science and Human Care' (1985); Leininger's 'Transcultural Nursing: Concepts, Theories and Practices' (1991); and Benner and Wrubel's (1988) 'Primacy of Caring'.

Two broad approaches in the contemporary North American literature are evident: a humanistic orientation, which is more significant, where caring is valued as an essence, having moral value, and represents the goal of nursing activity; and, to a lesser extent, a sociological perspective, where caring in nursing is linked to the history of women in society and their relative powerlessness compared to men. From a humanistic perspective Noddings (1984) and Watson (1990), claim caring to be grounded in women's experiences and focus attention on the subjective (feeling and experiences), affirming a naturalistic orientation of females towards caring and healing roles in society. Humanistic caring as the central concern of nursing activity and knowledge development, acts to ballast the perceived adoption of increasingly technical, rational 'positivist' values and practices in health care and nursing.

Hagell (1988), Reverby (1987) and MacPherson (1989) adopt a sociological perspective, still grounding caring in women's experiences, but exploring the social basis and context of caring within a history of women and of nurse caring. They draw attention to the shared history of women and nurses that struggled to promote the value of caring in a society that imposed a culture of male-based science, privileging positivist, empirico-analytical methodologies.

Australian scholars have not given as much attention to caring as a concept in nursing as their North American counterparts, but there are important developments in the local literature. A sociological perspective is taken by Dunlop (1988) and Speedy (1991), where caring is examined as a social product/activity in nursing, mainly done by women. Dunlop explores the historical changes in the social organisation of caring, highlighting how women were drawn into caring activities through the division of labour along female/male lines. Hooft (1987) is informed by humanistic/interpretative approaches, drawing upon moral philosophy to define caring as commitment by a nurse to professional outcomes based on the health of a client.

Poststructuralism

The theory informing this chapter is poststructuralism, a sociological theory that enables, through a genealogical method, the exploration of the social and historical basis of nursing knowledge and practice. Poststructuralism developed out of the work of French cultural analysts, including Foucault, Derrida, and Lacan, who focused on the role of language in the study of social organisation. Poststructuralist theory is not a cohesive whole, but has produced a wide range of literature informing a range of disciplines. Broadly, poststructural literature has challenged the ontological adequacy of logical empirical and interpretative positions in science, and refers to the production of truth as socially constructed. What is challenged is the notion that truth, the subject and reality are separate and independent from the social conditions that made them possible. The key theoretical concepts adopted in this chapter are from the work of Foucault and include; discourse, knowledge/power, pastoral governmentality and genealogy. Cultural imperialism, as articulated by Said (1993), is also employed in this chapter. Though not strictly a poststructuralist theoretical concept, imperialism has relevance for evaluating the degree to which discourses from one country can come to dominate discourses in another.

A discourse, Foucault (1970) argued, is produced by a series of statements forming a representation of a subject or object that is given force by its setting or utterer. Patterns of statements are termed 'discursive formations'. Caring as such is a discursive formation made possible under certain social 'conditions of possibility'. Foucault argued that discursive formations are hierarchical, having 'thresholds of epistemiologisation', the category of science having the highest level. A pattern of statements, setting out the conditions in which a discourse is regarded as true, under rules and laws, can become regarded as constituting a science.

'Power' in a Foucauldian sense is relational, that is, it operates in conditions of resistance. Knowledge and truth are political in nature; a person is subject to the functions of discourses that socialise, describe, and shape the individual, yet are restraining, coercing and limiting (Racevskics 1988). When knowledge fails to command adherence, an injuncture (that is, a move, a shift) occurs and new knowledge is generated. Power/knowledge then is productive, not simply a system of domination or repression.

Pastoral governmentality denotes power relations, exercised in transactional terms, commanding the particular way people can speak of themselves (During 1992). The concept is derived from early Christendom where power relations that existed between the pastorate and their parishioners framed and classified identities and moulded practices in Christian discourses. The practice of confessionals produced the disciplinary power where parishioners came to understand themselves. Foucault (1971) argued that this form of pastoral power is now constituted in the identity of professions, and exercised in relationships of health, welfare and education. This new form of pastoral power moulds a particular kind of individual or professional.

In contemporary historiography, knowledge is portrayed as a progressive discovery, an objective activity to know the truth, including the truth about the past. Foucault (1972, 1980) has dismissed the apolitical claims of historians, asserting that texts of history are forms of knowledge and power at the same time, affirming the present and becoming self-validating. Foucault's ethic was to convey and expose the closed nature of history, the exclusion of other constitutions and narratives in history. Genealogy is a strategy that permits the 'opening' up and revealing of power and domination of particular discourses, disrupting the continuity of knowledge development and truth claims of professions as presented in science. Foucault claimed that genealogies are '...antisciences.. are opposed to the effects of centralising powers which are linked to the institution and functioning of an organised scientific discourse within a society such as ours' (Foucault 1980).

Genealogy, as informed by Foucault, offers nursing the opportunity to interrogate the historical formation of caring and the uniformity in which it is constituted. Genealogical analysis illuminates the struggles, resistances, discursive and non-discursive practices at the everyday level of nursing practice, that result in a particular discursive formation of caring. Submitting to this analysis opens up the possibility for other constitutions of caring.

Said's (1993) concept of cultural imperialism is employed in this chapter to examine the power of English and North American discursive formations of caring and practices over locally produced, Australian/Indigenous formations. His study of culture and imperialism highlighted the power to narrate and block other narratives, that were produced through the intercourse of trade and travel. He is critical of the immigrant settler society that assumed terra nullius in cultural terms. While not denying that imperial powers have brought benefits in terms of liberal ideas and technology, the violence on and lack of acknowledgment of local cultural identities is undesirable. Said employs Fanon (1968) to illustrate this point:

> The settler makes history; his life is an epoch, an odyssey. He is an absolute beginning. This land was created by us, he is the unceasing cause: 'If we leave all is lost, and the country will go back to the Middle Ages.' Over against him the torpid creatures, wasted by fevers, obsessed by ancestral customs, form an almost inorganic background for the innovating dynamism of colonial mercantilism.

History, Said argued, is trapped and captured in the Western system of knowledge and discipline by the massive force of ideas from one culture (North American) to another, confining the development of a cultural identity that includes 'otherness'—a mixture of cultures and identities. He states: 'Rarely before in human history has there been as massive an intervention of force and ideas from one culture to another as there is today from America to the rest of the world'.

The movement of ideas in nursing knowledge and practice from other countries is worth evaluating for its effects on the formations of local knowledge and practices. Australia has been a site of struggle where cultural identity has been contested amongst settler groups. The massive information and technology transfer flow from the United States and Britain to Australia has great significance on the social organisation of the professions and their practices. Their effect is traced through the periods. The first period examined is early colonial Australia, a part of the 'New World', where the British who had lost the Americas sought to develop a penal colony.

Colonial caring 1788-1870

Nursing care in colonial Australia was delivered primarily in the home, the only organised hospital care being available for the poor, government employees, convicts and soldiers. In the early days of penal settlement male convicts were assigned to the wards of hospitals and gave nursing attention initially. Hospitals were not provided for the free settlers, but, later, charitable organisations provided care for new immigrants suffering from ill-health. Nursing care in these government and charitable institutions was delivered mainly by wardsmen although the overall domestic supervision of these institutions was usually undertaken by the paid office of Matron.

The predominantly English and Irish settlers brought their values, knowledge and practices of health care to the 'New World', impinging upon and overlaying the Aboriginal caring practices with their own. Hansford-Miller (1990) remarks that Europeans at the time of settlement lived in an age of open sewerage and cesspits, and epidemics were common. The 'curing' capacity of physicians, surgeons and apothecaries was minimal. Voltaire had described the medical treatment of the 18th century, as the art of pouring drugs, of which one knew nothing, into a patient of whom one knew less (Keen et al 1976).

Care institutions in Europe had been mainly established in medieval times by religious orders that were informed by virtue ethics and a discourse of moral asceticism. Moral asceticism was constituted in the hope of moral redemption and was governed by disciplinary practices whereby all intellectual and moral effort was directed towards the spiritual and the afterlife (Tarnas 1991). Medieval understandings of human behaviour and purpose were contested by discourses of individual liberty and reason; science held the hope of discovering truth.

New forms of government were conceived, based on concepts of rationally ascertainable individual rights and mutually beneficial social contracts. At the time of colonisation of Australia, Europe was experiencing the consequences of individualism in the form of economic liberalism. The discourse of laissez faire doctrine, supported by Adam Smith and David Ricardo, produced social conditions that resulted in a growing educated group referred to as the bourgeoisie. Significant social disruption (including the French Revolution 1789 and Gordon Riots 1780s in Britain) at the beginning of this period, and the concern about the growing numbers of poor, gave opportunities for revisionist analysis of society that included the discourse of political liberalism.

Political liberalism, supported by noted British philosophers, Bentham and Mill, suggested that the state should take a wider benevolent role in providing for the welfare of its people (utilitarian role) and support for suffrage as a democratic right. Edwin Chadwick's theory, that disease was transmitted by miasma, or bad air, gained considerable adherence in this period. His view of the need for more state intervention in providing public sanitation was consistent with liberal, benevolent discourse. The role of the colonial authorities in providing care for the population was limited to providing accommodation for the 'benevolent', that is, those requiring medical and dietary attention. The 'official' history of caring begins with European settlement, a history constituted in the discourses of Christianity and civility, sanitation and cleanliness.

Civilised Christian caring

'They regard infirm people as a nuisance; it is difficult to follow a nomadic life if many cripples exist, and so these unfortunates are either left to die in some secluded spot, or tapped on the head with a waddy' (Davenport Cleland 1980). The indigenous populations were largely regarded as incapable of conducting themselves in a caring manner. This was explained in popular discourse as due to their lack of civility and christianity. Irish/Australian nurses reinforced the discourses of aboriginal people's uncivilised, pagan nature; Mother Margaret Mullaly commented on the onset of her 'mission' from Ireland to Australia that it allowed her the opportunity to 'sow the seeds of faith and piety in lands still hidden in the darkness of ignorance and error' (Priestly 1990).

Traditional medicine and caring/healing practices of the Aboriginal inhabitants were largely dismissed as superstitious (Hansford-Miller 1990). Their social organisation was considered primitive and savage; native people were held responsible for their own demise. The colonisers were largely ignorant of the complexities of Aboriginal culture and popularised the notion of their 'passing away'—a discourse supported by the science of Social Darwinism. This passing away notion was integrated into popular discourse; one colonial Australian commented:

> Much has been done by philanthropists in attempts to mitigate the hardships and sufferings which appear to invariably dog the footsteps of the savage as soon as he is brought into contact with more civilised men; but, despite the best intentioned efforts that have been made, the Australian native is slowly but surely passing away from the face of the earth (Davenport Cleland 1980).

Colonial Australia displayed the tensions between science and Christianity that still existed in Europe at this time. As the professional ethic of physicians and surgeons developed, religious notions of care and charity were marginalised by secular notions of nobility and care by the health professions. As there were no registration boards to regulate the professions, there was tension as to the legitimate 'right' of people to practise health care. Garrick and Jeffery (1987) describe a trained doctor's objections to a religious minister and his wife's 'right' to administer health care: 'Of course I am aware that Mr. Brown is at liberty to quack if he will, but I think he would be doing his duty as a neighbour if he attend to the bodily ones' (Garrick & Jeffery 1987).

Private caring roles

Concern was held by colonial Governments as to the moral character of former women convicts and the imbalance of the male/female population in general. Women in colonial Australia were encouraged into marriage to promote the stability of the colony and ensure their good character. Gender relations reflected a sexual division of labour—women largely involved in 'reproductive' and 'domestic caring' work and the men involved in the 'productive' work of the market place.

Caring activities centred around caring for children and adults in the home with infectious diseases that included whooping cough, scarlet fever, diphtheria, measles, influenza and typhus. Liberal benevolent discourse enabled women to take up limited public caring roles contesting the dominant private caring discourses of this period. This was mediated by the paternalistic social organisation that largely supervised their caring practices. Women of the upper classes saw charitable activities, and a concern for children's welfare, as part of their responsibility. These women had significant roles in setting up orphanages, homes for destitute girls and benevolent societies. Women could bring to public life 'female traits' and share in housekeeping the State without neglecting their own homes.

Imperial Victorian caring 1870-1901

English notions and systems came to dominate caring during this period. Britain, in particular, had benefitted from the secure resources and markets of its colonies. British imperialism, however, was not motivated simply by economic determinants, but Christianity, commerce and civilisation went hand in hand. The colonies' new inhabitants, whatever their origin, benefitted considerably from the liberal ideas and technologies brought through trade, but the devastation and destruction of indigenous peoples continued.

The role of religious institutions in regulating education, welfare and health diminished throughout the Western world, as governments increasingly intervened in these matters. The Royal Commission into charitable institutions of this period (1890) reflected the government concern of paying patients and who was deserving of welfare, which inevitably had implications for nursing (Cushing 1993). The economic liberalist discourse that had dominated was blamed for the world wide economic recession of the 1890s and social theories and discourses of justice and state intervention were elevated.

As the colonies' population expanded, the number of benevolent societies and hospitals increased to support the indigent. Lucy Osburn, a Nightingale trainee, had arrived in Sydney in 1868, and the influence of the Nightingale system of training, though expensive, began to permeate the colonies. Institutional care was marked by the gradual replacement of male wardsmen with female nurses.

Dedicated supportive philanthropic care

'With reference to female nurses, you can always trust them; you can rely upon having your instructions carried out. When you have male nurses, very often you have them away from duty, and neglecting their duty' (Royal Commission into Charitable Institutions 1890). Despite concern about the suitability of nursing work for females, and its danger to women's 'nature', the government and doctors were persuaded that women's natural nurturing, loyalty and caring characteristics would be advantageous to all. A snippet from the *Argus* newspaper reads: 'There is no work which becomes a woman better than nursing the sick, giving full scope as it does for head, heart and hand, the more intelligent, educated and gentle the woman is, the more likely the work is to be well done' (*Argus* 13 August 1897). The conviction grew in popular discourse that there was a need for 'respectable women' of a 'higher standard' to nurse, with a commitment to rigorous techniques and duties to provide skilled care. The popular representation of Dickens' Betsey Prigg and Sara Gamp, the drunken slovenly nurse/servant, was promoted in a campaign to reform nursing. A correspondent in the Argus newspaper supported the reformation in the Nightingale tradition and stated:

> No longer would our sick and suffering dear ones be at the mercy of Mrs Gamps and Betsey Prigs, whose very presence in the sick room is often worse than the disease they are supposed to combat..No longer should we have to bow down before a temporary tyrant, placating her tantrums, watching with her, and over her, in mortal terror of her too-palpable incompetence (Inglis 1958).

These discourses discounted the religious nursing of Catholic traditions that provided care. The Nightingale tradition broached English middle class values that care of the sick was a natural and acceptable vocation for gentle women of a 'respectable' class. Standards of British nursing were promoted as better than the existing arrangements in the colonies. Mrs Gaffin, an English nurse, giving evidence at the Royal Commission declares: 'The women who nurse, although good and honest, belong more or less to the class they nurse, and see things from much the same point of view. They may, and no doubt do, bring much comfort to legs and rheumatic joints, but there their influence ends' (Royal Commission into Charitable Institutions 1890).

The philanthropic discourse dominated the service of caring. Philanthropy developed in the Christian and liberal ideas of European society and was constituted in duty, charity, and welfare. The centrality of moral ideals in defining behaviour were consistent with paternalistic Victorian notions of femininity. The growing popularity of the Nightingale nurse and the influence of these romantic philanthropic notions shaped nursing practices and allowed nursing to become a worthwhile occupation

The British Victorian notion of care became firmly embedded in nursing and excluded other discursive formations—despite the influx of non-British immigrants during the gold-rush years. Again, notions of civilised care marginalised other formations. Practices of benevolence were exercised by nurses and doctors in care for migrants and indigenous Australians, and examples of missionary zeal can be found. The conceptualisation of illness as disease and the organisations for care, that came with European settlement, were not congruent with the social and sacred explanations of indigenous peoples: 'The hospital would make room, if necessary for the natives; but since a patient who was hopelessly ill, and was sent to the native camp, died, the natives have a suspicion against coming. The natives receive relief as outpatients' (Report of The Royal Commission into Charitable Institutions 1871).

Applied housekeeping

'...women of education like the work from a scientific point of view, whereas it often becomes a drudgery to people of the other class'(Royal Commission into Charitable Institutions 1890). There developed a 'domestic technology' of plumbing, gas lighting and cooking, and the nurse was depicted as being a household manager of the hospital economy. Nurse caring during this period followed the Nightingale sanitary doctrine, promoting the order and cleanliness of the environment to allow healing to occur. Theoretical and practical nursing knowledge was introduced whereby the Lady Superintendent instructed nurses in the domestic management of the wards. Observation of patients was loosely formulated; there was some charting of temperatures. Instruction had more moral significance. The discursive practices of sanitation and cleanliness were supported by Listerian techniques of antisepsis and microbiology which were gradually adopted and adjusted to improve the outcome for patients and reduce the risk of morbidity.

Caring, however, involved tremendous hard work and there was considerable risk to nurses from infectious diseases and the harsh working conditions. Nurse Marie Magill describes her duties nursing in the fever tents at the Alfred hospital:

> I was called from my sleeping tent by the night nurse at 5.30 a.m., after dressing with only the most primitive and sparse toilet accommodation (no bath) I proceeded with the others to a room 10 feet by 10 feet, made my own cup of tea, waited in turn for cup and saucer (it was useless to provide our own); if night nurse left any bread, we had some with butter, if not, we had none. Thus refreshed, we went on duty at 6.00 a.m. We began by extinguishing night lights, got large brooms from an adjoining yard, swept, rolled up, and removed the long, heavy pieces of coconut matting. Left these on the grass outside until we swept the floors, and dusted; then carried back and relaid the matting. Then began the sponging of the patients with warm water we had prepared and carried from a kitchen near, made the patients' beds, took their temperature, and marked their charts. It was never specified how many tents I had to do, I frequently swept three, carrying the dreadful weight of matting, and was always responsible for eight patients at least—often sixteen—that they were sponged, etc., and ready for breakfast at 8 a.m. While these were served with their food by the wardsmaid I was supposed to go for my breakfast...(Royal Commission into Charitable Institutions 1890).

The hardships of nursing were considered compensated by the respect that surrounded the occupation and, despite evidence of dissatisfaction with the conditions of work, the discourse of dedication and devotion to duty predominated. The authorities and nurses argued for the maintenance of existing conditions of employment, supporting this production of nurse caring.

Post-Federation care 1901-1945

The adoption of the Nightingale system of nurse training was almost complete by the time of Federation in 1901. With the growing expectations of middle class women now seeking qualifications demand for places in nursing was high. Teaching hospitals were able to institute selective entrance policies and require initial unpaid probation periods. Trainees' salaries were low. Often, they needed to be augmented by other means, to meet basic necessities. Increasingly, nursing became professionally organised. In 1899 the Australasian Trained Nurses Association was formed, which successfully sought and obtained state registration for nurses. Nursing was a respectable occupation for those women who made it their career. Besides that, nursing was regarded by many as a good preparation for wifehood and motherhood. Most trainees went on to do midwifery.

Although nursing savoured status, there was little recognition for the long hours of work, often for less pay and less personal freedom than any female domestic servant would tolerate (Kingston 1975). Nurses were not militant and did not accept assistance from other bodies involved in labour reform. Uniform standards on hours and better salaries weren't finally established until the late 1930s.

People were seeking greater access to medical and nursing care at hospitals. Institutionalisation of the 'sick' in hospitals became the norm during this period and the 'right' to health care became embedded in social discourse. Almoners were introduced into hospitals to assess the financial status of patients seeking admission. Medical and surgical intervention became more frequent as medicine was recognised as a powerful weapon against disease and trauma. The poverty, unemployment and wars of this period contributed to the expansion of public hospital utilisation, and concomitantly a growth in the numbers of health professionals occurred. Increasingly the management discourse infused government activity as the government extended their financial responsibility for health care. The tenor of Christian, charitable discourse for caring no longer approximated the scientific and economic organisation of social life.

Disciplined and obedient care

'The probationer nurse did all the cleaning, sweeping, polishing and washing up. No one objected to this work. We believed that Florence Nightingale had never complained about anything she was required to do and we followed her footsteps' (Mortimer 1986). Trained nurses took up supervisory and administrative roles, while trainee and probationer nurses staffed the wards and engaged in direct care. This was not universally applauded by nurses, but security of employment was dependent on their superior's approval. As one nurse reminisced: 'At the Alfred hospital in the early thirties, nurses still whispered about the nurse who dared to write a book about the endless hard work, the unduly strict discipline, and the strange hospital hierarchy. She was instantly dismissed "as a warning to others", and in those depression years the threat of instant dismissal was indeed a deterrent' (Ogden 1990). Practices and regulations governed the behaviour and moral conduct of nurses, who were required to reside at their hospital work places. Living-in arrangements, leave passes, lights out at 10 p.m., hours of duty, uniform inspection and dress regulations, rules for visitation in each other's rooms, punctuality, respect and deference for higher rank, were some of the strict rules that related to conduct and etiquette.

Although the model of disciplined, obedient care dominated this period, there is considerable evidence of spirited and independent care provided by nurses. In contrast to the rules and regimen of the hospital, nurses aspired to becoming self-employed, perhaps as a home nurse, which provided better working conditions. Generally, however, there was a decline in the need for private nursing during this period, as patients now travelled to hospitals to access the medical facilities.

Providing loving, skilled and heroic care

Care provided by nurses has been often portrayed as an act of love, whether in peace-time or war-time. Patients were often hospitalised for long periods and cut off from their families by distance and by hospital regulations that restricted visiting. A nurse recalled an example of loving care: 'She was nursed under a full length bed cradle with electric lights attached to dry her dressings and keep her warm as she was nursed naked until the wounds began to heal. We all loved her and were overjoyed when she got better' (Lee 1986). In times of suffering nurses were often portrayed as tender and loving, providing the soft touch of a mother's or sweetheart's hand. Nurses themselves became seriously ill caring for those debilitated by the pandemic influenza (1915) and endemic infectious diseases.

Involvement in the war effort brought renewed contact with British nurses and Nightingale's discursive practices of regulation, discipline and obedience. Of course, the wars required nurses to care for wounded soldiers. Nurses were popularised as angels of mercy and lauded in songs such as 'The rose of no man's land'. A stretcher bearer described the work of nurses and their softening effect at the Western front in the First World War:

> The tragedy here was the tragedy of youth. There was beauty too in the presence of the nurses. One was like an angel...as she went from stretcher to stretcher. She sent the men on their last journey with a flicker of a smile...their gaunt and furrowed faces now lined and aged with suffering. She was there sixteen hours a day in that ward (Barker 1989).

Under the extreme conditions of the First World War, the 2692 nurses who served developed an independent spirit, and an increasing sense of Australian identity, resisting at times the strict designation and social roles that the British nurses displayed (Barker 1989). Tales of 'heroic care' have been documented for both world wars and these discourses reinforced those produced from Nightingale's Crimean war efforts, the representations of the 'lady with the lamp'. The romantic notion that nurses were safe and sheltered in war-time is discounted by the fate of nurses in war and as prisoners (Murphy 1983).

A war on infectious disease and establishment of scientific care

Medical science's increasing specialisation shaped care by producing a number of discrete forms of nursing. The following description of the scientific task orientation of theatre nursing is illustrated in this nurse's statement: 'The most important thing, in my opinion, that "Fay" taught us was that when you were "scrubbed" either as instrument nurse or swab nurse you never took your eyes off the site of the operation. You had to learn to pick up instruments by feel, not sight...'(Martin 1990). The development of community health nursing supported the pro-natalist position of governments with the establishment of baby health centres focusing on hygiene, pure milk campaigns and scientific parenting. At the same time, public health programs were developed for supervising and monitoring infectious diseases, in response to the concerns about the high levels of preventable illness in the community.

Nursing became increasingly identified with scientifically managed hospitals and less with domestic service. An emphasis on close observation and surveillance of patients shaped nurses as skilled observers of changes in their 'medical condition'. In times of crisis, the world wars and epidemics, the differentiation between the medical and nursing roles in the delivery of treatment and care became less differentiated; as Asher (1987) verified: 'We poulticed mumps patients with the dreaded orchitis, set up rectal glucose and saline drips when no doctors were available to give intravenous ones and tried hard to stop them developing complications which would keep them in hospital for months'.

However, autonomous practices were severely limited by the etiquette and disciplinary power of doctors and senior nurses who 'policed' the enforced divisions between doctors and nurses. Increasing numbers of medical and surgical procedures were undertaken by nurses who took up assisting roles and, in some instances educational roles to doctors (Gill 1989).

Scientific task caring 1945-1970

Hospitals, patient populations and health professionals grew significantly in number after the Second World War and specialisation of tasks both nursing, administrative and medical dominated the organisation of health care. The use of hospitals doubled between 1960 and 1970 (Radford 1979). Governments took over a significant portion of health care funding through taxation, and established more direct control over their administration. A number of factors contributed to nurses caring for an older population. They included: the success of public health policies, an improvement in pharmacologic treatments, an increase in the standard of living and a decrease in infectious diseases and infant mortality.

A nursing discourse of efficient scientific task care constituted in concepts of objectivity, rationality, responsibility, documentation and economy challenged earlier discourses. The notion of nursing as an ideal 'female activity' was contested by this constitution. Women sought different opportunities in the work place and there was an increase in the numbers of male nurses to more senior management positions in nursing. Psychiatric nursing developed as an occupation that was populated mainly by men, and in 1952 the first mental health nurse graduated. Nursing provided the opportunity for women to achieve a degree of financial independence but it was still widely felt to be a good preparation, an interlude for the development of the discipline needed to become a wife and mother; confirming women's reproductive and domestic roles.

A bland picture is often portrayed of the postwar period in Australian social life, 'marked by a sentimental attachment to Britain, comfortable affluence, ideological consensus, and cold war suspicions' although this picture changes for the 1960s (Bell & Bell 1993). This was the industrial era of the assembly line in factories, development of widespread welfare functions of the Federal government, and the introduction of communication technologies that resulted in increasing Americanisation of popular culture. This Americanisation of Australian social life was constituted in the discourses of liberalisation, modernisation and Westernisation. Caring was similarly shaped by these discourses as the nursing 'profession' was developed.

Caring with METHOD

'How we managed to get so much done in so little time I can't now imagine It must have been because we worked with "METHOD"!' (McInnes 1987). Scientific caring resulted in an extension of observation and documentation of the physical aspects of patients. Technological equipment provided the opportunity for increased mapping of changes in patients conditions and nurses honed their skills in surveilling bodies and diagnosing 'cases'. A nurse commented '...we could identify the symptoms of shock from half a ward away' (Hudson 1992).

Every aspect of the nurses' caring tasks was recorded: medical order books, temperature books, procedure books were filled with acronyms validating the tasks of nurses completed and of patients' activities. Care was allocated according to the seniority of nurses, slushy jobs going to the probationers. Whilst management was defined this way, nurses still found themselves undergoing a range of activities according to the availability of staff in their care situation. A general practitioner commented on the diverse work requirements of the nurse: '...something of an administrator, house keeper, telephonist-receptionist cum secretary, while at any time, she may be called upon to deliver a mother, assist in the theatre, supervise a drip, or lay out the dead—all in addition to her normal ward duties' (Clement 1966). Specialisation in medicine, availability of new medical technology and an increase in pharmacologic agents, led to an increased range of tasks in caring and complex organisational changes. These changes shaped many new nursing situations; the range of tasks are outlined in this quote:

> There seemed to be hundreds of sponges for the juniors to do. Considerate seniors would try to help between treatments but they were terribly busy with their own work; busy wards could be chaotic! Antibiotics were given

three hourly with needles which were re-used after sterilisation. There always seemed to be trolleys to set. We fought for sterilisers, heavy bowls and instruments out of the boiling, splashing water. We set up for dressings or IV cut downs...Sometimes we catheterised females with glass catheters and indwelling rubber catheters were guided by ferocious steel stillettes. We also coped with soap and water bowel washouts (Affleck 1992).

Senior nurses supervised the work of their junior nurses whilst they all surveyed the behaviour of their patients. A nurse reflected on this regulation and measurement of tasks in the period: '...sister would tape measure the top sheet turnover, it had to be a specified number of inches, I was recalled from breakfast to remake all of my five beds on one occasion' (Poynton 1986). The nurses' work was caring, but caring for each other was restricted; the stories of harsh treatment of each other (by senior to junior staff) are well documented.

Responsible caring included absolute adherence to medical instructions. Whilst their caring was constituted in observation this did not include initiation of treatment. Closer links and increased education for doctors drew nurses to assist and support that education and took them away from their educational role with their 'junior nurses'. Resistance and resentment to this development was evident even though the nurses acknowledged that medical education sometimes brought prestige to their institutions. One nurse recounted how patients toileting needs were 'suspended' during medical ward rounds; these rounds were dubbed by some nurses as 'Royal Progresses'. 'The patients were expected to contain their needs (i.e. toileting) while the honoraries round was in progress' (our own parenthesis, Goward 1992).

Patient-centred care

The discursive practices associated with scientific task care were not universally endorsed. Some nurse commentators were concerned at the increasing de-personalisation and fragmentation of caring tasks and others questioned the tremendous increase in surgery. A resistant discourse of patient-centred care developed in the 1960s, promoting a nurse-patient relationship recognising the emotional and social needs of patients. Shaw, the Chairman of the Student Nurses Association, argued that by focusing on the orderly and efficient routines and technical tasks '...we regard the relatives and friends as extraneous to an orderly routine...the routine of performing technical tasks with skill and efficiency...we have joined force with men and their emphasis of doing rather than being...this is the current image..brusque and efficient...' (1966).

Preliminary training schools and the need for new educational courses developed out of these changes. The inception of the Lister Home in Bendigo and Melbourne School of Nursing in the 1950s was an important break from hospital based education, elevating theoretical discourses for nurses' professional caring roles. The Melbourne School met with considerable resistance which eventually lead to its demise; theoretical scientific discourses were contesting the 'practical' discourses of caring that had dominated nursing for so long. Nurses' work was not constituted in autonomous professional practice and its constitution as an intuitive but practical endeavour that supported medical scientific practice of doctors held firm.

Caring in a liberal era

'The whole world should adopt the American system...the American system can survive in America only if it becomes a world system' (Harry S Truman in Bell & Bell 1946). Liberalisation and modernisation brought a focus on education for professionals and, in turn, these professionals ascribed more and more meaning to every aspect of people's lives. Adopting scientific rational processes for caring was promoted in nursing literature as a means to achieve the goal of professionalism. The Kellogg nursing scholarship holders, who visited the United States in the 1960s, educated Australian nurses in the use of 'the nursing process'. The nursing process was a problem-based framework for nursing practice and fulfilled scientific criteria of rationality and objectivity. The nursing process was considered to give coherent form to the vision of nursing, not only as being scientific, but also to legitimise and convey the complexities of nursing practice.

Liberalisation was given further shape in health care by the notion of 'patients rights' and consumerism. Rights in health care were constituted in recognition of and respect for the autonomy of an individual's ability to make decisions. Rights were also being extended in social life to groups that had been excluded in earlier periods due to their perceived lack of being civilised (note: Aboriginals were granted voting rights in 1966).

The adoption of the ICN Code of International Nursing Ethics in 1953, marked a significant shift from a focus on the character of the nurse and their etiquette to an ethic of care based on a moral code (Johnstone 1993). Hall (1959) promoted the use of a 'moral code' as foundational to professional practice and stated: '...nurses should be encouraged to do some thinking about moral principles...Nurses are professional people and among essential qualities of members in a profession is a certain breadth of vision of liberty of thought' (Hall 1959). Consideration of ethical issues was limited and constrained by paternalistic discursive practices that dominated health care. Informed consent, suffering, culturally sensitive care and malpractice were not substantial issues until the 1980s. Consumer issues were limited to accessibility to services; patients tending to be treated as an homogenous mass. Martin's (1978) study into migrant health care in this period supports this in relation to cultural care, asserting that only in the 1970s did there develop a discourse that elevated 'difference' and 'ethnicity' in health care.

Professional caring 1970s to present

The move away from the apprenticeship system of training to tertiary preparation was completed in this period and nurses were finally granted the title of 'professional'. In July 1989 the N.S.W. Industrial Court ruled that nurses were professionals; this event capped a period that saw a push for recognition of the nurse professional. The professional nursing associations argued that nurses possessed complex knowledge and skill that could meet the health promotion and ill-health needs of people.

The 1970s brought significant changes to the conditions of work, and the opportunities for tertiary education for Australian women. In 1969, came a landmark decision on the granting of equal pay for equal work for women workers. Women were also encouraged through various equal opportunity bodies and programs to engage in non-traditional work. Nurses seemingly shunned the early feminist activism of the 1960s and 1970s, preferring to adopt rationalist, objectivist standards that established their scientific credentials. Part of this 'professional scientific push' included the de-genderisation of nursing work and knowledge.

Alternative discourses of caring were disseminated through tertiary nurse education and a wider range of practice settings. Individualised humanistic care that appropriated the notions of 'caring science' and 'holism' were increasingly favoured in nursing texts. New holistic thinking in academic scholarship was encouraged by the re-evaluation of the mechanistic causality of Newtonian physics. The concept of the universe as a dynamic, indivisible whole, 'as a hologram made up of waves and quanta' (Griffiths 1993), has gained adherence in nursing scholarship. These concepts are incorporated into the discursive formation of 'holistic' caring.

Many social commentators have marked this era as post-industrial or postmodern. Positivist science, although largely retaining its attraction as a method of providing material wellbeing, has lost its allure as being reliable and as being humanity's liberator. The postmodern, Western mind is viewed as open-minded, indeterminate and shaped by a diversity of influences, the nature of truth being ambiguous and contradictory. Tarnas (1991) has described it as the era of the 'deconstruction of naive understanding' and the 'age of uncertainty'.

Professional humanistic care

The unique position of the nurse in the health care system, (as well as her/his traditionally inherent intimate position with the client), enhances the nurse's ability to develop an interactive/interpersonal therapeutic relationship that permits her/him to gain knowledge of the whole person and the ways in which each person defines their experience of illness. It is this 'insight', this knowledge, along with the nurse's theoretical knowledge of disease and her therapeutical skills that provides a basis for the humanisation and 'holistic' nursing approach to patient care (Marles 1988).

A discourse of 'professional humanistic care' focused less on the characteristics of nurses and more on the 'processes' that nurses engaged in delivering 'scientific' caring practice. Explication of, and interpretation of patient problems and needs have become institutionalised in the nursing process. Information for responding to the needs and problems of people is continually extended; the determination of risk and need is self-perpetuating and produced through further inquiry. Care interventions and actions are planned according to the information generated. This formed the 'objective database' for the development of protocols and strategies of care.

Professional humanistic care established the therapeutic relationship as embedded in a 'holistic' view of the patient. In holistic discourse the patient is affirmed as a 'subject', the experiencing patient, the whole patient, and not just as an 'object'. Nursing the 'subject' required communicative competence so the nurse could understand the social and personal needs of patients. Caring for the psych-social dimensions of the patient required the collection of information to support this realm of practice. The nurse then needed to 'know' the patient; that is to define the physical, social, psychological and spiritual aspects of the patients, so as to give holistic care.

Humanistic/interpretative caring discourses emphasised the subjectivity of patients and their 'illness experiences'. This humanistic caring continues to be promoted by some nurse scholars (Bartjes 1991, Wilkes 1991) as being able to 'uncover' the truth, the essences behind the patient's disposition. These nurse scholars consider the personal dimension of a patient's life as a target of intervention by nurses. This widens the discursive field of nursing caring from a scientific task orientation of the previous period. Nurses have integrated into their practice ideas about what constitutes psychological and social wellbeing, thus constituting a 'new' field of power/knowledge and modifying the way in which the patient understands the health-illness experience.

Instrumental rationality

Humanistic caring discourses have gained general acceptance as central goals of nursing activity. Paradoxically, today nurses' caring activities are being evaluated by managers as caring technologies and are measured as 'inputs' to the health industry. Enormous efforts are being made to define human services in rational economic discourse. The activities, techniques and processes of these services are included in measures of dependency ratios and diagnostic-related groups. Instrumental rationality, valued in economic discourse, is constituted in the concepts of measurement, flexibility and globalism. Furthermore, the information generated from the measurements of health and ill-health services provides the consumer of health care products and 'providers' of health resources with data to make 'rational' decisions. This discourse is seen by many to be destructive to 'traditional' cultural communities. The 'rationalisation' of health care facilities in the 1980s and 1990s is lamented by many nurses, because their caring culture was devalued. One nurse expressed her grief towards the closure of her hospital: 'I feel grief-stricken when I think of all the wonderful people, doctors, nurses and others who devoted their lives to make this hospital a place of special caring, often with limited funds, using mainly the human resources and exploiting the natural environment to produce excellent and exceptional results' (Arthur 1988).

Knowledge, as the intellectual 'commodity' specified in economic discourse, disrupts organisational arrangements for care. Nursing professionals are specified further into care managers and direct care is passed on to lesser 'educated' people (personal care assistants) while technologists handle the information processing activities. The person who is desired is the one who thinks in a economic way, a flexible multi-skilled, mobile person.

Caring as a social/political and cultural activity

'Community health nursing...developed my creativity. I came alive ...Working in community health also exposed me to the politics and economics of the health care industry...' (Savage 1992). Australian nurses and scholars have increasingly resisted a nursing identity that seeks to exclude the social, cultural and political aspects of nurse caring. Feminist groups have proclaimed their capacity to represent the position of women in society and provided alternate discourses which now occupy a highly salient position in nursing texts and courses. Revisionist postmodern, poststructuralist philosophies challenged the basis of empirical and interpretative positions of science that claim truth.

A discourse of frustration, powerlessness and complaint dominated inquiries and reports into nursing in the 1980s. Nurses incorporated professional humanistic care as their 'ideal' mode of practice, but found resistance in a world that increasingly adopted technological, rationalist values. The professional relationships of the time cast them in discursive roles as handmaidens and housewives, and as subservient. As a maternal and child health nurse suggests in a Victorian report: 'It is still apparent that doctors have a 'handmaiden' attitude to nurses. They do not appreciate the nurse's high level of knowledge and skill' (Marles 1988). Further, while nurses have welcomed widening caring practices informed by social, psychological and cultural discourses, disciplinary practices exist to limit their caring roles, as this nurse complained:

> M&CH nurses have expressed concern about being excluded from case conferences convened by social workers... With the introduction of tertiary courses which broaden the M&CH nurses illness/health theoretical knowledge base to include sociology, health education and human relations many social workers are unaccepting, and in some instances threatened by the nurse's ability to take on a broader role' (Marles 1985).

It would be incorrect to claim that the political/social and cultural discourses dominate caring practices and scholarship, but they have carved out an important place. They offer resistance to the totalising influence of scientific and professional discourses; they also enable an evaluation of unwanted imperial effects of discourses. Lawler's (1991a, 1991b) contribution is significant in this effort. Her literature on caring for the 'body' (somology) has contrasted the local production of knowledge with extant imported knowledge. Whilst it is undesirable to 'concentrate' efforts on parochial, nationalistic discourse, there is a need for greater reflexivity. This is the case at both the micro-level of nursing practice and in the broader epistemological project of developing nursing knowledge.

Conclusion

The new thrust towards humanism and its supposed liberating effects, relinquishes the expression of power and creates an epistemological position where knowledge is conceived as separate from power. Rather, in seeking to liberate patients from reductionist consequences of a bio-medical model of health, and in seeking to uncover the 'essence' behind a patient's disposition, dimensions of the person become a new field of power/knowledge. Humanistic caring does not challenge the normalising power of medicine, and its effects in the producing and specifying of the patient subject. This raises questions about the nurse's authority to scientise their personal encounters with patients, and the possibility of imperialistic tendencies where the representation of the 'other' may lead to a failure in differentiating the personal and social aspects in every nursing situation.

The nurse needs to ask the question: Is the nurse who conceives of humanistic caring, based on communicative competency, developing a true dialogue, or rather, is the nurse adopting humanistic canons, formalised in a 'caring' science, that do little more than reproduce that canon? Certain forms of knowledge are exercised over individuals and govern the nursing profession; the nurse and patient subjects are a product of the disciplinary practices and rationalising discourses of the 'modern' era.

In rejecting the truth claims of caring sciences and caring concepts, authoritative knowledge is not taken by the authors as fatuous. Rather, knowledge is seen in a different light; accounts of caring take place in the shared world of language and discourse. The conventions that produce a certain discourse of caring influence the accounts of the 'objective' world of the nurse. The emphasis here is on the meaning and conditions that generate and enable a discourse on caring. Each attempt at self-understanding (i.e. understanding one's discipline) takes one into the fuller social realm. This reflexive attitude needs to be a continuous undertaking. One of the chief propositions that this chapter advances is that the dominant discourse with nursing scholarship and practice contains and produces our understanding of care, and we learn to see our history of care as part of an already shared history of our social community. Our history and conception of care in nursing gains meaning only by its relation to its wider social context.

Poststructural analysis of the discursive formation of caring creates the epistemological space for other questions and does not confine or imprison caring (or knowledge) within any one representation. Rather, it promotes vitality, a plurality of ideas and opens the nursing identity up to new possibilities. This chapter does not offer to the reader the 'truth' about the place of caring in nursing, but offers an 'evocation'. The authors commitment is to a continued exploration of how nursing concepts are adopted to organise a set of practices which structure the relationship between nurses and patients.

REFERENCES

Affleck M 1992 Nursing narrative. In: Keane B, Goodwin R, Richmond J (eds) Mum me and TLC: narratives of nursing. Short Run Books, Melbourne

Argus 1987 In: Mackay M 1983 Handmaidens of medicine: hospital nursing in Victoria 1880-1905. MEc thesis, Monash University, Melbourne

Arthur D 1988 Speech. General Meeting Prince Henry's Trained Nurses' Association. In: Cordia M 1990 Nurses at Little Bay. Prince Henry's Trained Nurses' Association, Sydney

Asher J 1987 Letter book file. In: Cordia M 1990 Nurses at Little Bay. Prince Henry's Trained Nurses' Association, Sydney

Barker M 1989 Nightingales in the mud: the digger sisters of the Great War 1914-1918. Allen & Unwin, Sydney

Bartjes A 1991 Phenomenology in clinical practice. In: Gray G, Pratt R (eds) Towards a discipline of nursing. Churchill Livingstone, Melbourne

Bell P, Bell R 1993 Implicated: the United States in Australia. Oxford University Press, Melbourne

Benner P, Wrubel 1989 J The primacy of caring. Addison-Wesley, Menlo Park, California

Chinn P L 1991 (ed) Anthology of caring. National League of Nursing, New York

Clement D M 1966 The general practitioner view. UNA Nursing Journal LXIV(July):186

Cushing A 1993 The origins of female nursing in Victoria, 1850-1890. Conference Proceedings. Australian nursing: the story. First national history conference, Royal College of Nursing Australia, Melbourne

Davenport Cleland E 1980 The Aboriginals. In: Morris E E Australia's first century. Child & Henry, Hornsby

Dunlop M 1988 Science and caring: are they compatible? Conference Proceedings. Shaping nursing theory and practice: the Australian context. Lincoln School of Health Sciences, La Trobe University, Melbourne, p. 16-22

During S 1992 Foucault and literature: towards a genealogy of writing. Routledge, London

Fanon F 1968 The wretched of the earth. Farrington C (trans). Grove, New York

Foucault M 1970 The order of things. Tavistock, London

Foucault M 1971 Madness and civilisation: a history of insanity in the age of reason. Tavistock, London

Foucault M 1972 The archaeology of knowledge. Tavistock, London

Foucault M 1980 In: Gordon C (ed) Power/knowledge: selected interviews and other writings, 1972-1977. Pantheon, New York

Garrick P, Jeffery C 1987 Fremantle Hospital: a social history to 1987. Fremantle Hospital, Western Australia

Gill I 1989 The lamp still burns: nursing in Victoria 1936-1981 an autobiographical account. Bendigo College of Advanced Education, Bendigo

Goward Z 1992 Narrative. In: Keane B, Boodwin R, Richmond J (eds) Mum me and TLC: narratives of nursing. Short Run Books, Melbourne

Griffiths V 1993 A phenomenological study of inner knowing amongst critical care nurses practitioners. MNsg thesis, Royal Melbourne Institute of Technology, Melbourne

Hagell E I 1989 Nursing knowledge: women's knowledge. A sociological perspective. Journal of Advanced Nursing 14:226-133

Hall I 1959 The importance of nursing ethics. Australian Nurses Journal 55(3):54-56

Hansford-Miller F 1990 Aboriginal and English medicine in the Swan River Colony in 1829. Abcado, Perth

Hooft S V 1987 Caring and professional commitment. Australian Journal of Advanced Nursing 4(4):29-38

Hudson R 1992 Nursing narrative. In: Keane B, Boodwin R, Richmond J (eds) Mum me and TLC: narratives of nursing. Short Run Books, Melbourne

Inglis K S 1958 Hospital and community: a history of the Royal Melbourne Hospital. Melbourne University Press, Melbourne

Johnstone M-J 1993 The development of nursing ethics in Australia: an historical overview. Conference Proceedings. Australian nursing: the story. First national history conference, Royal College of Nursing, Australia, Melbourne

Keen J, Jarrett J, Levy A M 1976 Triumphs of medicine. Paul Elkin, London

Kingston B 1975 My wife, my daughter, and poor Mary Ann: women and work in Australia. Nelson, Melbourne

Lawler J 1991a In search of an Australian identity. In: Gray G, Pratt R (eds) Towards a discipline of nursing. Churchill Livingstone, Melbourne

Lawler J 1991b Behind the screens: nursing somology and the problem of the body. Churchill Livingstone, Melbourne

Lee B 1986 Letter book file. In: Cordia M 1990 Nurses at Little Bay. Prince Henry's Trained Nurses' Association, Sydney

Leininger M M 1991 Culture care diversity and universality: a theory of nursing. National League for Nursing, New York

McInnes S F 1987 Nurses at Little Bay book file. Prince Henry's Trained Nurses' Association. In: Cordia M 1990 Nurses at Little Bay. Prince Henry's Trained Nurses Association, Sydney

MacPherson K 1988 Looking at caring and nursing thought: a feminist lens. Conference Proceedings. Caring and nursing: explorations in feminist perspectives. Denver, Colorado

Marles F 1988 Report of the study of professional issues in nursing. Victorian Government Printer, Melbourne

Martin J 1978 The migrant presence. George Allen & Unwin, Sydney

Martin G 1990 Reminiscences. In: Alfred Hospital reminiscences 1927-1947. Melbourne, Victoria

Morse J M, Soberg S, Neander W, Bottorff J, Johnson J 1990 Concepts of caring and caring as a concept. Advances of Nursing Science 13(1):1-14

Mortimer N 1986 Nurses at Little Bay book file. Prince Henry's Trained Nurse's Association. In: Cordia M 1990 Nurses at Little Bay. Prince Henry's Trained Nurses' Association, Sydney

Murphy E 1986 Nurses at Little Bay book file. In: Cordia M 1990 Nurses at Little Bay. Prince Henry's Trained Nurses' Association, Sydney

Murphy F 1983 Desert, bamboo and barbed wire: the 1939-45 story of a special detachment of Australian Army nursing sisters, fondly as the 'Angels in Grey' and their fate in war and captivity. Ollif, Hornsby

New South Wales parliamentary debates 89:2769-71

Noddings N 1984 Caring: a feminine approach to ethics and moral education. University of California Press, Los Angeles

Ogden R 1990 Reminiscences. In: Alfred Hospital reminiscences 1927-1947, Melbourne, Victoria

Poynton E 1986 Nurses at Little Bay book file. In: Cordia M 1990 Nurses at Little Bay. Prince Henry's Trained Nurses' Association, Sydney

Priestly S 1990 Melbourne's mercy: a history of Mercy Private Hospital. Hyland House, Melbourne

Racevskics K 1988 Michel Foucault, Rameau's nephew, and the question of identity. In: Bernauer T, Rasmussen D (eds) The final Foucault. MIT Press, Cambridge, Massachusetts

Radford A 1979 Health and illth in Australian homes. In: Walpole R (ed) Community health in Australia. Penguin Books, Ringwood

Reverby S 1987 Ordered to care: the dilemma of American nursing. Cambridge University Press, New York

Royal Commission on Charitable Institutions 1871. Victorian parliamentary papers. Government Printer, Melbourne

Royal Commission on Charitable Institutions 1890. In: Victorian parliamentary papers Vol. 4. Government Printer, Melbourne

Said E 1993 Culture and imperialism. Chatto Windus, London

Savage P 1992 Nursing narrative. In: Keane B, Goodwin R, Richmond J (eds) Mum me and TLC: narratives of nursing. Short Run Books, Melbourne

Shaw R 1966 Patient or person. UNA Nursing Journal. LXIV(February):43

Speedy S 1991 The contribution of feminist research. In: Gray G, Pratt R (eds) Towards a discipline of nursing. Churchill Livingstone, Melbourne

Tarnas R 1991 The passion of the western mind. Ballantine Books, New York

Watson J 1985 Nursing: human science and human care. Appleton-Century-Crofts, Norwalk, Connecticut

Watson 1990 The moral failure of the patriarchy. Nursing Outlook 38(2):62-66

Wilkes L 1991 Phenomenology: a window to the nursing world. In: Gray G, Pratt R (eds) Towards a discipline of nursing. Churchill Livingstone, Melbourne

16

Primary health and nursing: strange bedfellows?

MARGARET DUNLOP, JANE JACOBS

Two scholars

There was a day when Jane and Margaret sat talking about nursing and primary health care. 'Why is it' Jane asked, 'that although there is much written about the central role of nurses in primary health, nurses themselves appear not to have moved into the role of advocating for client groups, like the self-help groups I've been studying? It bemuses me that we readily grasp the "new speak" and talk about it as the change that we need to turn health care around, but we have not as energetically entered into the analytical process of asking ourselves, who, what, when, where and more importantly "why" primary health care.

'When I approached small self-help groups, I found myself as a nurse welcomed with open arms. I think this is because nurses are viewed as practical, knowledgeable but approachable professionals who often have that commonsense approach. Nurses are seen as more down-to-earth, perhaps, as Taylor argues, "more ordinary" (Taylor 1993). Why is it that with such practical knowledge and skills, we never seem to see beyond the words of the policy documents or question the philosophies that are being advocated?'

'That's very interesting', Margaret said, 'because it has often seemed to me that nursing's relationship with primary health care today mirrors the earlier relationship between the developing nursing profession and the 19th century public health movement'. As Dean and Bolton (1980) argue, the developing profession, as it functioned outside the hospital, became the individualised arm of the public health movement, teaching the poor clean habits and orderliness. Nurses thus became integrally involved in the administration of poverty, rather than addressing its alleviation.

'When I read Dean and Bolton, I connected this outcome with the way nursing always conceptualises itself ministering to individuals, providing "individualised care". Where family and community come into this conceptualisation they do so by extension out from the individual who remains the primary focus. It seems to me that this is a central process shaping nursing as an apolitical group.'

... in conversation

Jane: That reminds me of a wonderful couplet I came across the other day from the nineteenth century sanitation movement:

> Do you wish to be healthy?
> Then keep the house sweet;
> As soon as you're up,
> Shake each blanket and sheet (Wohl 1983).

Margaret: Oh yes, this sort of advice, directed to the poverty-stricken denizens of England's industrial cities during the 19th century, must have been as wildly irrelevant as it would be in a refugee camp today. But this is the sort of individualised approach to public health through health education that developed alongside more broad measures directed at improving sanitation, water supplies, and, eventually, housing. Dean and Bolton argue that it was this individualised approach that the developing nursing profession embraced.

Jane: You use the analogy of today's refugee camps and in many ways that must have been what life in England's industrial cities was like. The migration from rural to urban areas resembled a refugee movement as agrarian reform closed down living opportunities in the country. As new work opened up in the industrial cities they became magnets for the uprooted agrarian working class. The developing factory system was only gradually able to absorb the army of labour which tramped the streets looking for work. The vast majority did not find the streets paved with gold, as rural mythology had promised.

Margaret: Quite the contrary, I imagine, the streets must have been paved with filth! You know, I have usually looked at the 19th century health movement from the perspective of nursing's involvement. Tell me something more about this movement from a broader perspective. How did the earlier public health movement come about and what did those involved think they were doing?

Jane: The impact of rapid economic change and industrial development together with the migration from rural to urban living gave rise to major public health problems, experienced as a dramatic increase in infectious diseases and work related illness and disability. Poverty and overcrowding in the lower class areas of the major industrial cities exacerbated sanitation and food supply problems, leading to poor nutrition and grossly inadequate disposal of human and other waste (Wohl 1983). Rapid urbanisation placed unprecedented pressures on air, water and living space. It was in this cauldron of change that the public health movement was born, formed in an attempt to respond to mounting social concern about the spread of infectious diseases and high mortality rates, especially among the poor.

Margaret: But why did people become concerned about this sort of thing? It was only 'the poor'!

Jane: But it wasn't only the poor. Although reference is usually made to Victorian philanthropy, a degree of self-interest on the part of the monied classes was undoubtedly involved (Wohl 1983). The lives of the rich and the poor intersected to a much greater extent than today (as Charles Dickens' novels demonstrate) and communicable diseases spread out from the ghettoes of the poor through the connecting link of the household servants. Moreover, the rich, like the poor, had to put up with the filth of the city streets, the toxic plumes of the factories, the tons of manure dropped by the transport system and the collections of human and other waste in cesspools, often not far from their own fashionable homes (Wohl 1983).

Margaret: Yes, I can see that sanitation measures may have been able to garner wider support, but the measures advocated by the public health movement seemed to go beyond simple cleaning up of the urban mess to focus on improving the health of the deserving poor and working class people.

Jane: Well, as the developing factory system absorbed an increasing amount of the available labour, concern for the health of the work force also appeared to increase. At the turn of the century, the poor health of Boer War recruits also provided impetus for public health measures. As Lord Rosebery said, 'it is of no use having an Empire without an Imperial race' (in Wohl 1983).

Margaret: That's British philanthropy speaking!

Jane: Yes, we also get an interesting perspective from an MP in 1909. He was speaking on the Trades Boards Act, a bill to control sweated labour which he claimed '...to be applied exclusively to exceptionally unhealthy patches of the body politic, where the development has been arrested in spite of growth in the rest of the organism. It is to the morbid, diseased places—to the industrial diphtheria spots that we should apply the anti-toxins of the trade boards' (H Tennant 1909 cited in Harrison 1991).

Margaret: How fascinating! The metaphor of the body politic is combined with reference to the newly fashionable germ theory to justify state intervention in industry!

Jane: Yes, despite much opposition, the state had intervened at an increasing pace, legislating to compel local authorities to carry out sewerage and water works, to set housing standards, to prevent adulteration of food and to vaccinate against smallpox. Factories, mines and public building came under increasing state control through an inspectorial system. District medical officers of health ensured that local authorities implemented state policies and controlled the activities of district nurses, community midwives and (from 1893) health visitors (Farrow 1987, Wohl 1983). Throughout the second half of the 19th century and into the 20th century, the state continued to raise its level of intervention in the interests of public health, changing the relationship between individual and state, family and state, industry/business and state.

Margaret: So what you're saying is that, from the mid 19th century on, legislation was used increasingly to control individuals and companies in the interests of public health?

Jane: Yes, but it was often reactionary legislation. For example, the Nuisance Removal Act of 1846 levelled penalties at the victims of the processes that produced 'unwholesome' dwellings (Wohl 1983). It was re-actionary also in being 'after the fact'. Harrison (1991) quotes one 19th century activist as saying that legislation was the 'reflex of public opinion, the moral thermometer of the community'. As she points out, although the activist was referring to criminal law, the metaphor can be extended to legislation more generally.

Margaret: Yes, a medical metaphor at that! If we follow the metaphor, the moral thermometer seems to have been shaped by the Sanitation Movement which, I understand, campaigned tirelessly for the sort of measures the State eventually put in place.

Jane: But the Sanitation Movement would not have succeeded unless it was coherent with pushing the concerns of the dominant classes. The situation appears similar to that of the 'green' movement of today. Although greens were initially dismissed as cranks, green concerns are now becoming incorporated into the mainstream of civil life. Much the same appears to have occurred with the Sanitation Movement.

Margaret: It is probably within the Sanitation Movement that Nightingale's activities and writings can best be understood. She identified the role of dirt, noise, smells and absence of light in impeding recovery. The twin themes of sanitation and the healing power of nature pervade her writings. Nightingale was firmly convinced that the miasma theory was correct and that the fashionable germ theory detracted from necessary sanitary reforms (Rosenberg 1979). By locating disease in the individual, the germ theory shifted the focus away from the urban mess that gave rise to 'miasmata' shifting in the direction of individual responsibility and victim blaming. It was the principles of sanitation she ensured were put into practice in the Crimea, dramatically reducing mortality rates at the military hospital at Scutari. It was sanitation principles she ensured were inculcated into probationer nurses at St Thomas Hospital and it was sanitation principles she applied to the sickroom in her *Notes on Nursing* (Nightingale 1860).

Jane: What seems to be happening here is that sanitation principles are being given an individualistic focus. It is true that while the Sanitation Movement pressed for reform of sanitary conditions through legislation, it also endeavoured to reach the poor with 'good advice' about 'healthy living', as exemplified by the couplet I mentioned earlier, however impractical (and ineffective) that advice at times may have been. There was certainly a strong interest in reform of the housekeeping standards of the poor.

Margaret: Which reminds me that a major change was happening to house-keeping itself. Davidoff (1976) explores the elaboration of housework which occurred in middle and upper class homes with the transition from country to city. The 'clean dirt' of the country (what is tolerable under dispersed living conditions) became the 'dirty dirt' of the city and the housework required to control such dirt became increasingly elaborated. A standard of cleanliness was thus produced by servants which ended at the front steps. It was these practices that well meaning ladies sought to teach to the poor, who lacked, among other things, the servants to carry them out. It was also these practices which probationer nurses learnt as part of their training.

Once trained, many nurses moved outside the hospital into the homes of the sick and the poor to provide nursing care. But they had a larger mission, as Nightingale herself put it: 'the district nurse may be the forerunner in teaching the disorderly how to use improved dwellings— teaching without seeming to teach, which is the ideal of teaching' (cited in Dean & Bolton 1980).

The disorderly were thus to be made orderly by the modelling and coaching behaviour of the district nurse.

Jane: And this went even further with the creation in 1893 of the health visitor who became a 'hands off' community nurse (Symonds 1991). With this move the giving of nursing care was split off from the giving of nursing advice. This split endures today, seen in Australia as the split between domiciliary and community nursing. In her research, Symond's British respondents tagged the two groups 'angels and interfering bodies' (Symonds 1991).

Margaret: I wonder which is which! But what seemed to be happening was that a discourse was created in which the poor themselves were made responsible for their lack of order and their practices were opened up to the kind but critical inspection of the nurse who benignly led them from chaos to order, from darkness to light. It would be little wonder if the poor saw them as busybodies!

Jane: Yes, and nurses themselves took on the victim blaming. Symonds cites the example of Miss Loane who worked as a district nurse in the area in and around London and wrote about her experiences. Loane herself placed the blame for the problems of the poor, including ill health, bad housing and under nourishment, firmly on their own ignorance and fecklessness.

By applying the growing understanding of sanitation principles to the individual, nursing fixed its sense of locus of responsibility at the level of the individual patient and his/her family—occasionally stretching to the friendship circle. Miss Loane suggested that the role of the highly skilled trained nurse was 'to organise and direct the labour of the patient's friends' (Symonds 1991). So even the inclusion of friends was part of the 'busyness'.

Margaret: As I mentioned earlier, this application of sanitation principles to the individual is seen in the book widely regarded as the first book on nursing theory, Nightingale's *Notes on Nursing*. Further theoretical development of nursing, seen as emerging in the United States with Peplau from 1952 onward followed this same individualised pattern, losing even the remnants of the broader understanding which Nightingale had inherited from the Sanitation Movement.

Fawcett (1984), after the fact, identified nursing's 'metaparadigm' as consisting of man (sic), environment, health and nursing. However, examination of Nursing Theory's use of environment reveals that the environment to which Nursing Theory refers is the micro-environment that surrounds the patient-nurse dyad (Dunlop 1992). This is true even of Rogers (1970) who ostensibly starts from a position of universal interconnectedness.

'Man' (usually now changed to 'person' in deference to feminism) is the bearer of his/her own health and illness with whom the nurse interacts as an individual to set up conditions for healing. When, as in King (1971), the family and community come into the picture it is the terms of their relationship to the individual, in a fairly similar way to that envisaged by Miss Loane.

What disappears from view in this individual focus is the wider socio-political and economic framework in which the nurse-patient dyad and its micro-environment are situated—increasingly a world order. Out of this new world order has arisen the ideology of primary health care which nurses are now being encouraged to embrace.

Jane: But primary health care as a policy framework challenges the organisation and structure of the biophysical tradition of health care which has largely shaped nursing and other health professionals by its individualised cure focus.

Primary health care's central tenet, health promotion, demands that nurses engage in a political process to achieve social justice. Thus health promotion is more than health education, providing primary care or participating in community development. It asks nurses to find creative and effective ways to address the social inequalities that contribute to ill-health and to become change agents.

Margaret: It seems to me that the political process that primary health care requires is in stark opposition to the relatively apolitical activities of nurses in the early public health movement. Although Nightingale had called upon health reformers to address the social chaos that besieged the poor and working class, nursing advocacy for social reform has been and is, a slow and fragmented process. Nurses often still view politics with disdain and deem policy making the responsibility of bureaucrats. Archer's (1984) research on nurses' political participation indicated the low level of political involvement and a strong tendency to see political action as discordant with the professional role of the nurse. The apolitical position of nurses continues to disempower those in society to whom nurses minister. It also ensures that the status of nursing remains static against a background of a dynamically changing health care industry where other health professionals jockey intensely to secure their status as credible, valuable and skilled health care workers.

Jane: Well, Keleher (1994) argues that the socialisation of nurses and the pursuit of professional status of nursing are two reasons for the political inaction that has resulted in nurses becoming 'somewhat insular ...attempting to introduce collegial models of modus operandi within the treatment model rather then focusing on more global issues of social justice in health'. This gives some explanation to the current place of nursing in the health care system. More importantly, professionalisation becomes an ideology that distracts us from tackling the social and political issues that surround health care. We remain within the treatment model, with our place made comfortable by our acceptance within the health care team. As in *Animal Farm* (Orwell 1954) we overlook the fact that some are more equal than others in that team!

Margaret: Yes, indeed. The voices and values of the dominant groups within health care, specifically doctors, health economists and medical administrators remain robust, ensuring their large measure of social control. Nurses knowingly or unknowingly assist in maintaining the status quo and promote health behaviours that society prescribes as being good and proper. So have things really changed?

Jane: Well no, I don't really think so. While nurses have willingly adopted primary health rhetoric and engaged in related processes they have failed to challenge the dominant values that underpin the biomedical model. Broom (1989) argues that the mechanisms underpinning the biomedical model are 'more powerful and more difficult to dismantle, especially when the social understandings that hide them are widely held beliefs about the naturalness of illness and the neuter benevolence of medicine'.

283

Margaret: I like that! The myth of the neutered system! I think it is true that if we attempt to implement primary health without challenging that neuter benevolence we shift the responsibility for health care to the community, creating new inequalities, while the mechanisms under-pinning the biomedical model continue their control. Responsibility, but not authority, is shifted, although admittedly the discourse of responsibility for health is an ambiguous one dithering among individual, community and government responsibilities. Responsibility thus becomes a veiled and vexed issue, possibly because no shift of authority has occurred.

If nurses do not take up the challenge of primary health care, they will be seen as supporting the current distribution of power and the biomedical model. But, by participating in primary health care in an apolitical manner, nurses may help to de-politicise primary health, unquestioningly shifting the burden of responsibility to under-resourced communities and individuals who are in no position to respond to government demands to be individually or collectively 'more re-sponsible'.

Jane: This is just what I found in my study. Community genetic disorder self-help groups shoulder an increasing responsibility for service provision for their members and the community at large. But they are unable to secure adequate resources because resource allocation criteria set by government demand that output be measurable. Informal support and information sharing, the principal activities of these self-help groups, do not meet such criteria (Jacobs 1994). The stated needs of particular communities may thus be at odds with the type of output measures demanded by government. So although primary health claims to have a bottom up approach, top down accountability measures continue to drive the show. What has changed?

Margaret: Yes, it is certainly ironic that there is so much talk about devolving responsibility, yet quality assurance and accountability demands by government continue government's strong central control. Of course, we are told that quality assurance measures provide opportunities for the work force to engage in continuous quality improvement, total quality management or whatever the most recent buzz phrase is, but it seems all of a piece with the demand for increasing surveillance of the self which Foucault (1977) sees as integral to the modern world. The intention is to convert accountability measures into shopfloor ideology, in much the same way as primary health philosophy seeks to convert health care decisions into 'community decisions'. Both moves effectively conceal who is running the show.

Wass (1994) distinguishes selective primary health care from comprehensive primary health care. What differentiates one from the other is that a selective approach deals with low cost medical intervention to the majority of the population. Wass suggests this approach might be seen in the short term to reduce prevalence rates of selective diseases, but in the long term it does not deal with the root cause of ill-health, nor does it generate community control over health service provision.

A comprehensive approach, on the other hand, is a community controlled process of change where medicine may play a lesser role. Government support of primary health tends to degenerate toward the selective approach (Newell 1988).

Jane: It seems that any intervention favoured by government, be it at primary, secondary or tertiary intervention level, will be driven by the political and economic agenda and not necessarily by concern for the social, cultural, biophysical or psychological determinants of the collective or individual. Currently, primary health espouses an holistic approach but it fails to challenge openly the established politico-economic order which supports its implementation. Instead, the political and the economic are disguised in structures such as quality assurance, incentive for best practice and supposed devolution of administration and service delivery at a regional or area level. These 'accountability' measures seem to be imposed in an endeavour to maintain quality during times of funding decline. They deflect responsibility from central government, passing it down the line without concurrent delegation of authority and control. In a way this is analogous to 'victim blaming'.

Margaret: As nurses, we also need to recognise that the values underpinning the primary health model may be unduly ethnocentric, reflecting those of the developed world and generated to deal with the revolution of rising expectations in the third world. Is there a universality of these values or is primary health another example of post colonial imperialism? That is a paper in its own right.

Jane: Well, you could certainly argue that the developed world ideas about access and equity may not be congruent with or sensitive to all cultural and social groups.

I found that genetic disorder self-help groups experienced a sense of helplessness and invisibility in a health care system that espoused primary health philosophy. If we do not analyse the reasons for this sort of situation, we are selective rather than comprehensive in our approach to primary health care. In other words, if some groups are disenfranchised, no matter how small, we have moved away from primary health philosophy.

Margaret: Talking about moving away from primary health philosophy, what is it anyway? The literature surrounding nursing and primary health care suggests that there is no universal understanding of what primary health care is, but more a continuum of understandings and practices. St John (1993) identifies a blurring of boundaries in nursing practice between primary care, an epidemiological approach to public health and community development. Each point along the continuum is determined by the social and political organisation of the health care system in which the nurse works.

Primary care is the first contact with individuals and/or families in a specified community. St John (1993) describes primary care as 'holistic, individualized care incorporating health education and promotion...in a community setting'. This common understanding of primary health as primary care is blinkered and fails to look at the broader community issues that may influence the health and well being of the specific community. But it is the sort of the understanding that largely informs nursing.

The epidemiological approach to primary health care has a broader population focus usually defined in geographical and/or disease risk terms. Wass argues that an epidemiological approach lacks the sensitivity to measure and quantify the micro-environment factors that contribute to health (Wass 1994).

The community development approach has a community driven element that encompasses a process of community participation in the prioritising and management of health issues identified by that community. St John (1993) argues that community development has a greater social focus and is better able to deal with identified issues in the context of health care. But what is a community?

Jane: Yes, indeed. This is where the comprehensive approach to primary health advocated by Newell (1988) and Wass (1994) starts to appear very idealistic. Originally, community meant those within a geographical area, those who held land 'in common'. But, as Thompson (1971) argues, that sense of community has almost disappeared from the modern world. Nevertheless, this author suggests that the word itself is used 'as being synonymous with a highly desirable way of life in which co-operation, harmony and personal attachment to a place and its people are characteristic'. What is forgotten are the intense antagonisms, intractable family feuds, xenophobia and narrowed choices which were also part and parcel of traditional communities.

Margaret: I agree. Community is one of those words to which I sometimes refer as 'passing smoothly over the cerebrum without raising a ripple'.

Jane: So, given the problematics of community, is it wrong for nurses to become involved with individualised health promotion, as they often do?

Margaret: Of course not! There is strong evidence for some lifestyle modification practices (e.g. quitting smoking), reasonable evidence for others (weight control, particularly in men), and equivocal evidence for others (cholesterol control, exercise). There are also some measures, like exercise and weight control, that improve the person's sense of well being and help to retain mobility. However, there are other prescriptions which appear, on balance, to add more to the total sum of human misery than is gained in life expectancy. As Crawford (1984) argues, our culture plays off health as self control against health as release. As an example of the latter, a participant in his study defined health this way: 'It's being able to do what you want to do when you want to do it. It's nice to be able to eat and drink what you want, not worry about being overweight or sticking to the diet the doctor told you to stick to'.

Another participant suggested that 'worry itself can cause more problems than actual illness' (Crawford 1984). Moreover, health advice itself keeps changing as the following extract from a 1917 Domestic Medicine Practice Book written by 'learned physicians' illustrates. 'Scientists agree that sexual intercourse should not be indulged in by strong and healthy persons more often than twice a week, and by a more delicate person more than once a week. Health and strength lie in the direction of its control and rightful use while weakness, nervousness and illness follow its immodest sway' (Miller et al 1917).

It seems that health education is inevitably intertwined with the morality and fashion of its time!

Jane: Yes, that sort of statement is bound to breed scepticism. Also, on balance we know that our advice is most often taken by those who are already advantaged in the quantity and quality stakes—those with the best education and highest family incomes. The disadvantaged have more to worry about than shaking 'each blanket and sheet'.

Margaret: However, the danger in the individual behaviour approach for nurses as for doctors (Keleher 1994) is that it becomes the end-point of our concerns. We become unaware of the conditions which create poverty and blame the poor themselves. As William Blake wrote

Pity would be no more,
If we did not make someone Poor:
And Mercy no more would be,
If all were as happy as we; (The Human Abstract).

We should not just glorify the virtues without seeing the background which is the condition of their existence. We can so easily become the 20th century version of the Victorian Lady Bountiful.

In addition, as in the 19th century, health promotion as health advice is only part of a wider movement for health improvement. Individualised cure, care and lifestyle advice makes a difference only around the edges. While often greatly appreciated by the individual receiving them, their effects on mortality and morbidity are actually rather small.

Jane: So we need to move to the political level and replace concern for a healthy lifestyle with concern for 'healthy public policy'—the 20th century equivalent to the Sanitation Movement.

287

Margaret: But then, somewhere in the middle, we've got things like advocacy for disadvantaged groups, consumer participation in decision making and community development. These measures could be regarded as a sociocultural approach to health improvement. But advocacy so easily becomes paternalism, consumer participation purely symbolic and community development an attempt to impose the past on the present. Even if it were possible to identify communities, say communities of interest, it is clear that they will vary in their ability to articulate their health needs and to access the resources necessary to meet them— which is, I suppose, why they need developing!

Much of the material on consumer participation and community development seems to hark back to the simpler times and less complex societies, easily tipping over into an elaborate form of victim blaming as 'communities' are expected to 'take responsibility' for their own health care.

Jane: So you could say that 'healthy public policy' attacks the issue of health improvement at the political level. As with the legislation on sewerage, drainage, food, housing and work in the 19th century, the aim is to create the preconditions for health at the level of the physical and social fabric. As with the 19th century legislation, such an approach can be expected to have a much greater impact on mortality and morbidity than individualised or 'community' approaches. But it is also an area where nursing's voice has been weak.

Margaret: In the past, so has the voice of the organised medical profession been weak, although there have certainly been individual doctors, just as there have been individual nurses, that have made a mark. However, increasingly the voice of organised medicine is being heard on issues of healthy public policy, particularly (recently) smoking and Aboriginal health. It seems to be part of a deliberate campaign to exhibit their 'social responsibility' at a time when they have been subject to considerable criticism.

Jane: Yet nursing, whose organisations have prepared 'a comprehensive and committed policy about the relationship between nursing and primary health care' (Keleher 1994), has appeared relatively silent. This may partly illustrate Keleher's point that the voice of nursing is generally not heard when more powerful voices speak. But where were we when Bronwyn Bishop made her famous statement about supporting cigarette advertising at sporting venues. Where were we when Graham Richardson and then Alexander Downer were decrying the poor state of Aboriginal health. These are just some of 1994's examples of nursing voices not being heard.

Margaret: But there is also something beyond healthy public policy as it is generally construed. Too easily the concept of 'healthy public policy' can slip into the sort of social engineering that remedies deficits here and there within the acceptable framework of existing inequalities between individuals, between communities, between cultural groupings and between nations and states. The effect is to try to remedy the deficiencies of the current system without disturbing it unduly. Just as the effect of the focus on the individual is to render invisible the social and cultural determinants of health and just as the effects of the focus on the 'community' is to render invisible the political and economic determinants, so the healthy public policy approach obscures and mystifies inequality, poverty and disadvantage.

In closing

The conversation must draw to a close, as inevitably happens in books. In real life, of course, conversations go on until the participants part.

In books, conversations are selected and constructed out of the discontinuous conversations of life—the purposeful talk, the chat over coffee, the word in the corridor, the exchange at a meeting.

We started with the idea of a dialogue to cope with the different perspectives and different writing styles of Jane and Margaret. But as we went along we discovered, as good conversationalists do, the Margaret in Jane and the Jane in Margaret. We also discovered that what we were saying was not new. Others had expressed concerns about the utopianism of primary health, the woolly use of community and primary health's functional role within the emergent new international order (or disorder!). Others, notably Keleher (1994), had expressed concern about nursing and other health professional orientation toward individualised care. Where appropriate, we incorporated them in the conversation.

Running short of time, we then tried Margaret writing the nursing, and Jane the primary/public health, material. We went back to rewrite the introduction and, in doing so, the dialogue began to emerge again. This is a true story of how this chapter was written, and like all true stories, it is a fiction. So what do we want to draw out of this conversation, reconstructed and fictionalised as it is?

Jane came to the conversation from the discomfort of trying to fit her research on genetic disorder self-help groups into a primary health framework. Margaret came to the conversation from the experience of trying to teach primary health philosophy and nursing theory within the same unit. It had seemed a good idea at the time!

For Jane, the groups (or communities) were too small to even raise a blip in a primary health landscape. The membership of the group was shaped within a biomedical model, conferring on them a uniqueness and individuality with which they were loath to part, even to join forces with other genetic self-help groups. They were afraid that their own unique problems and concerns would be lost within a collective organisation, dominated by the groups with stronger public appeal, whose disorders usually manifest at birth or in early childhood. Margaret had simply felt like a split personality trying to pull primary health and nursing theory into some sort of coherent whole. From these discomforts arose our title Strange Bedfellows which we still retained enough sanity to query. But, yes, we would agree that there is a decided lack of fit between the biomedical model, nursing models of individualised patient care and primary health philosophy.

Since they are all in bed together, it seems important for the future of health to explore the disjunctions and discomforts. While primary health is usually seen as a relatively new idea, most of its tenets were already developed within the Sanitation Movement and 19th century public health. These ideas were submerged for a season by the biomedical model, only to emerge in recent times as the 'new' public health.

The only thing new about the new public health is the apparent commitment to shifting the locus of control to 'the community' rather than having control exercised by the state and/or health professionals. It is a brave dream, resembling other 'power to the people' dreams. But it can also be seen as a cynical move on the part of the state to shift responsibility for the defeat in a battle which they no longer feel they can win. It was, after all, the failure of the malaria eradication campaign which spawned Primary Health (Newell 1988). It is not the state but 'the community' which has failed. Health professionals, in a similar move, pass the buck to the individual. But individual and community are both convenient fictions.

Like Newell (1988) we would agree that the primary health approach has succeeded in getting thinking about health out of the rut it was in. We would also agree that primary health with all its problems, is the most promising program we currently have to address the mounting health issues, but it needs to be seen as pointing a direction for change rather than providing a recipe. In Newell's words 'the continuing evolution of Primary Health Care is the nearest thing we have at present...' (1988).

Nurses are envisaged as occupying an important place in this program (Morrow 1986, Maglacas 1988). Yet, given our individualistic focus, it is evident that this nursing place may rapidly become that of 'the individualised arm of the primary health movement'. The importance of nursing to primary health is usually seen in terms of our numbers, which suggests that we are to be the foot soldiers rather than the generals! Ah, but of course, there will be no more generals. How silly of us! Foot soldiers traditionally work on the front line, carrying out the orders of their superiors. The Chinese Revolution gave us a new metaphor of them swimming like fish among the people, although this did not disturb the leadership of Mao Tse Tung et al. What primary health envisages goes much beyond that, almost to the withering away of the state. At the very least, the state becomes the servant of the people. But power is not yielded up so easily, except for promise of greater power. The era of the nation-state is drawing to a close as the era of empires earlier did. At one level, the world is disintegrating into increasingly small units which we might even be tempted to call communities. But at another level, the world is being bound ever more tightly together in a universal economic system with its accompanying political forms.

Within this larger context, primary health makes sense. Each community will take responsibility for its own health and welfare within a system of control so encompassing as to be well-nigh invisible, using primary health care as the lever to make desirable changes. The ideology of primary health will endeavour to ensure that communities are made to believe that they have the choice and they have the control. However, the range of choices will be limited to those made available by the dominant order and the control communities are permitted to exercise will be similarly circumscribed. Should nursing therefore dismiss out of hand primary health as an oppressive ideology? No, but we should start critically evaluating it as such. Within any ideology, there are features that are potentially useful, that can help to achieve the sort of ends which we as nurses say we are about.

When a system subscribes to an ideology, opportunities arise for using that ideology to get leverage on the system. It is done by saying to the system, 'We are taking you at your word. If you have, as you say, a commitment to primary health, then...' The ideology of democracy is often used in exactly this way to secure desirable change (say, in the position of women or of non-white races). Of course, we are not immune from ideology and self-interest ourselves—we do not stand in a privileged position outside the social order. Nurses seem to have embraced primary health speak through some degree of discontent with the place we occupied in the biomedical model. That discontent had already given rise to our ideology of individualised patient care which was, however, developed in complementarity to that biomedical model. The adoption of the primary health model thus demands as much of a shift of ideology for us as for the medicos. The shift is as great, but the will to make the shift is possibly stronger, since we have less stake in the biomedical model and our nursing models are relatively underdeveloped. (There are no huge research and technology industries entwined with them.)

Nursing cannot adopt primary health philosophy without profoundly shifting both its theory and its practice. To date, we have simply nibbled around the edges of the problem, adopting those aspects of primary health which fit with our traditional theory and practice. In this way, we are in the process of becoming the individualised arm of the primary health movement—useful angels and/or busybodies. With a bit of a squeeze, we could also incorporate 'community development' and join in the game of trying to find communities to develop (as in Nurses versus Social Workers).

It remains to be seen whether we can move beyond that point, making the changes to our theory and practice which create for us a powerful voice in the development of healthy public policy within the primary health model. Beyond this, can we create a praxis which makes a powerful contribution to the evolution of the primary health model and, perhaps in time, its revolution (or overturning) in favour of a more promising program? The way we, as nurses, take on board primary health care will largely shape the answer to that question.

REFERENCES

Archer S E 1984 Australian nurses' political participation 1982. College of Nursing, Australia, Melbourne

Blake W Songs of experience. Any edition

Broom D 1989 Masculine medicine, feminine illness: gender and health. In: Lupton G M, Najman J M (eds) Sociology of health and illness: Australian readings. MacMillan, Melbourne

Crawford R 1984 A cultural account of 'health': control, release, and the social body. In: McKinley J B (ed) 1984 Issues in the political economy of health care. Tavistock, London

Davidoff L 1976 The rationalisation of housework. In: Barker L, Allen S (eds) Dependence and exploitation in work and marriage. Longman, London

Dean M, Bolton G 1980 The administration of poverty and the development of nursing practice in nineteenth century England. In: Davis C (ed) Re-writing nursing history. Croom-Helm, London

Dunlop M J 1992 Shaping nursing knowledge: Interpretive analysis of curriculum documents, Royal College of Nursing Australia, Melbourne

Farrow S 1987 The public health challenge. Butler & Tanner, London

Fawcett J 1984 The metaparadigm of nursing: Present status future refinements. Image: The Journal of Nursing Scholarship 16(3):84-87

Foucault M 1977 Discipline and punish. Trans Alan Sheridan, Allen Lane, London

Harrison B 1991 Women's health or social control? The role of the medical profession in relation to factory legislation in late nineteenth century Britain. Sociology of Health and Illness 13(4):469-491

Jacobs J B 1994 A qualitative study of the experience of genetic disorder self-help group members in the Queensland health care system. How best can their needs be met in the context of a primary health care model of service development and delivery. Unpublished dissertation

Keleher H 1994 Chapter public health: challenges for nursing and allied health. In: Waddell C, Petersen A R (eds) Just health: inequalities in illness, care and prevention. Churchill Livingstone, Melbourne

King I M 1971 Towards a theory of nursing. John Wiley, New York

Maglacas A M 1988 Health for all: nursing's role. Nursing Outlook 36(2):66-71

Miller F E, Lyons C, Hunt H, McCormick F J, Burr B, King M L (eds) 1917 Domestic medical practice: a household adviser in the treatment of diseases, arranged for family use. Domestic Medical Society, New York

Morrow H 1986 Nurses, nursing and women. WHO Chronicle 40(6):216-221

Newell K W 1988 Selective primary health care: the counter revolution. Social Science and Medicine 26(9):903-906

Nightingale F 1860 Notes on nursing. What it is and what it is not. Reprinted 1971. Dover, New York

Orwell G 1954 Animal farm. Penguin, Harmondsworth

Peplau H E 1952 Interpersonal relations in nursing. A conceptual frame of reference for psychodynamic nursing. Putnam's Sons, New York

Rogers M 1970 Introduction to the theoretical basis of nursing. F A Davis, Philadelphia

Rosenberg C E 1979 Healing and history. Dorsen, New York

St John W 1993 Primary health care: a clarification of the concept and the nursing role. Contemporary Nurse 2(2):73-78

Symonds A 1991 Angels and interfering busybodies: the social construction of two occupations. Sociology of Health and Illness 13(2):249-264

Taylor B J 1993 Being human: ordinariness in nursing. Churchill Livingstone, Melbourne

Thompson F 1971 Suburban living and the concept of community. Australia & New Zealand Journal of Sociology 7(October):23-27

Wass A 1994 Promoting health: the primary health care approach. Harcourt Brace Jovanovich, Sydney

Wohl A S 1983 Endangered lives: public health in Victorian England. Dent, Guildford

17

Scholars in dialogue

CAROLYN EMDEN

Introduction

Just as the private world of scholarship tempts the imagination, so too does the communal world. What a treat it would be to have some scholars, having lost their way (say, in the Tibetan high country or the London subway), knock on one's door seeking lodgings and then overhear their conversation far into the night. Imaginations aside, generally, the 'talk' of our nursing scholars is couched in the careful language of professional journals, or lost all too quickly in the fleeting moments of a good conference. What do nursing scholars talk about, and how does what they say impinge on a nursing discipline and wider philosophic ideas? Such was the curiosity behind the study reported here in part, which in effect, eavesdropped the conversations of four pairs of nursing scholars in three Australian states: Beth and Tina; Robyn and Gloria; Elaine and Cherie; and Mary and Jan (not the scholars' real names).

The backdrop to these conversations is important. There have been no other nursing times like the present (and final) decade of the 20th century in Australia: the transfer of nursing education to universities is complete—culminating 20 years of unrelenting effort by nurses and their professional organisations—with the result that Australian nurses have never experienced better educational opportunity; and nursing scholarship is at an all-time high with the advent of at least four new scholarly journals and a veritable feast of conference options continuously available—to name just two significant features of the times. While these are highly prized achievements, they have not easily been won and the toll on nursing leaders and many others has been, and continues to be, considerable. The economic and political milieu of the times also is noteworthy: the national economy has been depressed for several years, placing increased pressures upon funding bodies, from the Federal Government to families with members wishing to pursue university study on reduced incomes. On the national political scene, a Labor Government is enjoying power for a record period. Noted for educational reform, this government has overseen a major reorganisation of the Australian national higher education sector including the redesignation of colleges of advanced education and institutes of technology to universities, and numerous amalgamations of institutions. These developments have markedly affected nursing education in terms of offerings and curriculum changes within universities. In the settings from which the scholars in this study were drawn therefore, one could expect a prevailing sense of satisfaction with what has been achieved by nurses; a sense of anticipation about what is still to be attained; and, reasonably, a sense of weariness from the very hard intellectual and physical work involved. Faced additionally as they are with the day to day ramifications of the economic recession and the restructuring of higher education, the generosity of these nursing scholars to agree to take time to audiotape themselves in dialogue with a co-scholar begins to show itself.

Four high standing nursing scholars (each holding both a doctoral degree and a professorship of nursing) were invited to participate in the study on the understanding they would engage in one hour of taped dialogue with a co-scholar of their own choosing, about issues affecting the advancement of a nursing discipline. Listening to the tapes of the scholars' conversations was a special research experience. The dynamics of the situation differed from an interview in terms of intimacy and spontaneity and I found the resulting conversations totally engaging by way of content and panache.

Initial approach to the data was by way of a thematic analysis, the outcomes of which are presented here. Despite the conversations following quite different pathways in their original formats, the dialogue of the scholars was found to focus around issues to do with nursing knowledge, nursing research and scholarship, nursing education, and clinical nursing practice. In relation to each of these topics, the scholars talked about how matters currently stand, problematics, and possibilities for advancement. The format for presenting the scholars' ideas also follows this schema using largely their language. A network of ideas about a discipline of nursing thus emerges from the dialogue. It is important for readers to appreciate that at no time did the pairs of scholars actually meet together and so consensus between pairs of scholars should not be assumed; nor indeed, consensus at all times within pairs. To begin, a brief introduction to each of the conversations is presented.

Beth and Tina have some exacting ideas about the most useful focus for nursing research (Beth holds that what nursing 'is' matters most, while Tina holds it is what nurses 'do' that matters), as well as about the construction of knowledge and where nursing knowledge fits. Both scholars indicate some frustration and powerlessness in expressing their concern about an erosion of nursing practice by other disciplines, and the seeming inability of nurses to make a stand on the domain of their field, in both university and clinical practice settings. Although clearly disappointed about some aspects of nursing, both scholars hold a basically optimistic view of the future.

Robyn and Gloria have ideas for undergraduate nursing education in particular (including national core curricula and increased credit transfer), and for developing nursing research, as opposed to other areas such as education. They are unhappy about the status of nursing within universities and practice settings; it is as if nursing is a discipline trapped in a web of economic and gender related constraints, whereby nurses are barely in control of their educational and practice processes. Despite these serious concerns, both scholars remain optimistic, albeit faintly at times, about the future of nursing as a discipline. Basically they see it as being a long slow haul for nurses collectively to reach their scholastic and professional goals.

Elaine and Cherie are particularly interested in interdisciplinary aspects of nursing: how nurses relate to members of other disciplines and how these relationships can strengthen nursing as a discipline; how nursing needs to be distinct from, and yet merged with, other disciplines; and how nurses must redefine their sense of cultural cringe about being nurses. Both scholars are frustrated about nurses' reluctance to name their discipline and promote it; their tendency to shelter within the parameters of other disciplines, and, linked to this, their lowered status within academic circles. They have clear ideas for bringing about change through research into clinical practice and hold out hope for nursing to be a stronger discipline in the future.

Mary and Jan have clear views about the actions nurses should take if nursing is to be advanced as a discipline, including: establishing areas of post-doctoral nursing research within universities; increasing the numbers of nurses holding PhDs; developing nursing research methodologies; and gaining good press for nursing. They are especially concerned about legal limitations placed on nurses' clinical practice and verge on a sense of helplessness as to how this situation might be changed. A further significant point is that they believe nurses need to develop and promote themselves within areas of specific nursing expertise. Both scholars see the immediate future as a time of tough decisions for nurses if they are going to advance nursing as a discipline.

Knowledge issues

Status of nursing knowledge

Beth and Tina consider that much nursing knowledge has been borrowed from other disciplines over the years, and that what makes it unique is how these various pieces are put together for the benefit of nursing. In addition, they believe there is a body of nursing knowledge yet to be discovered that clearly belongs to nursing. They see nurses as being philosophically disinclined to put people into boxes and categorise them; similarly, in advancing nursing knowledge, they consider many types of knowledge are needed, including positivist, phenomenological, and critical knowledge. The potential for other fields to use nursing knowledge for their own benefit is seen as a positive development. Elaine and Cherie consider there has been a significant breakthrough in the relationship between the fields of medicine and nursing, with evidence of medicine now valuing nursing as a discipline within the higher education sector; they also believe there is a growing recognition that a community of scholars does not have any disciplinary boundaries. Mary and Jan highlight that nursing as a discipline has developed dramatically over the past decade and any criticism that it lacks substance as a field of study in its own right does not hold up, as evidenced by the availability of study within nursing at doctoral level. Interdisciplinary developments include the crossing of disciplinary boundaries, for example members in one philosophy department were extremely pleased about having a nurse in their department because it brought an applied perspective and allowed a crossing over into the nursing discipline.

Problematics of nursing knowledge

Several problem areas were identified by the scholars. Scientific knowledge (to which nursing in part ascribes) is punitive in that everything is supposed to be generalisable—whereas in the human sciences it is necessary to select, by eclectic processes, the information relevant to a particular situation (Beth and Tina). A further concern held by these scholars is that disciplines that are already established in the university have laid claim to a lot of nursing language and nursing territory, and they cite health management and communication as being classic examples. Robyn and Gloria consider that nursing is primarily an oral culture, and because of this, nurses don't write their knowledge down to the same extent as other health professionals, which contributes to their work not being recognised. Elaine and Cherie are concerned that even though nursing is the largest health discipline, it is in danger of being subsumed under the broad title of 'health science'—possibly because of nurses' difficulty in articulating their discipline. They regard it a basic problem that people are ignorant of the discipline; they do not understand what nurses do, or are too afraid to talk about the things nurses do.

Ways forward in advancing nursing knowledge

All scholars see ways forward in advancing nursing knowledge: nurses need to be absolutely firm on what is nursing knowledge and why it is nursing knowledge (Beth and Tina); nurses need to identify the scope of the nursing discipline and to hang on to it (Robyn and Gloria); nurses need to name the nursing discipline and to value and promote it (Elaine and Cherie); and it is very important for nurses to identify a distinctive nursing perspective, for example, naming oneself as a nursing ethicist (Mary and Jan). Robyn and Gloria also consider that the development of a theoretical base and a research base is fundamental to advancing the discipline and further, that communication between nurses on a global basis will assist this. Elaine and Cherie are emphatic it is time for nurses to step out of other people's shadows—whether the shadows of scientists, the doctors, the social scientists, or the philosophers; they believe nurses need to locate themselves within the academy, and establish how they are going to articulate with, interface with, and do business with, other disciplines. They have found that studying outside the discipline of nursing broadens one's base; indeed they believe it is possible to learn more about nursing by getting completely outside it and into another discipline. For example, they have found it helpful in setting up structures within the nursing discipline to look at structures within sociology and psychology; the disciplines of history and economics also have proved very helpful in better informing nurses about nursing. These scholars further consider nursing will come into its own in a postmodernist era because it is not locked into any one frame of reference or paradigm. Mary and Jan make the additional point that 'provolution'—somewhere between evolution and revolution—is also a useful approach for nurses to utilise (after de Bono).

Research and scholarship issues

Status of nursing research and scholarship

All scholars have strong (and quite mixed) views on this topic. For example, Beth believes that pure nursing research is that which gets to the essence of what nursing is; Tina believes it is rather what nurses do; while both agree there must be some congruence between the two. Tina does not believe that nurses can talk about having a pure methodology; Beth suggests it is better termed an eclectic methodology. Robyn considers the focus of the study of nursing should be clients and their health status and not practitioners; Gloria suggests it should be a combination; both agree that the ideal research project is one on nursing practice with a nursing theoretical framework but that this is still to be realised. These scholars also agree that various definitions of 'scholarship' exist: Tina thinks that in the broadest terms, anyone interested in learning could be considered a scholar; Beth associates writing, research, and teaching with scholarship. Mary and Jan argue that research and scholarship are integral to one another and suggest it is increasingly being recognised that research is integral to nursing; they also see publication being linked very much to personal confidence.

Problematics of nursing research and scholarship

One pair of scholars believe nursing research has not focused on things that ought to make a difference to nursing (Mary and Jan); another scholar believes a lot of research done by nurses is medically oriented, such as clinical epidemiology (Cherie); while others feel frustrated because many nurses wish to pursue their higher degrees in the field of education, rather than nursing (Robyn and Gloria). Elaine is concerned that Australia has become an international dumping ground for much American nursing research that is not necessarily useful to Australian nurses. On scholarship, Elaine and Cherie believe nurses in universities are reluctant to own up to being nurses (to own the discipline) for fear of being regarded as a lesser class of scholar by other academics in the university; they see this as being exacerbated by the fact that nurses also are largely women who used to work in colleges of advanced education. Elaine believes the past oppressive system of nursing has detracted from the development of a community of nursing scholars because it has tended to punish free speech, debate, and disputation. The heavy administrative loads that most Australian nursing professors carry, in addition to the scholarly expectations of their roles, works against them engaging in dialogue with one another, according to Mary and Jan. Other scholars find that the university administration operates in a male, received, view of the world and that if women (nurses) challenge this male framework they usually lose out; thus, rather than trying to change the rules, they end up going over to the other side and operating by the male rules (Beth and Tina).

Ways forward in advancing nursing research and scholarship

Several views are forthcoming here, for example, if nurses research the practice of nursing, then its value will become self-evident (Elaine), and in a similar vein, if nurses get on and produce their research and scholarship, nursing will speak for itself (Mary). It is pointed out that philosophical and historical research is just as important as other nursing research (Mary and Jan), and indeed nurses should currently be collecting living histories of nursing academics for the benefit of future nurses (Robyn). Mary and Jan also are optimistic that a synthesis of presently available research approaches will produce some new methods, such as distinctive feminist research methodologies that provide a more contextually based approach that is grounded in the experience of women. These scholars further firmly believe that for the nursing discipline to develop, a high proportion of its doctoral students must explore the substance of nursing per se.

On scholarship and matters of university structure, Robyn and Gloria consider it essential that nurses use the political process to influence decision making about nursing within universities, and that they work at this from the inside. They also believe there is a need for an infrastructure in Australia to develop nursing scholarship. Mary and Jan speak about the advantages of an Australian Council of Deans and an Australian nursing 'professoriate' whereby scholars can meet together.

Nursing education issues

Status of nursing education

The scholars have several comments on this topic: Robyn and Gloria state that the advent of the nursing degree has advanced the discipline by producing graduates on equal footing with graduates from other fields; also, they perceive that these nurses will bring about a gradual evolution of positive attitudes towards university nursing graduates. In addition they point to the political nature of tertiary institutions and their view that nurses encounter problems within them because they don't know the rules; they don't know the games people play. Beth and Tina consider knowledge is international and world wide and that nurses should be able to apply knowledge from other disciplines to nursing. Robyn and Gloria see education as being the way nursing theory is applied; they also consider, in relation to nursing competencies, that the student's total development should be looked at, not just pieces of behaviour. Elaine makes the point that nurses look for explanations about the human condition in their education, especially the human conditions of illness and disability.

Problematics of nursing education

Several issues emerge here. Concern is expressed that nursing academics have been bogged down with getting higher education for nurses established which has detracted from their leadership, that more nurses with PhDs are needed for supervision of research students, that service teaching can result in up to 40% of some curricula being taught by non nurses, and that the number of nursing Faculties in Australian universities is being reduced (Mary and Jan). Other scholars are concerned that educational practice in their university is being driven by economic rationalism with the consequence that nurses are not in control of their own programs; and further, it has been a tall order for nurses to meet university expectations of scholarship, teaching, and practice, all within a short time frame (Robyn and Gloria).

Ways forward in advancing nursing education

A number of ideas are proffered here. For example, firm placement of the control of nursing education, including curriculum content, in the hands of nurses, and clear establishment of post-doctoral nursing programs in areas of specific expertise within Australian universities, thus enabling PhD students to be referred to where the expertise lies (Mary and Jan). More integration between education and practice and exploration of the concept of practitioner-scholars or practitioner-educators, development of more creative and cost effective teaching strategies; and further debate about the concept of a national core curriculum for undergraduate students and the issue of credit transfer (Robyn and Gloria).

Clinical practice issues

Status of clinical practice

The scholars did not speak at length on this topic, however Beth and Tina make the point that whatever it is that nurses do in the provision of appropriate care for someone, then that itself must be 'nursing'; Robyn and Gloria highlight the importance of reflective practice in nursing, and the shift from task oriented to patient assignment nursing; Elaine and Cherie believe nursing is going to come into its own as chronic illness,which does not respond to medical treatment, increases; and Mary and Jan point to the relationship between control of practice and nurses' legitimated authority (or lack thereof) to practice.

Problematics of nursing practice

Gender issues are raised by three scholars: Tina (within a discussion about nurse managers) states that being female and a nurse goes hand in hand; Jan (within a discussion about the law discriminating against nurses) states that nurses are the third sex; and Mary speaks of the whole dominant area of male politicians and male doctors who are responsible for the shape of the Australian health care system. Elaine and Cherie comment on the clinical career structure and are concerned that it could backfire with the unwitting creation of a new hierarchy which is linked to monetary rewards. Robyn and Gloria highlight difficulties associated with the ANRAC competencies which are intentionally broad but hence difficult to assess. Elaine and Cherie, citing some telling evidence, are concerned that people have a mind set about nurses being relatively unskilled. In a discussion about the independent and interdependent functions of nurses, Mary proposes that nurses do not see their independent role as being important, while Jan points out it is one of the greatest frustrations for nurses, when they do make independent judgements, that they are either ignored or not taken seriously. Jan also is very concerned that (a) nurses lack the legitimated authority to match their professional responsibilities (that is, they are not free to nurse); and (b) that the trend in Britain to replace nurse managers with non-nurses will be followed in Australia, whereby, in effect, nursing at the bedside level is not controlled by nurses. In a discussion about the distinction between political awareness and militancy, Beth and Tina believe nurses have not been sufficiently politically aware and skilled. In a similar vein, Mary and Jan believe the professional organisations, the Australian Nursing Federation and Royal College of Nursing, Australia, have not adequately politicised important nursing issues, such as the devolution of nurse administrators.

Ways forward in advancing nursing practice

Several ideas are put forward, such as equipping future nurses with strategies to cope with micro and macro political systems (Beth and Tina), and equipping them not only with the language of nursing, but also the fiscal language of management (Mary and Jan). Mary and Jan also have strong views about the professional and public face of nursing: they believe more free press is necessary within the discipline, that is, within Australian nursing journals; they consider nurses should promote nursing through general avenues such as womens' magazines; and they consider it very important that nurses receive education in media relations. These scholars also suggest that nursing leaders need to have a broad vision of the whole, see where things are connecting and not connecting, and hold the interest of the profession at heart.

Research approach

Several theorists were influential in the conduct of the studies 'Scholars in dialogue' and 'On being a scholar' (reported in a separate chapter). From a phenomenological perspective, van Manen and Colaizzi were particularly helpful, as was Polkinghorne from a narrative perspective. The methodological ideas of these authors are increasingly apparent within nursing literature; thus I have chosen to highlight some of their key ideas aside from these, as follows.

Van Manen

Max van Manen (1990) is deeply immersed in the phenomenological tradition from an educational perspective. The immediate appeal of van Manen to both 'Scholars in dialogue' and 'On being a scholar' was his claim to bridge Anglo-American and European philosophical traditions (on the basis of his study and research on both Continents). He identifies phenomenology and hermeneutics as human science approaches that are 'rooted in philosophy' and because of this, he believes human science researchers need to be familiar with the philosophic traditions. Further, researchers should choose a particular research method only when it is in harmony with the 'deep interest' that they bring to the research. Van Manen purports that every phenomenological inquiry is driven by an abiding concern:

> phenomenological research is a being-given-over to some quest, a true task, a deep questioning of something that restores an original sense of what it means to be a thinker, a researcher, a theorist...It is always a project of someone: a real person, who, in the context of a particular individual, social, and historical life circumstances, sets out to make sense of a certain aspect of human existence.

He also provides the reminder that a phenomenological description is 'always one interpretation, and no single interpretation of human experience will ever exhaust the possibility of yet another complementary, or even potentially richer or deeper description'.

Van Manen's ideas about phenomenological inquiry were in harmony with my own thoughts and feelings about the research being reported: I brought an 'abiding concern' to the study from earlier research, about the thoughts of nursing scholars on advancing their field. This concern was firmly embedded in my interest in philosophic traditions which, van Manen claims, is a hallmark of quality phenomenological research. Further, I was attracted to van Manen's idea that hermeneutic phenomenological research is 'fundamentally a writing activity'. He notes a general neglect of the relationship between research and writing and deplores the notion that writing is something that enters the research process at the report stage. Van Manen believes writing is 'closely fused' into the research activity and that a 'certain form of consciousness' created by the art of literacy is required in phenomenology. As he points out, the object of human science research is 'essentially a linguistic project' and as such, for 'scholars such as Husserl, Heidegger, Sartre, and Merleau-Ponty the activities of researching and reflecting on the one hand, and reading and writing on the other hand, are indeed quite indistinguishable'. Not only does the writer produce text, but 'the writer produces himself or herself...to write is to measure the depth of things, as well to come to a sense of one's own depth' (van Manen 1990). Much of what van Manen says about writing and phenomenological research rang true for this research: writing was integral to the process from the beginning, whether making contact with participants, or transcribing their thoughts, or searching for meaningful approaches to data analysis—the whole project has been an experience of 'feeling my way forward' through writing. This process proved to be at times difficult and tortuous which may serve to shed light on van Manen's statement that 'in a society dominated by orality, phenomenology would be quite impossible'. As nursing increasingly is recognised as an oral culture, this may account in part for the sense of challenge posed by the research.

Colaizzi

Paul Colaizzi's guidelines (1978) to the collection and analysis of phenomenological data were valued for their explicit nature. Colaizzi writes lucidly of the difficulties and anxieties his field of psychology has experienced in coming to realise that it does not belong, philosophically or methodologically, to the natural sciences out of which it was conceived. Having identified human experience as the prime interest of the psychologist (in contrast to observable human behaviour), he seeks to provide some ways for the psychologist to objectively investigate human experience—objectivity from the phenomenological perspective being 'fidelity to phenomena'. Colaizzi's writing strikes an empathic chord to nursing readers; indeed one can substitute 'nursing' for 'psychology' in the text in many places and highlight nursing's own quest for research methods that are congruent with the kinds of research questions that nurses wish to ask. Perhaps psychology, like nursing, has felt the need to articulate its research methods with inordinate clarity in order to justify its research programs to adherents of more traditional scientific approaches; hence, perhaps, Colaizzi's explicit description of how one might approach a phenomenological inquiry. (Although Colaizzi refers, in 1978, to forthcoming writings by himself, these cannot be traced; meanwhile his chapter 'Psychological research as the phenomenologist views it' appears to have assumed classic status in that it continues to be cited regularly in social science and nursing literature.)

Colaizzi's recommended method of phenomenological analysis involving seven procedural steps has been widely cited within nursing literature and shall not be repeated here. Suffice to say the method proved largely workable although I would add the cautionary note that when applied to more than one data set (as in 'Scholars in dialogue') it can have the unfortunate effect of homogenising the data whereby the individuality of the participants is lost. I also consider that to fully implement Colaizzi's method as intended by him requires considerable skill on the researcher's part. Heeding Colaizzi's advice with the interviews in 'On being a scholar', I endeavoured to show a high degree of sensitivity to the 'full richness' of the other person, and to listen with the totality of my 'being and personality'. Importantly, the questions used tapped the participants' 'experience of phenomenon as distinct from their theoretical knowledge of it'. Of further value were Colaizzi's ideas about the frontier area of phenomenological research (the area 'fraught with controversies and problematics'), whereby he touches upon the following notions: neither by-passing, nor being strangled by, the literature; uncovering of presuppositions (held by both researcher and participants) by dialogical research; passing beyond research to existential insight through dialogical research; and realising that the phenomenological thesis can never be exhausted (1987).

Polkinghorne

Donald Polkinghorne (1988) believes the solutions to human problems will not come 'from developing even more sophisticated and creative applications of the natural science model' which he sees as having been largely the pattern of events to date. In the course of practice as a psychotherapist he has come to appreciate the significance and importance of people's 'stories' ('the patient comes to the analyst with a story to tell') and, consequently, the key argument he wishes to make is that 'narrative is a scheme by means of which human beings give meaning to their experience of temporality and personal actions'. Polkinghorne envisages a new kind of training will be necessary for scholars in the human sciences which includes 'study of the structures and relations of linguistically organized reality' and further, that the human sciences will need to conceive themselves as 'multiple sciences'—rather than natural sciences— because the human being exists in 'multiple strata of reality'. Polkinghorne's work carries the narrative style of philosophising through several stages, including research approaches, to a narrative approach to clinical practice. In doing so he provides a considerable challenge to the human sciences to reconceptualise their ways of theorising and practising. The appeal of narrative to 'On being a scholar' lay partly in its affinity with a Continental style of philosophy—that is, a non-analytic or argumentation style—and in its suggested approach to gathering and analysing narrative research data.

Narrative research, according to Polkinghorne (1988), can be of two forms: descriptive and explanatory. Descriptive narrative research produces 'an accurate description of the interpretive narrative accounts individuals or groups use to make sequences of events in their lives or organizations meaningful'; while explanatory narrative research constructs 'a narrative account explaining "why" a situation or event involving human actions has happened'. The concept of descriptive narrative research was relevant to 'On being a scholar' in that scholars in different disciplines used the narrative form to bring together the events of their lives as scholars into unfolding themes. Polkinghorne identifies the interview as the basic source of evidence about narratives which often take a form similar to a modern novel 'with flashbacks and with portions of the story out of chronological order'. He points out (citing Mishler 1986a) that in many survey situations the interviewer is seeking short answers and instead 'often receives long, storied responses' which subsequently suffer cumulative suppression within the stages of a typical study. In narrative research, the interviewer needs rather to 'move from the specific stories a person uses to account for particular episodes to more general life stories that provide self-identity and give unity to a person's whole existence'. In analysing such interviews, Polkinghorne refers to Labov's work (cited by Mishler) and suggests that transcripts can be 'broken down and particular statements identified according to the functions they serve in the narrative account', thus a 'core story' is abstracted from the interview content—which can then be compared with other core stories of a similar structure.

The data gathered within 'On being a scholar' were in storied form. As Mishler explains, stories are likely to be found in studies that use unstructured interviews, where 'respondents are invited to speak in their own voices, allowed to control the introduction and flow of topics, and encouraged to extend their responses' (1986a). He points out that respondents may also tell stories in response to direct questions 'if they are not interrupted by interviewers trying to keep them to the 'point'. In contrast to mainstream interview research which, according to Mishler, tends to treat stories as problems because they are difficult to code and quantify, narrative analysis seeks to identify the story and its sub-plots, or a series of different stories, within a response.

Mishler (1986a) suggests that much diversity can be found in narrative analysis as 'we are at an early stage in the development of this approach'. He goes on to identify three orientations to analysis that draw on various writers in the area: the textual (how parts of the text are connected); the ideational (meaning of what is said); and the interpersonal (relationships between speakers). Mishler brings these orientations together in an approach to his own research that involves creating a 'core narrative' (after Labov) and then identifying its constituents or themes to help understand it. Polkinghorne suggests that the value of core stories as proposed by Labov is that they can be 'compared to other stories with a similar structure but told in other contexts'. According to Polkinghorne: 'analysis is carried out using hermeneutic techniques for noting underlying patterns across examples of stories'. He also points out that 'the theme or point of a story is not usually directly presented by the text, for it requires inference and interpretation on the researcher's part' and hence the desirability of transcripts of interviews being available to other researchers so they can follow the moves from data to interpretation.

From narrative to core story

Specific advice on how to transform a narrative interview transcript to a core story is not provided by Mishler, Polkinghorne, or Labov except for mention that the core story may consist of about 25% of the original text (Mishler 1986b). This proved consistent with my own approach whereby I devised the following procedural steps:

1 Reading the entire text several times within a period of several weeks to grasp its content
2 Deleting all interviewer questions and comments from the text
3 Deleting all words that detracted from the key meaning of each sentence or group of sentences uttered by the respondent
4 Reading the entire remaining text for meaning
5 Repeating steps three and four until satisfied that all key meanings were retained and extraneous content eliminated
6 Identifying constituent themes within the text
7 Moving fragments of themes together to create a coherent core story, or series of core stories.

The procedure as it was carried out could be likened to 'combing' the data (my own term), whereby data were reduced in such a way that their underlying structure and meaning were not diminished. Core stories were then returned to the study participants and the following questions asked:

- Does the core story 'ring true'?
- Do you wish to correct/develop/delete any part?

As a result of feedback received from each participant, some minor amendments were made to the core stories. It is significant that all stories 'rang true' to their originators (despite a wide variance with the form of their original telling), indicating the procedure for arriving at the core story was sound—at least for this study. The procedure as adopted in 'On being a scholar' is offered here for testing and development by other nursing researchers.

Conclusion

While readers will wish to draw their own insights from the scholars' dialogue, their views about the status of the nursing discipline, its problems, and ways forward in advancing the discipline, may be expressed briefly as follows.

Views on the status of a nursing discipline

Nursing is an eclectic discipline that draws on and contributes to, many other disciplines. Increasing numbers of doctoral students in nursing attest to the maturity of the discipline, as well as the development of innovative nursing research methodologies. Research and scholarship are viewed as integral to one another and to clinical practice, where the client assumes a position of central importance. Interest in the human condition is central for nursing students, at all levels of preparation, and translates into reflective clinical practice and the development of nursing therapies.

Views on problematics of a nursing discipline

Scientific knowledge has not significantly advanced nursing as a discipline. Much research undertaken by nurses has tended to advance other fields such as education or medicine, rather than the nursing discipline. Several factors have helped reduce the control of nursing education by nurses: the oral nature of nursing knowledge has led in part to a lack of recognition of nursing by other disciplines; some university structures subsume nursing under titles such as 'health science'; other disciplines have laid claim to some of what nurses would consider nursing language and nursing territory; and service teaching arrangements enable a quite high proportion of curriculum content to be taught by non nurses. Nurses working within the largely male dominated frameworks of Australian universities experience difficulties both as women academics and nurses; with many nurse leaders at professorial level being additionally burdened by heavy administrative workloads. All nurse academics are feeling, at a time of rapid development in nursing education, challenged by university expectations of teaching, research, and scholarship. In the clinical practice arena, devolution is of major concern (if overseas trends are to be fully realised in Australia) whereby, in particular, nurse managers are replaced by general managers within organisational structures. Many nurses are suffering diminished authority in clinical practice settings in terms of their independent decision making—despite the advent of clinical career structures and clinical competencies—which impacts negatively on efforts to advance nursing as a discipline.

Views on ways forward in advancing a nursing discipline

Nurses are becoming increasingly confident about their field through research and scholarship. It is in nursing's interest for this search for meaning to continue via many approaches, including feminist research and the study of nursing from both within and outside the discipline. Postmodernism heralds unprecedented development of this kind in nursing because it frees nurses to pursue various frames of reference and paradigms. Nurses need to establish themselves firmly within Australian universities, creating strong and positive relationships with other disciplines in the process. By strengthening their political skills they are better placed to influence decision making within the higher education sector, as well as teach these skills to students who can in turn influence their spheres of practice. An infrastructure for developing nursing scholarship in Australia is a priority: forums for nursing professors and Deans would provide excellent opportunities for exchange; free speech and debate also must be facilitated via further multiple forums, as well as greater freedom of press encouraged in Australian nursing journals. Universities should move urgently to establish their areas of post doctoral nursing expertise, whereby higher degree and doctoral students can be assured of the best supervision available around the country. The issues of national core curricula and credit transfer deserve ongoing debate in the undergraduate area, together with the further development of creative, cost effective teaching strategies across all courses. Moving the nursing discipline forward also requires: visionary, committed leaders with a clear sense of direction; political will on the part of nursing organisations such as Royal College of Nursing, Australia and the Australian Nursing Federation to address key issues confronting the discipline; and, commitment on the part of all nurses, in all work places, to sharpen, and exercise, their political nous in the interest of achieving full nursing autonomy.

From the scholars

It is fitting that this chapter closes with some words from the scholars themselves. As can be seen, the thematic approach to analysing their dialogue tended to have both a depersonalising and fragmenting effect upon what they had to say. The following segments of dialogue therefore provide direct insight into their thinking and a sense of 'eavesdropping' their conversations. It is remembered that the conversations were held quite separately from each other; at no time were the pairs of scholars in joint dialogue. Four segments are presented (one from each pair) for readers' interest.

Elaine and Cherie on practice issues

Elaine: I think that one of the most important things we've got to do, this is top of my list, is to stop being apologetic about being nurses, that we have to name the discipline, own it, redefine our sense of cultural cringe about it, and to start both valuing it and promoting it—instead of promoting education or the social sciences or politics or physiology or some other...that relates to medicine. Because I think quite seriously that if we don't stop being apologetic about being nurses and doing nursing, we'll slip back into someone else's shadow.

Cherie: Yes, well I think that's something that would be on top of my list too; I'd have expressed it a little bit differently by saying that we have to put the practice of the discipline central to the discipline and discourse about the discipline.

Elaine: Does that mean naming it? I'm thinking about all those Deans of health science and Deans of other things who now presume to give advice on nursing, where I think nursing is in danger of simply becoming subsumed under that broad title 'health sciences' even though we are the largest discipline.

Cherie: Or just straight 'health'; like...I think there's a problem though in we as academics having an expectation that we can do this, because if you talk to clinicians and if you ask the clinicians what nursing is, they can't tell you.

Elaine: But if you ask them what they do, they can.

Cherie: Yes, but then they have difficulty differentiating what it is they do...to one of the other health workers; they know in themselves, in their hearts and their minds what it is; it's the articulation of the discipline that's the difficulty, and maybe that's why some academics are quite prepared to let it become 'health sciences' or 'health studies' or whatever, because they have difficulty.

Elaine: Or because, I'd argue, the language is deficient; deficient from its reality generally. I think there's another element here, I think there's this sense of not owning up to being a nurse, not wanting to own the discipline, for fear of all sorts of things—like being regarded as a lesser class of scholar, being regarded as a second class citizen in the university.

Robyn and Gloria on research issues

Gloria: I think one of the areas that we as nurses in Australia should be thinking of is whether nursing is any different in Australia than anywhere else and if so, what is the theoretical basis of that?

Robyn: I agree. I'm not sure how you go about testing that; it has always interested me as a research question because I tend to think that the proper study of nursing is people. I think Martha Rogers made a major contribution to nursing when she said that we should be focusing on studying people and not nurses; the focus of the study of nursing should be the client and not the practitioner.

Gloria: I think it has to be a combination.

Robyn: Well, you can study the practitioner in interaction with the patient or client; that is nursing, or look at people and their health, that is something we should be studying; but just to be studying how better to educate nurses, or something like that, I don't see as advancing nursing per se. except as very, very peripherally. Now I know that's not necessarily a popular point of view but I do believe...

Gloria: ...what you are saying, if I have understood you correctly, is that you don't see a connection between nursing research in relation to nursing practice and care...

Robyn: No, no, I'm saying I believe our research focus for nursing should be on people and their health status, or lack of health status, or the nurse caring for the patient, studying the process of nursing if you like; I believe these will advance the discipline of nursing. But I don't believe studying how to teach a nurse how to give an injection for example, or other such educational matters, is going to advance nursing. It might advance education but it isn't advancing nursing, and I believe very passionately about that as you know.

Beth and Tina on knowledge issues

Tina: What are my thoughts? A body of knowledge probably is something that is borrowed from a lot of other disciplines and yet we tend to try to argue that what is 'nursing' is unique; I think probably there is fairly little that is unique, it's the parts we take from other disciplines that make nursing unique.

Beth: I think we have taken a lot from other disciplines over the years but I also think we have our own body of knowledge waiting out there to be discovered, which, because the other disciplines are so oriented to who owns what, they can probably tap into virtually anything we talk about or think about and say it's theirs. And so apart from the competition, I think there is something that is ours, but what we have got to do is fight for it and say it is ours, and why.

Tina: I agree, I suspect that we haven't fought for it because we have been so busy trying to work out what is our unique body of knowledge; there may not be anything at the moment that is unique, so we have to capture what is everybody else's and lay claim to it, and we have been fairly hesitant to do that. Also, other disciplines are much more established in the university sector so they have laid claim to a lot of our territory; probably the health management area would be a classic example.

Beth: Yes. The other very interesting area where we argue we have one body of knowledge and the social scientists argue they have the body of knowledge, is the area of communication. Where we call it 'interpersonal processes', or 'nursing relationships', they talk about 'communication', and yet one of the areas of assessment with our students is what we call 'communication', but we are not using the word in the same sense as the communication theorist is using it. We are talking about interactive processes, and yet it means that if we can't use words from other disciplines, simply because they belong to the other discipline, then half our language is gone.

Mary and Jan on education issues

Mary: It seems to me that we are not moving fast enough in relation to establishing sound post doctoral areas of study in our Faculties of Nursing. I guess it is going to come over the next five years, I would hope so anyway, but I think that until we really bite the bullet, there have got to be a lot of hard decisions made...on what a Faculty can actually develop. There is no doubt that there is a push from Government as well as from our own universities, saying: 'Identify the areas of expertise that you are going to grow in and build up; not only breadth in those areas, but depth and really profound depth'. This is an area that nursing now has to move into; in the past we've wanted to be all things to all people.

Jan: I think it's also a hard decision, not just for all those reasons that you have cited Mary, but also for the reason: 'Are these really the right decisions professionally as well?' How do you know you are making the correct judgment in terms of the demarcations of specialised areas or areas where you have pooled expertise? I think it's a risk you have to take.

Mary: Yes, it is always a risky business; you have to take risks; you have to look at where you think nursing ought to be heading and then move in those directions. But on the other hand, you can really only go so far as your expertise on staff will allow you to go.

ACKNOWLEDGEMENTS

The eight nursing scholars who participated in this study are sincerely thanked for sharing their dialogue and for their sustained support. The advice of Professor Judith Parker also is gratefully acknowledged.

REFERENCES

Colaizzi P F 1978 Psychological research as the phenomenologist views it. In: Valle R S, King M (eds) Existential-phenomenological alternatives for psychology. Oxford University Press, New York

de Bono E 1990 I am right, you are wrong: from this to the new Renaissance, from rock logic to water logic. Viking, London

Mishler E G 1986a Research interviewing: context and narrative. Harvard University Press, Cambridge

Mishler E G 1986b The analysis of interview-narratives. In: Sarbin T R (ed) Narrative psychology: the storied nature of human conduct. Praeger, New York

Polkinghorne D E 1988 Narrative knowing and the human sciences. State University of New York Press, Albany

van Manen M 1990 Researching lived experience: human science for an action sensitive pedagogy. State University of New York Press, New York

18

Only connect...feminism and nursing

JULIANNE CHEEK, TRUDY RUDGE

Introduction

The term feminism was first introduced into the English language in the 1880s and since then has evoked, and continues to evoke, strong reactions amongst various sectors of society. It is variously shunned by some as extreme and subversive, whilst others have embraced it as offering a possibility for shifting women from the margins to the centre frame of social analysis thereby allowing for the possibility for woman to be defined in her own right, not as 'Other' (see de Beauvior 1972). However, too often supporters and critics of feminism alike assume that their audience shares common understandings of what feminism is. Such an assumption is problematic given that feminism itself is a contested concept. As Shulman reminds us, 'Feminism is not a monolith; there are many different, even at times contradictory positions which may spring from good feminist motives' (1982).

There are however, some common features of all feminist approaches. Weedon (1987) succinctly summarises some of this commonality when she writes, 'feminism is a politics. It is a politics directed at changing existing power relations between women and men in society...[which] determine who does what and for whom, what we are and what we might become.' Patriarchy was a term coined by Millet in 1970 to describe the existing power relationships between men and women in contemporary Western society. Patriarchy literally means the rule of the father. Weedon provides a useful working definition of patriarchy when she writes that patriarchy 'refers to power relations in which women's interests are subordinated to the interests of men' (1987). However, again a word of caution is needed at this point. Like the definition of feminism itself, patriarchy has many different inflections and emphases. It is important to be aware of this and not assume common understandings.

The starting point for much feminist analysis is a critique of the patriarchal nature of society in the quest to shift 'woman' as a category from the margins to the centre of social analysis. Indeed Luke (1992) posits that this is a central task for all feminist theorists, 'regardless of diverse disciplinary perspectives and theoretical standpoints.' In keeping with Luke's assertion, the major impact of feminist approaches on nursing thought has emanated from the attempt to trace the effect of the exclusion of women's knowledge from the essentially patriarchal arena of health care both on the production of nursing knowledge, and on the form of nursing practice (see Ehrenreich & English 1978, Hagell 1989, Doering 1992).

It is important to point out that in critiquing the social and political structures emanating from patriarchal constructions of reality, feminism has relevance and implications for men as well as women. Eisenstein points out:

> In my understanding of the term 'feminist' then I see an element of visionary, futurist thought...[which] encompasses a concept of social transformation that, as part of the eventual liberation of women, will change all human relationships for the better. Although centrally about women, their experience, condition, or 'estate'...feminism is therefore also fundamentally about men, and about social change (1984).

Such a view adds balance to what often has become a polemic debate setting up women against men, and in the process obscuring the fundamental issues at stake. Eisenstein reminds us that existing patriarchal structures also work against some men. This is particularly true of those men in the past who have chosen to pursue nursing or other so-called 'feminine' professions. Thus, by shifting and disrupting the place assigned to women by social structures the potential is there to shift and disrupt much else.

The nurse as feminist?

Historically nursing has been perceived as traditionally a female and feminine occupation. Hence, gender has played a significant part in the way that nursing has been, and continues to be, constructed. The low status of nursing and the way in which the work of nurses is devalued, especially when compared to other health professionals, can at least in part be explained by its gendered nature.

Given this, it may seem surprising that nursing and feminism have not articulated with each other well—in fact hardly at all. This is evident from the often gender neutral, or even gender blind, accounts of nursing put forward by nursing theorists such as Orem 1983, Roy 1984, Neuman 1989 and Watson 1985—to name but a few. However, an increasing number of contemporary nursing authors have begun to recognise the impact of the gendered nature of society on nursing and the nature of its practice base (Chinn 1989, Wheeler & Chinn 1991, Lawler 1990, Speedy 1991, MacPherson 1991, Doering 1992, Webb 1993). Concomitant with such a growing awareness of the potential of feminist analyses to illuminate aspects of nursing and nursing practice, there are emerging feminist based reappraisals of nursing knowledge (Doering 1992, Hagell 1989, Bunting & Campbell 1990, Gray 1992); nursing research (Webb 1993, Speedy 1991, Anderson 1991a); and professionalisation in nursing (Bruni 1991, Turkoski 1992, O'Neill 1992, Yaros 1991).

Yet despite this growing genre of feminist based nursing literature there is still considerable debate as to the appropriateness of feminist theorising for understanding nursing and nursing knowledge (Webb 1993, Allan 1993). Many nurses have not embraced feminism, and still are reluctant to do so, either finding feminism too radical or seemingly irrelevant. As Speedy (1991) notes 'explicit feminism seems to have been rejected by all but a few nurses. Nevertheless, an examination of the concepts which are currently guiding the development of nursing and nursing knowledge suggest that feminist principles, *whilst not necessarily recognised as such*, are becoming more and more influential' (our emphasis).

Webb (1986) points out that the ongoing tension between feminism and nursing has been to both feminism's and nursing's disadvantage, asserting that 'I am convinced that an exploration of feminist writings and participation in groups and campaigns would lead nurses to be able to practise real caring nursing instead of the alien and subservient forms of patient care they are often involved in at present.' In the same vein, Meleis (1991) argues that a feminist perspective has the potential to be 'utilised to understand, to explain, to raise consciousness, and to develop theories that enhance understanding of the situation, the daily experience, and the responses of clients'. Further, it is an often overlooked point that a feminist perspective can also be used to develop understandings and raise the consciousness of nurses themselves. Thus, whilst a gender sensitive framework can enable nurses to study phenomena grounded in the life and experience of the nursing client, it is an equally valid framework from which to explore the phenomena that 'represent and emanate from the lives' of nurses and which are 'related to the quality of their [nurses] lives..that may be seen as problematic from their [nurses] perspective' (Meleis 1991).

In light of the preceding discussion, this chapter explores the somewhat problematic relationship that has historically existed between feminism and nursing. There are a number of points of tension and resistance between feminism and nursing. However, if the theoretical tenets of each perspective are explored and grounded in terms of their relationship to the everyday reality of women and nurses, then it may be possible to shorten the distances between the domains of women and nurses, feminism and nursing, and theory and practice; in order to promote a multiple view of truth.

Such a multiple view of truth is imperative if nurses are to begin to counter the misunderstanding, marginalisation and manipulation by others that has characterised nursing's history in both the societal and practice setting contexts. Nursing marginalises and devalues feminism at its own peril for, as Bryson (1992) asserts, '...feminist political theory cannot be conveniently "ghetto-ised", for the issues it raises are of vital importance to any understanding of political power; in seeking to explain and challenge the situation of women, it increases our understanding of all areas of political life, any political theory that ignores it is inevitably partial and impoverished'.

Feminism—diverse disciplinary perspectives and theoretical standpoints

Given the preceding discussion, what are the diverse disciplinary perspectives and theoretical standpoints in feminism? A convenient and common means of grappling with such diversity has been to neatly package feminist theory into three main approaches—liberal feminism, socialist/Marxist feminism and radical feminism, all of which are discussed in detail later in this section. The essential difference between these approaches is the way in which they conceive of changing existing power relations between men and women in contemporary society. The discussion of feminism in nursing analyses (and not just nursing analyses, we might add) often almost mandatorily 'covers' these three approaches, and then having 'done' feminism moves on to apply supposedly generic feminist principles to the task at hand. This is problematic in two senses. The first is that feminism can not be neatly packaged and sanitised in this way. Secondly, in adopting such an approach it is very easy to over simplify each approach and gain at best a superficial grasp of their complexities and implications. Bryson (1992) asserts that such schema 'caricature complex theories which can not be neatly slotted into such distinct categories and which are constantly evolving...the classification of theories must therefore be approached with caution'.

Perhaps the tensions that do exist between nursing and feminism can be explained, at least in part, by the tendency of nursing literature to neatly package feminism into these various approaches without a full exploration of the basis and rationale for so doing. As a consequence one of two things often happens—either writers assume a certain 'type' of feminism in their work but do not make either the choice, or the reasons for the choice, explicit (e.g. see Chinn 1989, Webb 1993, Allan 1993); or nursing literature about feminism attempts to reduce feminism to its lowest common denominator thus stripping it of its theoretical integrity and richness (e.g. see Bunting and Campbell 1990, Turkoski 1992). In this second approach there is a tendency to promote an 'essentialist' approach or what Eisenstein (1984) terms 'a false universalism' which ignores, for example, the race, class and so forth of the individuals concerned. An essentialist conception of feminism actually works against the tenets of feminism itself.

Women, like nurses, are not a homogenous group. Indeed, Cott (1987) observes that 'the ruling fiction of feminism, the conception of "all women" is like the ruling fiction "all men" in democratic theory—always observed in the breach.' The danger is that if nursing literature about feminism attempts to distil an essentialist definition of feminism then the analysis may lose its potential to bring about real change in nursing. Further, such analyses will run the risk of alienating many nurses unable to identify with either the brand of feminism being posited and/or the position from which it is being asserted—usually a white, middle class orientation.

Thus, it is imperative that in any purported feminist analysis the 'multiplicity and the interconnectedness of the forces that maintain present inequalities, the inadequacy of any one dimensional attempt at change and the impossibility of isolating gender issues from other structured inequalities' (Bryson 1992) be recognised. Women, like nurses are drawn from diverse social settings and contexts. To ignore this is to accept another version of what is 'normal' female, or indeed nursing, behaviour albeit in a feminist guise. Feminism is not a closed or tidy concept. Consequently attempts to reduce it to neat categories will ultimately prove unsatisfactory both in terms of loss of theoretical integrity, and the limitations in the possible applications of the resultant attenuated theoretical stance. Acknowledgment of women's ways of knowing without recognition of the ways in which structural power relations impact on the expression of that experience, leave the analyses located within the personal experience of women, and concomitantly nurses. While there have been recent analyses, such as Doering (1992) that examine such poststructural feminist thought, even this sort of analysis rejects problematising or deconstructing 'knowing' or the meanings attributed to it by liberal feminism. With the preceding discussion in mind, we now turn to consider the main ideas inherent in each of these approaches to feminism and then move on to consider more contemporary developments in feminist thought which draw on poststructuralist perspectives.

Liberal feminism

Liberal feminism draws on the liberal traditions of the 17th and 18th century which were concerned with the rights of 'man' such as the right to vote, to own property and to hold political office. Liberal feminism seeks to extend the same rights to women. Thus, the emphasis in this approach is winning the right for women to participate in society to whatever extent they desire. However the emphasis is on individual women achieving 'success' in existing social structures—'women were to adapt themselves to the structure (patriarchal), rather than the other way around' (Eisenstein 1984). Thus liberal feminism posits an essentially conservative position in that achievement for women is viewed as gaining access within existing social structures. The structures themselves are not in question. Feminists such as Firestone (1970) are critical of this approach arguing that it 'concentrates on the more superficial symptoms of sexism—legal inequities, employment discrimination, and the like' and conceptualises success as the 'production of women who were merely clones of their male counterparts'. Gavey (1989) succinctly encapsulates much of the critique of liberal feminism when she writes, 'although liberal humanist values are not unworthy, the absence of meta-theoretical concerns about power render them insufficient'.

Marxist/socialist feminism

Marxist feminism recognises that liberalism is somewhat hollow and limited if women do not have the economic means to realise their aspirations

(Eisenstein 1984). Thus there is a need to examine the intersection of gender with class. As in all Marxist analyses the emphasis is on women's relation to the economic basis of production in society. Of course, locating women in the class system, based as it is on one's relation to the economic sphere in terms of paid work, proves problematic with respect to women who work at home and who are not paid. To which class do these women belong? How in a Marxist analysis can we determine the worth or value of their labour in a labour system that is essentially patriarchal and therefore into which they do not neatly fit? Furthermore, it is difficult to apply a strict Marxian concept of class to those women who either work part time or who do not work continuously due to family commitments. Many nurses fit into these two categories. Partly in reaction to these concerns about the limitations of a strict Marxist approach to feminism, a socialist feminist perspective developed. Socialist feminism, whilst having much in common with a Marxist analysis, does not afford primacy to the economic sphere alone but rather,

> socialist feminism goes beyond conventional definitions of 'the economy' to consider activity that does not involve the exchange of money. Within its concept of productive activity, therefore, it includes the procreative and sexual work that is done by women in the home. In analysing all forms of productive activity, socialist feminism supplements the analytic tool of class with the additional conceptual tool of gender (Jaggar 1984).

Thus socialist feminism challenges the 'private/public distinction embedded in Western thought...to reveal the gender asymmetry underpinning the conceptual frameworks and categories of Western thought' (Felski 1991). In so doing socialist feminists have much in common with radical feminists.

Radical feminism

Radical feminists hold that the most fundamental form of oppression in society is the domination of men over women. Such oppression applies equally to the public and the private realms. Thus for radical feminists a catchcry became 'the personal is political'. The goal of radical feminism is not the elimination of difference (as is the case with liberal feminism and to a lesser extent Marxist feminism) but rather to celebrate difference and an overt 'women centredness'. Being equal does not mean being the same. Weedon (1987) succinctly summarises much of the project of radical feminism when she writes, 'in the short term, for radical feminists the only way in which women can assert their autonomy from men and recover their true and natural femininity is in separation from men and the patriarchal structures of society'. Thus radical feminism advocates fundamental social change and a withdrawal from patriarchy until this is achieved. 'The contemporary radical feminist position...refuses to accept the existing leftist analysis not because it is too radical, but because it is not radical enough' (Firestone 1970).

However, one of the inherent problems in radical feminism's assertion that difference is to be celebrated is that the risk is run that 'woman' will again be relegated to 'other' or 'different to'—once again perpetuating the 'normality' and 'naturalness' of essentially patriarchal Western society. This is particularly evident if we consider contemporary feminist thought which draws on poststructuralist perspectives. These perspectives challenge the very nature of language itself with which we construct our world and expose its role in constructing and perpetuating gender based inequalities. As yet nursing has not explored these perspectives and what they might reveal and explain about why nursing has been slow to embrace feminism and why feminism has at times seemed to have had little to offer nursing. It is to this task that the discussion now turns.

Poststructural feminism

Poststructural or postmodern feminism is a feminist perspective which seeks to provide an analysis of women and women's lives that remains women centred, as did the earlier feminisms. However, it differs on several fronts in both its form of theorising and its practical and political applications. These differences arose from the realisation that feminism, as it had previously been constructed, had not fully explored differences between women themselves and the impact that such differences have on the political voice of feminism (Weedon 1987, Game 1991, Smith 1990). It must be noted however, that these changes did not occur in a vacuum. They were, in part, in keeping with changes occurring in other disciplines. Further, they were also a response to criticisms concerning feminist knowledge arising from within the feminist perspective itself. As Weedon (1987) contends, feminist knowledge which continues to constitute a unitary view of 'woman' as the object of that knowledge will not allow analysis that takes account of the continuing actions of 'women', especially when women's actions appear to be contrary to their interests as defined by that knowledge. Such difficulties have arisen because earlier feminist perspectives failed to recognise the often contradictory positions which women can take towards their lives. Furthermore, the political implications of poststructural feminism are such that feminism can no longer 'challenge from within the structures of the institutions [as this] is fraught with contradictions. Many feminists are subject to the danger of co-option and the reproduction of knowledge as power over rather than for most women' (Weedon 1987).

Feminist analyses illuminated by such perspectives are very different from the feminism we have discussed previously. Code (1990) highlights that contemporary feminism now confronts the power and knowledge which continues to silence and exclude the knowledge of women. Simultaneously, feminism is increasingly viewed as a contested arena, not a monolith based on a unitary view of woman's experience of gender or womanhood. Stanley and Wise (1990), writing of their own changing perceptions, state that 'while accepting that these analytic categories were important and useful to feminism, we felt the ways they were used unexplicated failed to unpack the assumptions and generalisations embedded within them'. Further, as with the generalisations associated with analyses of the meaning of 'woman', they consider that the category 'feminism' itself was used in monolithic terms, without fully exploring the *academic* implication of the political, ethical and epistemological differences that existed 'within feminism' as 'between women' (emphasis in the original).

From this perspective, while it is useful to identify and categorise the different ontological and epistemological assumptions which underpin the various feminisms this is not to delineate arbitrary boundaries (see Speedy 1991, Bunting & Campbell 1990). Poststructuralism would question such setting of boundaries. Instead, poststructural feminism asks how such boundaries define and limit both feminist knowledge and women. To question such formulations, poststructural feminism focuses on key aspects of knowledge; namely language, power and subjectivity and the interactions between them.

Language and its use to communicate or limit understanding is a key element of poststructural feminist analyses (Weedon 1987, Game 1991, Gavey 1989). As Gavey suggests poststructural feminism questions the humanist traditions which have viewed women and the language used to explain women's experience as both universal and ahistorical. Gavey (1989) further contends that while feminist discourse privileges women's language 'as transparently reflecting women's unique experience...the importance of language as a constitutive process remains largely unrecognised'.

The analyses of women's experience obtained by applying such perspectives problematises women's experience, and the language used to describe it. For example, Weedon (1987) highlights the different definitions of a concept, such as femininity, which arise when used in the differing fields of advertising, pornography or indeed the family. She contends that different aspects of femininity are selected as definitive depending on these various contexts. The result of such analysis is that even concepts such as femininity, which present as absolute in one context, may emphasise other aspects in another. Such analysis allows that even within the concept of femininity itself there is a constellation of understandings which are not fixed but instead are contextual. Poststructural analyses therefore do not seek to present unitary explanations of women's experience, described in language which is assumed to present reality. Instead, they question the impact of the context on that experience and the language used to express it.

Hence, the very notion which has been sacred to liberal feminism, that of uniting women under the banner of one unitary experiential banner, cannot be claimed in poststructural feminism. Significantly, as Gavey (1989) asserts 'this does not mean that experience does not exist or is unimportant', but instead there is a recognition 'that the ways in which we understand and express it are never independent of language'. Furthermore, as language is not construed as the innocent communicator of experience, then language usage is viewed as closely interwoven with the power relations embedded within the context of social experience. As a consequence of this, Weedon (1987) argues that language needs to be considered from a Foucauldian perspective (Foucault 1977, 1980). From this perspective, it is possible to identify how language, as either written texts or talk, becomes discursive fields which structure the way we both think and talk about events in our lives. Discourses, and the discursive fields they form, are 'system[s] of statements which cohere around common meanings and values....[that] are a product of social factors, of powers and practices, rather than an individual's set of ideas' (Hollway 1983). Such a conceptualisation of language allows for analysis that remains aware of the interplay between power and language.

Discourses frame the power/knowledge structures of any discursive field or framework. For poststructural feminist scholarship, 'rather than 'discovering' reality, 'revealing' truth, or 'uncovering' the facts, feminist poststructuralism would, instead, be concerned with disrupting and displacing dominant (oppressive) knowledges' (Gavey 1989). Since at any one time in history there are a number of competing discourses, the goal of poststructural analysis is to compare the way such discourses compete for dominance. Such analyses also indicate how some discourses come to dominate, and appear as 'natural'. At the same time, this perspective explores how such discourses deny the authoritarian effects they have by appealing to notions such as 'common sense' (Code 1991, Weedon 1987, Gavey 1989). Discourses also provide frameworks from which individuals are able to position themselves within society. The positions available to individuals and the power accruing from such positions are set by the existing power relations implicit within such discourses. For example, the discourse of medical science is a dominant discourse in the health care arena. It is rational and objective in character and nursing has aligned itself with this discourse and position in its own discourses (see Parker & Gardner 1992, Cheek & Rudge 1993).

As Gavey (1989) contends, the variety of positions open to individuals are multiple and often 'potentially contradictory'. Unlike 'the subject' of humanistic liberalism or objective science, the subject in poststructural analysis is capable of taking up many positions, some of which will be supported by dominant discourses, while others may not. Subjectivity, or the experience of being an individual is likewise, as Weedon (1987) suggests, the site of conflicting forces. Just as language mediates meaning and experience, subjectivity is constituted in and by language. Hence subjectivity is open to difference, silencing and conflicting interpretations. However, unlike the notion of subject portrayed in individualist humanist discourse, this subjectivity is not privileged as a site of power but instead is viewed as 'the site of this battle for power' [and] 'it is a battle in which the individual is an active but not a sovereign protagonist'. Street (1992) has outlined just such a battle over the subject positions available to nurses; such positions as technical nurse, managerial nurse, nurturant nurse, authoritarian nurse or educating nurse.

To return to the notion of femininity and the female subject, it is important to note that the female subject of poststructuralism is not passive in relation to the position she takes vis a vis femininity. Instead, she actively chooses from the range of positions available to her in the discourses of femininity. Previously we noted how the concept of femininity is contextual. Furthermore, similar to other forms of discourse in society, it is also mediated by the texts which seek to define femininity as a social reality. Smith (1990) asserts that femininity is textually mediated in that the texts which represent femininity in a variety of ways, at the same time produce within women the desire to be feminine as it is constituted in the text. Smith used various forms of texts such as etiquette books and the like to show how such texts form the basis of how the female subject can position herself in relation to the concept of femininity. By such positioning, she can monitor her own behaviour in terms of the text, and also the behaviour of others. Smith further argues that such texts concerning femininity not only represent femininity but result in the female subject taking up the feminine position itself.

Nursing has texts which also seek to define the reality of nursing, such as case notes, care planning documents, procedure manuals and the like. Such texts form the discursive frameworks which allow nurses to position themselves in relation to nursing. These texts represent nursing, and as Smith suggests with etiquette books and women's magazines, produce the desire to take certain positions vis a vis nursing. Just as texts on femininity allow self-monitoring, or monitoring of others, so do nursing texts. Also such texts represent nursing and simultaneously produce various subject positions for nurses. Such analyses highlight the importance of choice and the active role that individuals take towards their positionality. Central to this is the notion that such choice leads to a subjectivity which is defined by that individual with/in their social context. However, as Ellsworth (1992) warns, 'social agents are not capable of being fully rational and disinterested; and they are subjects split between the conscious and the unconscious and among multiple social positionings'.

Therefore, poststructural feminist analysis does not rest with the acknowledgment of the multiplicity of positions open to women, as does liberal feminism, for example. As Weedon (1987) suggests, it is also the role of poststructural feminism to account for how 'women tolerate social relations which subordinate their interests to those of men and the mechanisms whereby women and men adopt particular discursive positions as re-presentative of their positions'. Subjectivity is not a unitary concept, instead it is fractured and structured by the variety of ways that discourses structure our sense of self. Weedon further suggests that 'language, in the form of socially and historically specific discourses, cannot have any social and political effectivity except in and through the actions of the individuals who become its bearers by taking up the forms of subjectivity and the meanings and values which it proposes and acting upon them'. Specifically, discourses offer subject positions and in so doing they manufacture desire to achieve certain forms of subjectivity (Game 1991, Smith 1990, Weedon 1987, Hollway 1989, Coward 1984).

Central to this argument are the power relations which ensue from the battle over contested subjectivity. Previously we argued that discourses were not equal in terms of their authority. Similarly, subject positions taken in respect to particular discourses are unequal. Further, due to differences in authority attributed to such positions, some subject positions are more attractive than others. For example, subject positions with which we grow up, appear more 'natural', and dominate those positions which we may come to through later educational or social experience. Certainly, these alternative positions and their accompanying discourses have less power accruing to them. Weedon (1987) and Gavey (1989) suggest feminism is just such an alternative discourse. But there are also more seemingly mundane ways in which we can take up multiple positions with/in subjectivity.

In an analysis of popular culture and the manufacturing of female desire, Coward (1984) explores the perfect female body, and she asserts that while 'the ideal' tyrannises women, because to so many it is unattainable, at the same time, because its focus is on areas of fatness, it fragments the female body. Such fragmentation, as with subjectivity, allows women to maintain 'an ambiguous relation to the ideal image' (Coward 1984) and while they seek bodily transformation according to the dominant discourse of body shape, women are also capable of finding fragments of their bodies which they value. In this ambiguity, Coward finds a point of resistance, an alternative discourse awaiting its political time. Hence, the power to define the female body which resides within the dominant discourse, also allows for the potential for development of resistance to such hegemonic discourses. Such reconceptualisations of power relations in society also foster the creation of more complex understandings of concepts such as empowerment (Gore 1992). If power is not a characteristic of an individual but instead the outcome of assuming strategic positions in relation to specific discourses, then the personal and collective power that is seen to arise from processes of empowerment as they are conceptualised at present in nursing are rendered problematic.

As Gore (1992), Ellsworth (1992) and Lather (1991) suggest, the very notion of empowerment espoused in much of the literature is predicated on a universalised and universalising, rational individual. Much of the nursing literature is predicated on just such a position (see Chinn 1989, Mason, Backer & Georges 1991, Emden 1991). As poststructural feminist analysis emphasises, such understanding as we have of our experience is both partial and partisan. Because of this partiality, it must also be recognised that the results of empowerment will be both partial and inconsistent. Empowerment may not lead to freedom from oppression through rational action. Such conceptualisations destabilise the inherent optimism which dominates much of the rhetoric surrounding empowerment. Furthermore, Ellsworth (1992) suggests that empowerment predicated on rational humanism 'treats the symptoms but leaves the disease unnamed and untouched'.

The notion of empowerment which is gaining the ascendancy in feminist writing is not empowerment which is highlighted in 'the current fashion of individual self-assertion, upward mobility and the psychological experience of feeling powerful' (Lather 1991). This is directly in contrast to works such as Belenky et al (1986) which Lather contends offer an analysis of women and their experiences which remains located in such psychologistic reductionism. Instead, using Gramsci, Lather views empowerment as the ability to analyse 'ideas about the causes of powerlessness, recognising systemic oppressive forces, and acting both individually and collectively to change the conditions of our lives'. Poststructural feminism allows for the production of knowledge and hence scholarship which permits the variety of voices and sources of women's knowledge to be expressed. This is done, not through the grand narratives of 'Theory', but through acknowledgment of the position that 'provisionality and undecidability, partisanship and overt politics replace poses of objectivity and disinterestedness' (Hutcheon 1989).

This perception of empowerment allows that the forms of scholarship are based on both ontological and epistemological bases very different from those espoused by earlier forms of feminist theorising, such as ways of 'knowing'. For example, Lather (1991) and Martin (1988) both contend that resistance and feminist practice must recognise the displacement of power and hence develop strategies for resistance and empowerment which displace rather than confront. This is necessary to overcome the complexity of powerlessness so that the different levels can be acknowledged and resisted. Locating its critique at the sites of the taken-for-granteds, such as language, subjectivity and power, poststructural feminism seeks to question epistemological bases of both mainstream and feminist knowledge. As Spivak (1989) suggests, its task is to 'deconstructively critique something which is so useful to you that you cannot speak another way'. Consciousness raising is one such way that feminism found to address issues such as empowerment in the 1960s and 1970s. The discussion now turns to consider both consciousness raising and consciousness raising for nursing.

Towards a critical consciousness raising

Simone de Beauvior (1972) declared that women do not say 'we'. The feminists of the 1960s and early 1970s argued that it was because of such a lack of consciousness by women of both their individual and collective identities that patriarchy could continue to parade as natural, normal and even inevitable (Millett 1970). Consequently women needed to have their consciousness raised in a 'process of transforming the hidden, individual fears of women into a shared awareness of the meaning of them as social problems, the release of anger, anxiety, the struggle of proclaiming the painful and transforming it into the political' (Mitchell 1971). The notion of consciousness raising itself drew on the Chinese Maoist tradition of 'speaking bitterness' to express and share personal feelings and experiences in order to work on political strategies for change (Cohen 1970).

Feminists asserted that in such a process women could affirm that what happened in the realm of their personal, everyday reality was important and that others shared similar frustrations, experiences and feelings. Indeed, 'the heart of consciousness-raising was the discovery that one was not alone, that other women had comparable feelings and experiences' (Eisenstein 1984). Further, it was essential that women be able to recognise that their individual frustrations, disappointments and failures were not isolated phenomena but rather 'they were the symptoms of a society-wide structure of power and powerlessness' (Eisenstein 1984). The personal was thus political—to use the well known catchcry attributed to Carol Hanisch in 1971.

Indeed, MacKinnon (1983) declared that 'the feminist method is consciousness raising' in that it enabled a rejection of the distinction of the knowing subject and the known subject, thereby enabling women to 'grasp the collective reality of women's condition from within the perspective of that experience, not from outside it'. The notion of 'raising' is a metaphor for the emergence of an awareness that, once it had surfaced, allowed the possibility for action to occur. In nursing's case, one of the possible benefits of consciousness raising is to enable nurses to see the multiplicity of points at which they can resist the various forms and guises of power that are embedded in nurses' oppression.

Like women, nurses (the vast majority of whom are women) historically have lacked a sense of identification and consciousness as a group. Consequently nurses have tended to remain a loosely aligned group of workers without a strong collective or political voice. Thus when nurses went out on strike in 1986 in Victoria it was indeed a momentous event, as well as being a time of much soul searching and the need for collective support and affirmation. Sally McManamny (1986) has written an unique, first hand account of consciousness raising in action when she describes her individual thoughts and feelings whilst on a picket line in the Victorian strikes, and intersperses this personal reflection with text that outlines the political dimension of what nurses were collectively striking about and hoping to achieve. She reveals the surfacing of both a personal and collective consciousness when she concludes, 'there is so much more we have to consider. One thing is clear however, nurses are learning'.

Why have nurses been slow to realise a collective consciousness? One reason possibly relates to the fact that in its drive for professionalisation, nursing has drawn on a patriarchal model of professionalism (see Turkoski 1992). Furthermore, such a model is based on the hegemony of the analytic discourse of the 'expert' which is viewed as being derived from a legitimate knowledge base which is then used to legitimise the power and practice of that professional group (Donzelot 1980). However, Street (1992) asserts that the discursive field which resides in the oral culture of nursing has been overpowered by this requirement for extensive nursing documentation, increasingly computer-generated. Furthermore, along with the pressure to document care, has been the concomitant development of a plethora of standards of practice, procedure manuals, competency statements and the like which, following Smith (1990), can be construed as another form of textually mediated reality of and for nursing.

In such development, the personal has been largely ignored and un-acknowledged. Street speaks of the need to validate the oral culture, that is the personal. However her analysis enters the realm of the political when she reveals the mixed messages that nurses receive from management about the legitimacy of their oral culture. On the one hand extensive written 'objective' documentation is required, yet on the other, time is allowed for the oral exchange of information in the 'handover'. Simultaneously, many nurses resist the pressures to document, considering it to be tedious, often trivial, and time consuming. However, it is our contention that, while they resist the pressure to document, nurses fail to connect the source of such resistance as emanating from contestation between the dominant scientific-medical discourse, with its emphasis on so-called objective data, and the alternative but less powerful discourse of the subjective, oral culture of nursing.

Further, the development of a collective consciousness is problematic given that nurses operate in a number of contexts. The diversity of settings for nursing may have the effect of creating seemingly disparate concerns predicated on differing areas of specialist expertise. By using the patriarchal model of professional expertise, which is premised on notions of objectivity, rationalism and autonomy, it is possible for nurses not to recognise, and therefore acknowledge, the very real commonalities within nursing. Such lack of recognition has the potential to result in tensions between different 'types' of nurses, each claiming to have rights over various areas of expertise. The danger is that nurses may be split into various factions represented by specialist domains, arguing over power/knowledge issues. The power and ideology embedded in such specialisations are often based on the special–isations within hegemonic medical discourse, and are supported by the bio-technical structures within the health system. Again, this draws on the hegemony of the patriarchal model of expertise, not on the nurturance/knowledge axis Street (1992) has identified as the key source of nursing knowledge and practice.

How do nurses build a dialogue which counters the hegemony against which nursing must assert its identity? The recognition of commonality is not to deny difference but to build understanding from respecting what has brought about the difference. In other words, it is to acknowledge the validity of the first person understandings people bring with them, without using these differences as a means of denying the right to an authoritative voice. In this process of acknowledgment trust can be built from the recognition of the other's different, but in many ways similar, experience. Nurses need to listen to each other's experiences yet at the same time remain cognisant of the effects that nursing's structural position can have on what is heard and understood.

Thus, in acknowledging the validity of difference it is essential to recognise where the differences come from, to value difference, and to search for common experiences within such differences (Luke 1992). From the building of trust and support networks across and within contexts, nurses will be able to move from the personal to politically determining action based on a belief system which acknowledges the political dimensions of oppression. Poststructural feminist analyses open up fields of possibility for action rather than closing off discussion prematurely because, finally, we can 'understand' the sources of such oppression. As Ellsworth (1992) suggests, the 'situation makes it impossible for any single voice...to assume the position of center or origin of knowledge or authority, of having privileged access to authentic experience or appropriate language'.

Without such understandings nursing's relentless quest to gain professional status and recognition is problematic, in that whatever gains are made will be within parameters set by powerful others. Such authoritarian parameters and structures dictate, and will continue to dictate, nursing's path to professionalism by limiting the system of possibilities for real change. The danger is that nurses will continue relentless self-surveillance, demanding more and more of themselves in the pursuit of the unachievable—unachievable in the sense that the rules constantly change and are made by others. For nurses to connect both with each other, and to the sources of power implicit in certain of their positions, nursing must recognise that 'the master's tools will never dismantle the master's house' (Lorde 1984).

Conclusion

Connections between nursing perspectives and feminist perspectives have not been strongly forged, despite some nurses arguing that such links are both necessary and logical. The impact of feminist theorising and perspectives on both nurses and their clients has been limited by the essentialist understandings of 'woman', and hence 'nurse', that have so characterised nursing 'feminist' analyses.

This chapter has posited that poststructural feminism allows for analyses of nursing which recognise the complexities of the variety of positions assumed by nurses. Furthermore, this perspective, because of its openly political stance, offers the potential for nurses to explore the often contradictory and inconsistent nature of such subject positions in the variety of contexts in which they work. Such an exploration is essential if nurses are to ever be truly empowered for as Gore (1992) writes 'while the desire may be to move from the conception of power as repression to em-power-ment (in a dichotomous fashion with great optimism and human agency), the institutional location (context again) of much [nursing]...practice may militate against it'.

If nurses use strategies such as consciousness raising, underpinned by the insights afforded by critical and poststructural feminist perspectives, the variety of voices that constitute nurses and nursing will not be subsumed under often unexplicated unitary explanations. To continue to pursue and promote such unitary and essentialist explanations and understandings of nurses and nursing is to continue the silencing and exclusion of certain voices within nursing itself.

By connecting the personal realm with the political and epistemological stances opened up by poststructural feminism, nurses have the potential to develop strategies which will enable the acknowledgment of both the complexity and political nature of nurses and nursing, thereby offering the possibility of truly empowering all nurses.

REFERENCES

Allan H T 1993 Feminism: a concept analysis. Journal of Advanced Nursing 18:1547-1553

Allen D G 1992 Feminism, relativism, and the philosophy of science: an overview. In: Thompson J L, Allen D G, Rodrigues-Fisher L (eds) Critique, resistance and action: working papers in the politics of nursing. National League of Nursing Press, New York, pp 1-19

Anderson J M 1991a Current directions in nursing research: towards a poststructuralist and feminist epistemology. Canadian Journal of Nursing Research 23(3):1-3

Anderson J M 1991b Reflexivity in fieldwork: towards a feminist epistemology. Image: Journal of Nursing Scholarship 23(2):115-118

Belenky M F, Clinchy B, Goldberger N, Tarule J 1986 Women's ways of knowing: the development of self, voice and mind. Basic Books, New York

Bruni N 1991 Nursing knowledge: processes of production. In: Gray G, Pratt R (eds) Towards a discipline of nursing. Churchill Livingstone, Melbourne, pp 171-190

Bryson V 1992 Feminist political theory. Macmillan, London

Bunting S, Campbell J C 1990 Feminism and nursing: historical perspectives. Advances in Nursing Science 12(4):11-24

Cheek J, Rudge T 1993 Discourse analysis: a methodology for turning nursing texts into critique. In: Book of proceedings, Research in nursing: turning points. National conference of Centre for Nursing Research. Adelaide, South Australia, pp 47-56

Chinn P L 1989 Nursing patterns of knowing and feminist thought. Nursing and Health Care 10, pp 71-75

Code L 1991 What can she know? Feminist theory and the construction of knowledge. Cornell University Press, New York

Cohen C B 1970 Women of China. In: Morgan R (ed) Sisterhood is powerful. Vintage Books, New York

Cott N F 1987 The grounding of modern feminism. Yale University Press, New Haven and London

Coward R 1984 Female desire: women's sexuality today. Paladin, London

de Beauvior S 1972 The second sex. Penguin, Middlesex

Doering L 1992 Power and knowledge in nursing: a feminist poststructural view. Advances in Nursing Science 14(4):24-33

Donzelot J 1980 The policing of families. Hutchinson, London

Ehrenreich B, English D 1978 For her own good: 150 years of the experts' advice to women. Anchor Press, New York

Eisenstein H 1984 Contemporary feminist thought. Allen & Unwin, Sydney

Ellsworth E 1992 Why doesn't this feel empowering? Working through the repressive myths of critical pedagogy. In: Luke C, Gore J (eds) Feminism and critical pedagogy. Routledge, New York, pp 90-119

Emden C 1991 Ways of knowing in nursing. In: Gray G, Pratt R (eds) Towards a discipline of nursing. Churchill Livingstone, Melbourne, 11-30

Felski R 1991 American and British feminisms. In: Beilharz P (ed) Social theory. Allen & Unwin, Sydney

Firestone S 1970 The dialectic of sex: the case for feminist revolution. Bantam, New York

Foucault M 1977 Discipline and punish. Tavistock, London

Foucault M 1980 Power/knowledge, Gordon C (ed.). Harvester Press, Brighton

Game A 1991 Undoing the social: towards a deconstructive sociology. Open University Press, Milton Keynes

Gavey N 1989 Feminist poststructuralism and discourse analysis: contributions to feminist psychology. Psychology of Women Quarterly 13:459-475

Gore J 1992 What can we do for you? What can 'we' do for 'you'? Struggling over empowerment in critical and feminist pedagogy. In: Luke C, Gore J (eds) Feminism and critical pedagogy. Routledge, New York, pp 54-73

Gray D P 1992 A feminist critique of Jean Watson's theory of caring. In: Thompson J L, Allen D J, Rodrigues-Fisher L (eds) Critique, resistance, and action: working papers in the politics of nursing. National League of Nursing Press, New York, pp 85-96

Hagell E I 1989 Nursing knowledge: women's knowledge. A sociological perspective. Journal of Advanced Nursing 14:226-233

Hanisch C 1971 The personal is political. In: Agel J (ed) The radical therapist. Ballantine Books, New York

Hollway W 1983 Heterosexual sex: power and desire for the other. In: Cartledge S, Ryan J (eds) Sex and love: new thoughts on old contradictions. Women's Press, London, pp 124-140

Hollway W 1989 Subjectivity and method in psychology: gender, meaning and science. Sage, London

Hutcheon L 1989 The politics of postmodernism. Routledge, New York

Jaggar A 1984 Feminist politics and human nature. Harvester, Brighton

Lather P 1991 Getting smart: feminist research and pedagogy with/in the postmodern. Routledge, New York

Lawler J 1991 Behind the screens: nursing, somology, and the problem of the body. Churchill Livingstone, Melbourne

Lorde A 1984 Sister outsider. The Crossing Press, New York

Luke C (1992) Feminist politics in radical pedagogy. In: Luke C, Gore J (eds) Feminism and critical pedagogy, Routledge, New York, 25-53

MacKinnon C 1983 Feminism, method and the state: an agenda for theory. In: Abel E, Abel E (eds) The signs reader. Chicago University Press, Chicago

McManamny S 1986 Nurses' work, nurses' worth. Arena 77:119-128

MacPherson K I 1991 Looking at caring and nursing through a feminist lens. In: Neil R M, Watts R (eds) Caring and nursing: explorations in feminist perspectives. National League of Nursing Press, New York, pp 25-42

Martin B 1988 Feminism, criticism and Foucault. In: Diamond I, Quinby L (eds) Feminism and Foucault: reflections on resistance. Northeastern University Press, Boston, pp 3-19

Mason D J, Backer B A, Georges C A 1991 Toward a feminist model for the political empowerment of nurses. Image: Journal of Nursing Scholarship 23(2):72-77

Meleis A 1991 Theoretical nursing: development and progress, 2nd edn. J B Lippincott, Philadelphia

Millett K 1970 Sexual politics. Avon Books, New York

Mitchell J 1971 Women's estate. Vintage Books, New York

Neuman B 1989 The Neuman Systems Model: Applications in nursing education and practice, 2nd edn. Appleton-Lange, Norwalk

O'Neill S 1992 The drive for professionalism in nursing: A reflection of classism and racism. In: Thompson J L, Allen D J, Rodrigues-Fisher L (eds) Critique, resistance, and action: working papers in the politics of nursing. National League of Nursing Press, New York, 137-147

Orem D E 1983 The self-care deficit theory of nursing. In: Clements I, Roberts F (eds) Family health: a theoretical approach to nursing care. Wiley Medical, New York

Parker J, Gardner G 1992 The silence and the silencing of the nurse's voice: a reading of patient's progress notes. Australian Journal of Advanced Nursing 9(2):133-156

Roy C 1984 Introduction to nursing: an adaptation model, 2nd edn. Prentice Hall, Englewood Cliffs

Shulman A K (1982) Dancing in the revolution: Emma Goldman's feminism. Socialist Review 62:32-33

Smith D E 1990 Texts, facts and femininity: exploring the relations of ruling. Routledge, London

Speedy S 1991 The contribution of feminist research. In: Gray G, Pratt R (eds) Towards a discipline of nursing. Churchill Livingstone, Melbourne, pp 191-210

Spivak G with Rooney E 1989 In a word—interview. Differences 1(2):124-156

Stanley L, Wise S 1990 Method, methodology and epistemology in feminist research processes. In: Stanley L (ed) Feminist praxis: research, theory and epistemology in feminist sociology. Routledge, London, pp 20-60

Street A 1992 Inside nursing: a critical ethnography of clinical nursing practice. State University of New York Press, New York

Turkoski B B 1992 A critical analysis of professionalism in nursing. In: Thompson J L, Allen D J, Rodrigues-Fisher L (eds) Critique, resistance, and action: working papers in the politics of nursing. National League of Nursing Press, New York, pp 149-165

Watson J 1985 Nursing: human science and health care. Appleton-Century Crofts, Norwalk

Webb C 1986 Feminist practice in women's health care. John Wiley, Chichester

Webb C 1993 Feminist research: definitions, methodology, methods and evaluation. Journal of Advanced Nursing 18:416-423

Weedon C 1987 Feminist practice and poststructuralist theory. Blackwell, Cambridge

Wheeler C E, Chinn P L 1991 Peace and power: a handbook of feminist process, 3rd edn. National League of Nursing Press, New York

Yaros P S 1991 The feminist movement and the science and profession of nursing: analogies and paradoxes. In: Neil R H, Watts R (eds) Caring and nursing: explorations in feminist perspectives. National League of Nursing Press, New York, pp 77-83

19

Searching for the body in nursing

JUDITH PARKER

Introduction

Nurses work in the context of concrete involvement in and connection with fundamental predicaments and expressions of the human condition; threats to embodiment and mortality, expressions of hope and despair. Nurses are there when people are at their most vulnerable; they are witness to life's most profound events, those of birth and death and significant bodily change. They work on a daily basis with people who are dealing with issues stemming from and surrounding their perishable body; issues of pain, suffering, disfigurement, confusion, disturbance. They work with people whose worlds have been reduced to chaos (Sacks 1986).

Nurses provide intimate body care. They manage embarrassment, shame and nakedness (Lawler 1991). They deal on a daily basis with what Kristeva (1982) describes as the abject body. That is to say, they deal with bodily secretions and excretions, with vomit, pus and blood. They work at the ambiguous border between the 'clean and owned' or hidden body and the 'defiled' body rendered visible through loss of form and integrity (Creed 1993). People and their embodiment are the heart of nursing practice.

In medicine too, the body is central. But here it has been constituted as a scientific anatomical and physiological object rendered amenable to investigation and treatment. In medicine the person as subject fades into the background and the focus is upon reducing complex, variable and diverse human experience to diagnostic categories. In our era, the medical body has been constituted and sustained in the context of the modern hospital through particular networks of practices, institutions and technologies that have ensured positions of medical dominance and nursing subordination. Thus the focus has been upon the scientific medical body, and the relational incorporative ambiguous body of nursing practice has been marginalised and reduced to a pale shadow of the medical body, to a set of procedures stemming from medical directives.

This chapter traces out a search for a fuller expression of the body in nursing. It starts with an exploration of the historical context in which the medical body was constituted with the rise of science in the early 18th century, and which saw the emergence of the modern hospital and professional nursing in the 19th century. This places the search in the context of the imperatives of the modern era in Western society. This is to say, the search is located in the context of Cartesian epistemology, which resulted in the split of being into subject and object and the consequent emergence of the rational autonomous subject. It is located as well within the context of the sovereignty of abstract decontextualised generalised knowledge over situated embodied practical knowledge, and the authority and technologising impulses of science. The search is also placed in the context of disciplinary techniques imposed upon the female body (nurses), how these are related to the history of the male subject (doctors), and how both relate to other changes in society, particularly advances in medical technology.

From the late 1950s nursing theorists attempted to define the domain of nursing as separate from that of medicine and to shift nursing away from its medically derived focus on procedures and diseases. Most of these theorisations came out of the United States and in varying ways drew upon the scientific and humanistic thinking of the era. These theorists believed that nursing required a scientific knowledge base in order to claim disciplinary credibility. Furthermore, this knowledge had to be unique to nursing, so that nursing could claim status as a profession independent of medicine.

The search thus moves on to an exploration of nursing theoretical literature which has attempted to conceptualise the person as more than an object of medical intervention. One strand in the literature broadens the medical object body to incorporate psychological and social dimensions. I am calling this the bio-psycho-social body. The other emphasises holistic transcendent qualities and the power of the person as subject to control the object body. I am calling this the etherealised body. In neither, however, is the givenness of the unchanging anatomical body in dispute. Both bodies are constituted in modern scientific and humanistic terms and are linked to technologies of therapeutic control. These provide means of limiting and containing the visible, out of control body and distancing the nurse from close involvement with the vulnerable hurting body of nursing practice.

The search then shifts to the practice domain and I draw upon data from an ongoing study to discuss the constitution of the body in practice; in written progress notes, at the end of shift collective handover and at the bedside handover. These data provide indications of aspects of the invisibility of nursing and its overshadowing by medicine. They suggest that the nursing focus upon the body and the nature of the relationship surrounding nursing care have been powerfully marked with the imprint of prevailing forms of relationships of control and the exercise of power and authority.

I then consider these data in light of the work of three writers who have focused on the embodied practices and body practices of nurses. Each of these writers has emphasized the invisibility of nursing practice and has sought means of overcoming its hiddenness. One, Benner (1991), advocates public story telling by nurses as a means of making visible the embodied practices of expert nurses and the notions of good that are embedded in practice.

Another, Street (1991), considers issues surrounding the extent to which nurses are enmeshed with constraining forces through their habituated practices, thereby colluding in their own oppression. She advocates ideology critique as a means of helping to shape a transformative and constitutive practice. She argues that this will enable the unspoken and hence invisible values of clinical nursing practice to be opened up for debate and explicit formulation. Of particular concern to her are the unspoken values surrounding the written records and oral communication of nurses.

The third, Lawler (1991), hints at some of the darker, more primal and archaic forces which both empower and constrain nurses' embodied practices. She points out that nurses have a vast knowledge of the body in what she describes as their 'somological' practice which is not documented because people prefer not to know about it. She argues that the body is central to nursing practice but it is hidden. She suggests that more work needs to be done in theorising the body in practice so as to render nursing practice more visible. The search concludes with some speculations about the function of the nursing handover in facilitating nurses' management of the abject body.

The medical body

Central to an understanding of the historical context within which the medical body was constituted is the development of science as a method for understanding, controlling and manipulating nature. In the latter half of the 17th century, as Merchant (1980) points out, Baconian empiricism and Cartesian rationalism were combined in a program which sought to dissect nature so as to discover and achieve mastery over its secrets.

Several writers have referred to the chilling language of male dominance in which Bacon couched this scientific quest. According to Merchant (1980) and Capra (1982) nature had traditionally been thought of as female, both bountiful mother and chaotic disorderly force. However, within the context of the rise of science and the emerging concept of progress linked to a patriarchal structure of the family and state, nature had to be controlled, 'enslaved', constrained and moulded, and like a witch, her secrets 'tortured' from her. By the 19th century, as Merchant (1980) points out, nature had 'exposed herself to science'...and 'from an active teacher and parent, she has become a mindless, submissive body'. In medicine, the once sacred body which replicated the larger sacred active cosmos, came to be viewed in natural science terms, as the Cartesian 'res extensa', a passive and inanimate machine, structured by mechanisms requiring mechanical explanations of their functions.

Leder (1990) has pointed out the theme of mortality in Descartes work which recognises the body as a scene of decay and disease. The era in which Descartes lived was seeing the emergence of the individual (male) subject in

Western society and with this came the recognition of personal individual finitude and fears of mortality. According to Leder, Descartes believed that the existential threat posed by the perishable body could be overcome through the development of scientific knowledge of causes and treatments. It is perhaps worth noting that the historian Ariès (1974) has claimed that while death was accepted with passive resignation and mystical trust in the pre-modern world, this attitude was modified in the 13th to 15th century to become more intensely personal. With the emergence of the notion of 'self' in Western Europe around the 16th century, embeddedness of the human being in a timeless community, the organismic body corporate, began to give way to individual location of unique (male) subjects within a finite, vulnerable corporeality.

The separation of the body from its enmeshment in a sacred world and its objectification meant that it could be scientifically controlled and investigated as an object of nature. It became passive and determinate as Leder (1984) has noted, through 'purging...spontaneity, wilfulness and occult desires'. Leder (1992) has indeed gone so far as to argue that this image of the body is based 'first and foremost not upon the lived body, but upon the dead or inanimate body' and that this image is central to the metaphysics underpinning modern medical practice. This seemingly paradoxical position, given the therapeutic project of modern medicine to preserve life, stems from an understanding of the body as dead in the sense that it is understood as separated from mind and is thereby devoid of subjectivity and intention. Thus the once sacred, passionate, mysteriously productive and fruitful body, the epitome of life, was reduced, through fear of death, to the status of an inanimate dead object.

This medical body has been profoundly influential in our culture. Its dominance and power have been such that other ways of understanding and dealing with people have become silenced or confined to the fringes. This is especially true in health care settings. It can be difficult for doctors and nurses not to think of people in terms of physiological and pathophysiological concepts and for people generally not to define themselves in this way. As Illich (1986) has pointed out, the body of subjective experience is a 'unique enfleshment of an age's ethos' and the enterprise stemming from Cartesian dualism and scientific medical enquiry and intervention has engendered people who to a greater or lesser extent objectify themselves as medical bodies.

The impact of the hospital context on the body in nursing

In order to understand the particular ways in which the medical body has influenced the body in nursing, consideration needs to be given to the emergence of the modern hospital. Early hospitals made available to emerging medical science a kind of laboratory. Hospitals in those early days had nothing to offer that could not be provided in the home. They arose to meet the needs for shelter and care of the homeless sick. With the assemblage of large numbers of the sick in hospitals, doctors gained experiences which were unavailable to them in private practice. Thus the hospital served as a location within which diagnostic and therapeutic skills could be honed. Then when this clinical expertise was linked to the advances that took place in science and technology over the next hundred years, particularly in periods of war, significant advances in surgery and internal medicine were made possible (Inglis 1958).

Nursing work was structured, like the work undertaken in factories, according to the principles of scientific management with tasks broken down into units which could be undertaken by replaceable workers. Nurses were thought of initially as types of maidservants and housekeepers (Woodham-Smith 1951). However with the advent of the Nightingale era and the introduction of the hospital based system of nurse education, nursing was transformed and elevated from its maidservant status to a middle class 'wife or daughter' status within the hospital family which was dominated and controlled by the medical 'husband or father' figures (Parker 1990). Thus nurses were trained to be 'ladies' and to reproduce in the hospital context the structure of relationships and the patriarchal values of Victorian households.

It seems that by the time professional nursing arose in the 19th century, Descartes' dream of controlling mortality through the scientific control of the perishable body had still not been realised. Men became rational 'subjects', i.e. 'minds' in the quest for autonomous individuality, while women were banished to the realm of the frailties of embodied being. Women were defined as 'body' and distanced from 'mind' (Ehrenreich & English 1973). They were represented as the sum of human fears and frailties and thus exemplified the ambiguities of concrete embodiment (Kristeva 1982). As I have argued elsewhere (Parker 1990), 'the patriarchal culture in which modern nursing arose was deeply suspicious about intimacy and human caring nurturant functions. It seems these evoked fears about human frailties, vulnerabilities, defencelessness and the ultimate decrepitude of human embodiment'. Thus attempts were made to define and limit all of these to the female realm and then control them through family based authority and power.

In the hospital context, a setting which both sustained and threatened the ideology surrounding medicine's curative powers, there was considerable ambivalence towards nurses. As women, they were like the patients in so far as they represented the vulnerability of human embodiment, and like nature, they represented maternal fecundity and the potential for chaotic disorder. They were both desired and feared. It was thus important for them to be controlled and regimented. Nurses were therefore systematically disciplined to know their place relative to the (mostly male) doctors.

The first trained Matron of one Australian hospital pointed out the danger of, 'making too much of our knowledge...(for) we are in a great measure the handmaid of the medical man, and our function in this particular is to be obedient in every detail' (Trembath & Hellier 1987). Thus nursing knowledge was driven underground and rendered invisible through medical control and the collusion of nursing leaders.

Nevertheless, for nurses as for doctors, the bringing together of sick people into the hospital community provided opportunities for the development of clinical expertise and consolidation of knowledge and skills in the understanding and clinical management of people suffering from a variety of conditions.

With scientific progression and the expansion of medical technologies, nurses also had the opportunity to become skilled in using these tools.

I would argue that with the further development of scientific medicine over the last 25 years, patriarchal values have become less important within the hospital context as a direct means of controlling human frailties through controlling women. We live in a culture which sustains the belief that advanced medical science has begun to provide a much stronger defence against mortality through its technology. We can produce evidence to suggest that it has provided the weaponry whereby the inevitability of life processes can be challenged and 'attacked' in the battle to defy mortality. Thus, rather than being seen as doctors' handmaids, nurses within hospitals have gained status as physicians' assistants in the technologically based battle against the ravages of life processes.

But it has been a vicarious status. In the era of overt patriarchal medical dominance, nurses were rendered invisible and reduced to passive docility and controlled objects through being women, and therefore bodies, and the repository of the ambivalences surrounding corporeality. With the development of the defences provided by advanced technologies, nurses have gained status and prestige through taking on cast off medical tasks. But this has reinforced the understanding of the body in nursing as a shadow of the medical body.

The nursing theory challenge to the medical body

This search for the body in nursing now takes me to a consideration of the work of some nursing theorists from the United States of America who tried to conceptualise the person so as to capture the breadth of nursing's concerns. This section describes two broad approaches which can be discerned. One identifies the person in relation to a bio-psycho-social body and the other in relation to a holistic etherealised body.

The bio-psycho-social body

One early theorist, Johnson (1961), argued that while both doctors and nurses viewed man (sic) as a system, for doctors this was a biological system, whereas for nurses it was a behavioural system. She then proposed a behavioural sub-system model of the person with behaviour understood as the sum total of physical, biological and social factors/behaviours. In a somewhat similar vein Roy (1970) drew on interactionist, adaptation and systems theories to define the person as a bio-psycho-social being in constant interaction with a changing environment, i.e. as an open adaptive system.

Here the person is defined as a system that functions as a whole by virtue of the interdependence of its parts and which adapts behaviourally to environmental and organismic stimuli. The person comprises coping mechanisms and adaptive (effector) modes. The former are innate or acquired ways of responding to the changing environment with sub-systems of regulator (automatic responses) and cognater (learnt) mechanisms. The latter comprise

334

a classification of ways of coping that manifest regulator or cognater activity. Nursing is then seen as the science and practice of promoting adaptation through nursing diagnoses, nursing interventions and facilitating adaptation outcomes for persons and groups.

However, several nursing theorists of the time (e.g. Levine 1971, Rogers 1970) were claiming that the major distinction between medicine and nursing was that medicine was reductionist while nursing was holistic, that is to say that the person is more than and different from the sum of their parts. Johnson's and Roy's models were therefore both criticised on the basis of their implicit reductionist assumptions and their view of the person as a system constituted by the sum total of its parts (Meleis 1985).

Subsequently Roy tried to address this criticism by adding a philosophical underpinning to her systems adaptation model. This was based on principles of humanism and included notions of the person as having creative power, and behaving purposefully and not merely as a chain of cause and effect. However this addition emphasises even more the mechanistic understanding of the body inherent in the model. The body is seen as a passive inert mass, an anatomical given, responding reactively to stimuli. The person disappears and the patient becomes an object of nursing scrutiny. In promoting adaptive responses to stimuli this model thus shares with biomedical science the aim of controlling the body through behavioural techniques.

The holistic etherealised body

One writer, Levine (1971), challenged the Cartesian medical scientific orthodoxy permeating nursing, which she claimed had resulted in loss of wholeness and humanness through its mechanistic understandings of both body and mind. She believed that a holistic orientation could be achieved through using strategies directed towards the conservation of a person's energy and their structural and social integrity.

Another writer who defined nursing as a holistic science was Rogers (1970), whose ideas were based on concepts from general systems theory, microphysics and evolutionary theory. She conceived of the person as an energy field, co-extensive with the environment, identified in terms of unified wholeness, openness, unidirectionality, pattern, organisation and sentience. Her theory explicitly attempted to be holistic, non-causal and non-reductionist.

Nursing scholars have also attempted to differentiate nursing from medicine through emphasising the caring dimension of nursing science in opposition to medicine's curative function. A major writer in this field, Watson (1979), draws in part upon Roger's thinking and identifies nursing as a humanistic science with caring the central unifying domain of nursing (Cohen 1991). Watson (1988a) describes caring as a moral ideal and trans-personal caring as a spiritual creative union between two people which transcends 'self, time, space and the life history of each other'. She claims that caring occurs in a field consciousness of 'transpersonal caring-healing' which becomes dominant over physical illness, the curing ethic and the dominant treatment ideology (1988b).

The human caring ideology stemming from this holistic thought and assertions of the dominance of consciousness over matter is a not surprising reaction to the supremacy of the biomedical conceptual system which reduces persons to body parts and diagnostic categories. It draws upon the images and languages of music, poetry and art with the aim of capturing metaphysical aspects of ideas such as human centredness and trans-personal caring (Watson 1988a).

However this caring ideology shifts attention away from the concrete physicality of human existence. It is holistic and dynamic, but it is de-corporealised in its attempt to give dominance to consciousness over matter. There is little value given to the embodiment of the human condition other than the need to transcend it, or to the boundaries, limitations and contingencies of history, culture and language. The human body within this caring paradigm is not only ungendered, it is reduced to insubstantiality; it is decorporealised and rendered immaterial as focus is put upon extending human consciousness through space and time. It rests explicitly upon humanistic ideals of personal growth and development and the nurse's role in facilitating this. The formulation of this body fails to take account of socio-historical factors in the constitution of bodies or acknowledge human agency as a factor in knowledge development.

Thus it can be seen that both sets of nursing theorists conceptualised the body in conformity with scientific and humanistic imperatives of the modern era. Particularly apparent in their work is the Cartesian division between mind and body, the assumption of the autonomy of the subject and the search for technologies of control over the body. While Roy and the systems adaptation theorists have emphasised the object body, Watson and the holistic theorists have given more emphasis to the autonomous and transcendent nature of the subject.

The body in nursing practice

This search for the body in nursing now moves to practice, to nursing progress notes, the collective nursing handover and the bedside handover.

The body in progress notes—a pale shadow of the medical body

In a study of patient progress notes, a colleague and I examined the documented record of a woman's last days of life which were spent in a large metropolitan hospital (Parker & Gardner 1991). The focus of both medical and nursing entries in these notes was upon the patient's body; upon investigations, observations and treatments. The medical entries were extremely detailed and communicated many aspects of the patient's physical condition, investigations and treatment. They were often recorded in the active voice and acknowledged preceding medical entries, with thanks given for opinions expressed. On occasions they ended with an instruction to the nurses.

The medical entries were assured, confident and authoritative. Nursing entries were made in the passive voice, and by contrast, were unsystematic and discontinuous. They were weakly reflective of medical entries with seemingly ad hoc documentation of procedures undertaken and observations made. Thus a medical entry which commenced: 'Tired, lethargic, tongue dry...' is followed by a nursing entry: 'Condition remains the same, lethargic and tired, washed with full assistance'.

The lack of continuity in the nursing entries was in stark contrast to the medical entries. We noted that one nursing entry stated: 'Condition unchanged. 24 hour urine collection completed. Dressing to leg ulcer changed to BD with hydrogen peroxide as quite "sluffy" and doesn't appear to be improving at all. Observations stable. Remains on 1.5 litre fluid restriction'. The entry from the next shift made no reference to the preceding one. It simply stated: 'Voiding satisfactory amounts'.

The nurses reported observations ('epistaxis continues', 'leg ulcer looks clean', 'no respirations, no palpable pulse') but were careful not to include entries which might suggest they had made a medical diagnosis. They stringently observed legalities such as filling all the space on a line so that subsequent entries could not be inserted. The doctors by contrast wrote carelessly across the pages. The nurses claimed that they would like to write in more detail, but felt constrained by the medical view that doctors waste time if they have to wade through 'unnecessary' material. The nurses believed that their documentation was devalued and they were fearful of medical coercion and legal liability.

There appeared to be no attempt made in these notes to utilise a systematic form of documentation stemming from a nursing perspective. The use of a patient problem list, for example, with a subjective, objective assessment plan (S.O.A.P.) for recording information, would be consistent with Roy's problem focused approach stemming from a systems adaptation model of the person. Neither was there any indication that these nurses had been influenced in their documentation by the etherealised caring ideology as promoted by Watson. It is difficult not to conclude that the body which emerged in these nursing entries in the patient's record was a weak echo, a pale shadow of the dominant medical voice.

The body in the nursing handover

It is at the collective nursing handover that a sense of the nurses and patients as people rather than as cyphers and symptoms emerges. The nursing handover, which takes place at each change of shift, is clearly functional in a system of work practices that requires 24 hour nursing surveillance. It is the site at which nurses constitute their practice as an ongoing enterprise through talk. They exchange information about medical diagnoses and investigations in the particular shorthand language of medicine: 'Past history of COAD and CA lung, in ICU because he was PE. Had a VQ. It was NAD.'; make clinical judgements: 'large pressure area...granulating well'; pass on awareness of patient idiosyncrasies which have implications for nursing surveillance activities: 'he's a wanderer'; note indicators of improvement in morale: 'had her lipstick on today'; make moral judgements: 'This is a terrible diagnosis, they've got on here...pethidine seeking behaviour'; and identify themselves as separate and distinct from the medical staff: '*They* ordered...', '*They* think...'.

The following extract from a tape recording of a nursing handover in a major metropolitan hospital reveals the nurses as confident, relaxed, empathic and lively as they talk in everyday colloquial and imprecise language about a patient who emerges as an idiosyncratic personality in their conversation.

> *Nurse Giving Handover (NGH):* Bed 17 is Patient-x, 86, he had his turp on the 28th. He's on an incontinence chart, he's continent, he's gorgeous. (LAUGHTER) He was here, Sam, wasn't he? Sam, he's beautiful, he walks with his frame...

> *Response (RESP):* He'd probably been here almost a month when I went on holiday.

> *NGH:* Sometimes he walks without his frame, he's so pleasant, yesterday he goes can you go and get my clothes cos I've got this art smock and I'm not doing painting at the moment. So adorable, he's so cute.

> *RESP:* I vaguely remember him beating up two nurses and a doctor every time he had a catheter. (LAUGHTER)

> *NGH:* Oh, he's so beautiful.

> *RESP:* He's self-caring now.

> *NGH:* He's got MRSA in his urine and that's why he's in Bed 17. But he is continent.

> *RESP:* What's his groin looking like? That was rather nasty.

> *NGH:* No, it looks good, mmm, his leg's still red, cellulitis looking, but um he's off his IV anti's and he's on oral Keflex 500 QID.

> *RESP:* Oh good, it's nice to seem him really happy, even if he does have a tumour.

> *NGH:* Mmm, he is, he's gorgeous. (LAUGHTER).'

As this extract reveals, nursing observations are not dominated by the penetrating distancing reductive scientific medical 'gaze' described by Foucault (1972), but rather by a global incorporative and constitutive 'look' (Parker & Wiltshire 1995). The 'looking' of the experienced nurse involves highly skilled clinical judgments that incorporate not only an understanding of physiological and pathological bodily processes, of drug regimens and interactions, of infections and wounds and healing processes, but also at the same time include a responsive understanding and knowledge of the person and their manner of dealing with what is happening.

Thus in the handover both nurses and patients become visible, but only to the nurses. Their spoken words are vivid and communicative, but also ephemeral. The practice of the nursing handover shows aspects of the depth and breadth of nursing practice knowledge. It also shows how the nurses constitute the patient as a person through everyday talk. However, because the handover is communicated orally and only among nurses it tends to reinforce the invisibility of the nurses in the hospital context.

The body at the bedside handover

Some nurses have attempted to make their practice more visible and one means of achieving this is the bedside handover; where at the change of shift the outgoing nurse 'hands over' her patients to the incoming nurse at the patient's bedside.

At one bedside handover I observed, the two nurses went to the bedside of the elderly woman. I noticed that she was receiving a blood transfusion and oxygen, she was pale and sweaty and had her arms folded across her chest. She looked very sick. The nurses examined the chart at the end of the bed, checked the medical orders, and discussed the treatments that had been given and the ones that were to be given on the next shift. One nurse spoke to the patient briefly: 'You're supposed to have your arm out straight, Mrs X'. She then adjusted the patient's arm to the appropriate position, checked the rate of flow of the blood transfusion and gave further information to the other nurse, speaking about the patient in the third person.

They then moved on to another room, to the bedside of an elderly man with catheter drainage who was sitting beside his bed. He too looked very sick. This man was not addressed directly at all. 'He's very aggressive', the morning nurse said: 'not with it'. She then bent over, picked up the catheter and manipulated it to check that it was draining appropriately. Both nurses then left the room without another word. On another occasion the patient was not present. But it did not seem to matter; the nurses stood at the bedside and discussed the patient's condition and treatment in some detail, and when finished moved to the next bed.

However, at another bedside handover, the manner of the nurses was more personal. They went to the bedside and the morning nurse introduced the patient to the afternoon nurse. She said: 'This is Jenny who'll be looking after you this afternoon'. The nurses spoke first to and then about the patient and continued to alternate from one mode of address to the other. They would speak to each other in a fairly technical manner and then involve the patient in the discussion, checking out the patient's perceptions of what was happening to her. The patient appeared to find the interaction fairly difficult, not seeming to know where to look when she was being talked about.

Managing a bedside handover, I believe, is an extremely complex, multi-dimensional undertaking requiring a range of highly developed skills and understandings. It is to a certain extent a social event, a human gathering involving introductions and the pleasantries associated with social discourse.

The bedside handover is also concerned with the management of transition—the bringing to closure of one act or episode and introducing another in the ongoing drama of the patient's hospitalisation. Yet the context is a professional one wherein there are fairly specific sets of expectations held by each party about the appropriateness of the actions of each other. The nurse as the carer is expected to provide body comfort and care, and technical care, to assess and monitor the patient's condition, and to make judgments about intervention and maintain a safe environment. The patient, the cared-for, is vulnerable by definition, in bed, sick and uncertain, possibly anxious about outcomes of medical investigations and treatments, likely to be trying to cope with disfigurement, pain, disability. The bedside handover crystallises many of the inequities inherent in the nurse-patient relationship, all of which have to be managed at some level at this brief assembly.

In shifting the handover from the privacy of the nurses' gathering in a closed room to the bedside, from offstage to centre stage, as it were, the nurses became more visible. But on occasions the patient disappeared altogether. In the context of the dominance of biotechnical practices and patterns of management perhaps it is not surprising that the nurses modelled the bedside handover on the medical round with its focus on the technical and the instrumental dimensions of care. But while this mode of professional presentation may give nurses greater medically derived status, and make explicit the power they can wield over the vulnerable patient, it reinforces the nurse as a medicalised wraith. It also reinforces the patient as a medical commodity and gives only a glimpse of the possibility of a more fully engaged form of communication in the awkward patient-nurse encounter described above.

These data suggest that the nursing focus upon the body and the nature of the relationship surrounding nursing care have been imprinted with customary forms of relationships of control and the exercise of power and authority. In the public domain of written records the nurses were clearly fearful of legal liability and of overstepping medically defined boundaries of what they are permitted to document.

At the collective handover the nurses talk about their practices and the abject nature of nursing work. They also constitute the patient as a human being who is much more than a problem list. There is a hint of the depth and breadth of nurses' practice knowledge of the body but the structure of this form of communication tends to reinforce nursing invisibility.

At the bedside handover the nurses seemed to be constrained by the limits imposed by the prevailing model of the medical round. Some nurses apparently wanted to involve the patient but were unable to resolve the complexities of managing to exchange technical information in the context of a polite social exchange. In this context, the person appears to be constituted in conformity with the medical body and the nursing procedural care that flows from this understanding.

There is little evidence to suggest, in any of these forms of communication, that nurses have been influenced at all by nursing theorisations of the body, either as a bio-psycho-social object or as a transcendent etherealised subject.

Embodied practices and body practices

This search for the body in nursing now moves on to a discussion of the work of three writers in the nursing literature. These are Benner (1988), Street (1991) and Lawler (1991), who have taken a very different approach to writing about the body in nursing from that taken by those who theorized the body in either bio-psycho-social or etherealized terms. Benner and Street focus on nurses' embodied practices while Lawler's interest is in nursing and body practices.

Benner and embodied practice knowledge

Benner is a significant nursing writer who has been instrumental in shifting the debate in the nursing literature away from a focus on abstract theorisations towards emphasis on clinical knowledge and embodied practice expertise. In 1982, Benner and Wrubel put forward a critique of the limitations to knowledge imposed by abstract reason and theoretical knowledge. Drawing upon Heideggerian phenomenology, and Polanyi's work on the nature of personal knowledge, they argued for a revaluing of the knowledge gained through practice and experience. They concluded 'that clinical knowledge development has been largely ignored because neither the nature of skilled knowledge nor the relevance of experience to its acquisition is widely understood'.

In their subsequent work (1988) they continued to draw out the implications of Heidegger's thought for nursing and turned their attention to Merleau-Ponty's (1962) phenomenology of the body as well. Drawing upon this, Benner and Wrubel (1988) argued that through embodied intelligence people grasp situations directly and pre-reflectively and that as involved concerned participants, people are engaged in and constituted by the situations in which they find themselves.

Benner subsequently described the elaborate practical discourse of 'knowing a patient' nurses have, which she argues is central to an ethic of care and responsibility and can only be learnt experientially. This knowledge stems from the common human circumstance of embodiment which allows for understanding and protection of vulnerability and is guided by situated understanding of particular human concerns. She also describes the ethical discourse found in nursing narratives, which offer descriptions of embodied human characteristics of courage and dignity, notions of good which are threatened in specific situations and the wisdom stored in particular stories (1991). Benner draws upon the narratives of nurses as an explicit means of illustrating socially embedded caring practices and everyday ethical expertise, and uses public story telling as a medium for making various dimensions of expert nursing practice visible. She thereby emphasises the public and shared nature of language and its performative aspects.

Benner (1988) points out that nurses' embodied caring practices have been marginalised in a health care context which gives weight to managerial and technical relationships and primacy to a high technology curative approach to medicine. She sees that caring is central to nursing, but rejects the traditional decontextualising, operationalising social science approach to the study of caring which reduces it into discrete behaviours and therapeutic techniques. She takes the view that caring is not a sentiment, feeling or attitude of the private individual nor is it a psychological state. Rather emotions are tied to public meanings and embodied learning and knowledge, and thus caring arises within the context of a common world of meanings and practices. She sees that practices and traditions are embedded in actual communities and narratives and provide the basis for everyday ethical comportment.

In emphasising the notion of situated freedom and the limits to autonomy, she rejects the idea of the radical free subject defined as apart from and in opposition to others with attendant notions of rights, justice and utilitarian values. She argues for an ethic of care and responsibility based on a communitarian and relational notion of self.

Benner offers a critique of Cartesian epistemology and of the privileging of general decontextualised knowledge that can be applied to a wide range of situations. Her rejection of the dominance and supremacy of the concept as an isomorphic representation of nature enables exploration of other ways of knowing and understanding, such as pre-reflective embodied knowledge and narrative tales.

She challenges the authority of science through advocacy of strategies whereby nurses make manifest their practice through learning to identify, value and articulate their caring practices. She is thereby facilitating the emergence of a nursing discourse of resistance to the dominant technologising impulses of advanced medical practice which reduce the body to a medical object.

Benner's work epitomises the feminist aim of rediscovering and revaluing the experiences of women. She has opened up a world of embodied practices, of expertise embodied in these practices and wisdom contained in the narratives of ethical practice. She posits a corporealised relational self and describes engaged care as a moral source of wisdom. Her work offers a critique of Cartesian epistemology, extreme individualism, abstract knowledge and procedural ethics.

Benner positions the nurse structurally in opposition to the oppressive and constraining forces of instrumental managerial and technical relationships and high technology curative medicine. She makes explicit her view that the marginality of nursing can be addressed through opening up skilled practice for peer appreciation, and the constitutive generative transformative power of public story telling. Implicit in her work therefore is a view of power as exercised by those who conform to and support the demands stemming from technologically driven structures and systems. People whose work is not consistent with these technologising impulses, such as nurses, are therefore disempowered. Nurses become empowered through recognising, strengthening and articulating their unique knowledge and skills.

Benner recognises the extent to which people's embodied practices are embedded in relational networks, traditions and history, and that corporeality imposes limits upon the human capacity to act autonomously, rationally and freely. She makes reference to Heidegger's notion of the technological self which refers to the objectification of subjectivity, but she does not explicitly discuss the extent to which power relations are expressed in and through corporeality. That is to say she does not address the issue of the docile body (Foucault 1980), which is regulated by disciplinary power and which reproduces oppressive practices.

A feminist writer, McNay (1991), points out that Foucault's idea that the body is produced through power, and is therefore a radically contingent entity, is helpful to feminist theorisations of the body. This is because it provides a way of understanding the body as a concrete phenomenon without attributing a fixed biological or prediscursive essence to its materiality. However she makes the point that Foucault's emphasis on the means by which the relationship between power and knowledge reduces human agents to passive bodies cannot explain how people can act with any degree of autonomy. McNay notes further that Foucault has not analysed those disciplines which produce forms of subjection that engender the feminine body. Furthermore his analysis of disciplinary techniques focuses on those in control rather than on the voices and bodies of those being controlled. He therefore overestimates the effectiveness of disciplinary forms of power and fails to elaborate any notion of resistance on the part of those subject to disciplinary power.

Street and embodied rituals and transformative actions

Recently an Australian writer, Street (1991), has studied embodied practices of nurses from a perspective informed by feminist critiques of Foucault such as that offered by McNay (1991). She examines relationships between power and knowledge in the hospital context and focuses on the hegemony by which oppressive practices are maintained, accommodated or resisted. She argues that hegemonic relationships, particularly the doctor-nurse relationship, create nursing invisibility and enable it to be continually recreated and reconstituted in a context dominated by the privileged status and authority of medical power and knowledge.

She identifies through a range of examples how nurses' embodied knowledge can result in ritualised actions that contribute to the maintenance of oppressive technologies of power. She notes also, with some dismay, that when challenged nurses recognise their own embodied passivity but do not change their actions as a consequence of this insight. She points out that an analysis of the constitution and relationships of power/knowledge in the hospital context emphasises the disempowerment of nurses, thereby reinforcing the concept of the disciplined docile body. This is particularly apparent in relation to nurses' collectivist embodied rituals of routinised practices and lack of participation in the written documentation which provides the official records of patient care.

However, Street recognises the overly deterministic nature of the idea of the docile body. She therefore also draws upon feminist critiques to demonstrate transformative actions which can be analysed in relation to what she describes as nurturance/knowledge as opposed to power/knowledge. She indicates the extent to which nurses' embodied nurturance/knowledge contributes to transformative outcomes both for patients and for the medical/nursing team. She gives examples such as nurses' activities in interpreting medical jargon and procedures to patients, their judgement of and actions in relation to critical situations, and their refusal at times to accommodate themselves to demands stemming from the hierarchy if they feel patient comfort and safety is in jeopardy.

She draws attention to the resistance of clinical nurses to written documentation of their practice which adds to nursing invisibility and relative powerlessness within the wider institutional culture. As she points out, nurses' lack of written documentation of clinical knowledge also means it is not available for reflection and critiques among nurses and to this extent nurses contribute to their own powerlessness. She suggests, however, that this resistance to the development of a written nursing culture represents a counter hegemonic movement by clinical nurses, which is not formally organised but constitutes a taken for granted recognition that the written word cannot adequately capture the nature of the care nurses provide. It seems she is suggesting that nurses prefer to communicate verbally so as to ensure the transmission of a nursing culture which constitutes the person in a more fully incorporative way.

Street stresses the importance of making nurses' unspoken embodied power/knowledge and nurturant/knowledge values more visible through ideology critique. She suggests a range of strategies to enable nurses to engage in their own enlightenment and empowerment. These include systematic processes of reflection and collaborative critique of nursing actions, contexts and knowledge. She believes that collaborative discourse will enable nurses to utilise their oral skills and engage in systematic counter hegemonic actions.

Both Benner and Street thus stress the importance of making more visible nurses' embodied caring practices or nurturant knowledge. Benner argues for public story telling and analysis of nurses' narratives as a means of achieving this. Street argues more for an ideology critique, to make visible for debate and reconstruction the unspoken values of both power/knowledge and nurturant/knowledge inherent in clinical nursing practice.

Lawler and nurses' knowledge of the body

However, neither of these writers directly addresses the issue of the invisibility surrounding the nature of nurses' work with other people's bodies. Another Australian, Lawler (1991), is one of the first nursing writers to focus explicitly on nurses' particular knowledge of the body. She argues that this has not been well documented because nurses deal with what people do not want to know about the body, or may want to know out of perverse interest. She sees that nurses' knowledge of the body is extensive but because of the societal context in which the body and its functions are hidden, there is pressure on nurses to hide nursing and the work that nurses do. Nurses' work is intensely private and discussion of what nurses do makes people uncomfortable. Nursing work engenders embarrassment and ambivalence. She points out that nurses are constantly faced with the 'unnaturalness' of 'natural' bodily functions which are normally managed privately and with modesty.

She draws upon Elias' (1978) view that in our culture the body has been civilised, that is to say, it has become a private matter linked to internalisation of taboos which regulate body functions and exposure of the body. Thus, when body functions cannot be managed privately there is a threat to what it means to be civilised. The social order is threatened with disruption (Garfinkel 1967). Nurses work in the ambivalent context between the private and public domain, attempting to manage taboos and return social order (privacy) to the body. This involves working with aspects of the body about which the greatest fears are held, those to do with body products, death and sexuality. Nurses thus have to manage nausea and the 'aesthetically unpleasant' on a daily basis and also deal with their own fears of mortality and sexuality.

Additionally, Lawler argues that nurses are mostly women working in the context of a patriarchal society with gendered meanings of the body. Thus sexuality, masculinity and power are linked and institutionalised within the patriarchal system. Nurses therefore have to manage also the threat posed to the social order through the control they exercise over the dependent male body.

Lawler describes what she calls a system of basic rules which nurses learn from practice and which patients are expected to respect. She calls these rules of compliance and control, dependency, modesty and protection. However the rules are quite subtle, for while patients are expected to be compliant, co-operative and dependent, they are also expected to take an active interest in what is going on and to be as independent as is feasible. Patients are expected to be modest, and to maintain the borders of sexual propriety. They are expected to demonstrate a modicum of embarrassment but they should not be so embarrassed that a situation becomes awkward. She describes the protective and private social atmosphere that nurses create as a means of dealing with 'unnatural' situations concerning patients' bodily functions. She describes the low-key, unsurprised and matter-of-fact approach nurses take to the patient's situation and the minimising language they use, which facilitates an environment of permission to expose vulnerable bodies to nursing care.

In moving beyond accounts in the nursing literature about technical and procedural aspects of body care, Lawler has brought into the open previously hidden or merely hinted at dimensions of nursing body practices. She has opened up a world of complex, ambivalent experiences of nurses with dead and dying bodies, with body products and with sexuality.

Lawler recognises the limits to a purely sociological approach to the body. She refers to the mystery and power of sexuality of the body and points out that existing explanatory frameworks and methodologies do not adequately accommodate the body within the social sciences. She might thus agree with those feminists who adopt a psycho-analytical perspective and who argue that disciplines such as sociology which bypass the corporeal reality of the body, cannot adequately deal with the associated bodily issues of desire and psychic impulses (McNay 1991).

345

Nursing and postmodern critiques

The writings of Benner, Street and Lawler offer critiques on different aspects of the modernist assumptions about the subject and the object (body) which have rendered much of nursing practice invisible. To a greater or lesser extent, and in varying ways, their work is consistent with postmodern critiques which reject notions of an integrated unified self and which understand the subject as a discursively produced, historically changing, concrete, embodied, desiring and reflective being with situated freedom.

Similarly, either implicitly or explicitly, they reject the dualistic separation of the world into appearances and essences which results in the mind-body split, and the separation of the self from the natural world. Benner particularly makes explicit the understanding that this critique of the object makes untenable the notion that there is an objective, reliable, universal foundation for knowledge. In emphasising the embodied nature of knowledge these writers are in accord with postmodern views that knowledge legitimation can only be local, plural and immanent, i.e. constituted through practice (Fraser & Nicholson 1990). Street particularly acknowledges the embodiment of hegemonic forces and Lawler acknowledges the mystery of sexuality in embodied knowledge.

Benner recognises the postmodern critique of linguistic signs as private marks in stressing the performative aspects of language and its public and shared nature. Each of these writers sees knowledge as a discursive practice and emphasises the narrativity of modes of knowledge which have been repressed and marginalised by science. Each facilitates an understanding of the invisibility of nursing and the body in the context of medical dominance, hospital structures and nursing practice. Each offers a critique of various aspects of scientific and humanistic assumptions of modernism.

Speculations: the abject body and nursing

In this section of my search for the body in nursing I want to offer some speculations about the function of the collective nursing handover in facilitating nurses' management of the abject body.

I am of the view that Kristeva's (1992) work on the abject body, and the particular relationship of women to the abject, could offer useful insights into addressing the gap identified by Lawler in current understandings of the body in nursing. The Australian film theorist, Creed (1993) for example, draws upon Kristeva's work and identifies three ways in which the horror film illustrates abjection. I believe that each of these has direct relevance for understanding the body in nursing. She describes images of abjection such as the dead body and bodily wastes; the notion of the border between the symbolic order and that which threatens its stability (i.e. the ambivalent border between the hidden 'civilized' body and the 'polluted' body requiring nursing care); and the maternal (= nurturing = nurse) body which represents maternal authority and is therefore a site of conflicting desires.

It seems to me that these illustrations of abjection are relevant to nursing because nursing abounds with culturally constructed images of the horrific, and the shame and humiliation stemming from the vulnerability of corporeality. The closeness of nursing to the abject shows up the fragility of the symbolic order manifest in the rationalising and technologising impulses of advanced medicine. Nurses play a boundary role between culturally constructed notions of 'dirty' and 'clean', the out of control and the controlled, the visible and the invisible. They maintain boundaries to keep at bay monstrous images. They are also authoritative in relation to the abject and thus conjure up powerful archaic images of forces of both generation and extinction.

Nurses work at the boundary of the medical technologising culture that seeks to overcome death through technological control. They also work at the boundary of the patient's lost or unmade world (Sacks 1986). Their closeness to the patient's experience raises ambivalences within the medical culture, for nurses embody intimations of mortality and thus threaten the medical enterprise of overcoming death. Their closeness to the patient's experience also raises ambivalences within patients, for nurses become powerful mythical figures who evoke images of both terror and desire.

Perhaps it is not unexpected that nurses adopt an apparently subservient demeanour and a low-key unsurprised approach to care. As I have noted elsewhere, much of the culture of clinical nursing practice is about 'making ordinary' (Parker & Gardner 1991) what are in fact extraordinary events in the patient's life. The clinical nursing community of the ward or care unit promotes a culture of everydayness in the remaking of the broken chaotic worlds of patients. It does this through a taken-for-granted approach to the bodily invasions it inflicts, through touch, everyday talk, jokes, sharing of life experience and safe silences. It thereby routinises chaos and ritualises the technical dimensions of care. This is the nursing work of 'purifying' the abject.

I am arguing here that this boundary world of managing the abject, of returning the 'taboo' to the 'clean and owned' does not usually rest upon the establishment of a unique one-to-one relationship between the nurse and the patient. Patients may speak of 'my doctor' but they seldom speak of 'my nurse'. Rather nursing care is experienced by patients more as a collectivity or as a communal practice. The unique individuality of a particular nurse is experienced by the patient more as a sparkle of sunlight or a shadowy feature upon the communitarian face of nursing. Patients relate to nurses as a comforting corporate self which facilitates easeful management for both patient and nurse of otherwise shameful secrets, or embarrassing or disgusting situations. Thus, the presence of nursing facilitates the remaking of broken worlds and the incorporation of the abject into the community, i.e. into the corporate nursing self.

Furthermore, I would suggest that in the hospital context the nursing handover at the beginning and end of each shift serves as a location wherein the nursing collective, corporate self is constituted, deconstituted and reconstituted on a daily basis. It enables individual nurses to group and regroup as a team or collective self for the shift. It enables the collective self to dissipate its incorporation of the abject and deconstitute at the end of the shift.

347

I am arguing that managing the abject poses enormous threats to one's belief in the taken-for-granted everyday continuity of life and that as human beings we need defences against the abject. Advanced medicine provides powerful technologies of defence and nurses witness both the success and failure of such defences. The constitution of a collective identity provides a means of managing the abject through collective incorporation. The nursing handover is a longstanding ritual in hospitals which facilitates the daily constitution of a collective identity and its deconstitution at the end of the shift so that the nurses can go home to their everyday world and leave behind the ambiguities of the abject.

Nursing has long been identified with women and with the frailties of human embodiment. It has clung to a collective identity in the face of its own abjection, and the threats posed by its daily dealings and polluted objects and by the oppressive technologising impulses surrounding modern medicine. There is, however, much to be learnt from nursing about living with the abject body, about dealing with the unnameable and taboo dimensions of embodiment, and about humanising embodied caring practices in the context of oppressive structures.

Conclusion

This chapter has placed the search for the body in nursing within the broad socio-historical context of the dominance of Cartesian metaphysics in Western thought and the emergence of modern professional nursing in relation to medical dominance. It has argued that, in light of these influences, the body in nursing has been constituted in terms of the Cartesian split between mind and body and as a weak shadow of the medical body. It has shown that attempts by some North American nursing theorists to articulate nursing as distinct and separate from medicine have, nevertheless, retained notions of the Cartesian split between mind and body in their formulations. One school of thought has tended to emphasise the body as a passive object responding reactively to stimuli, while the other has focused on the dominance of the mind over the body, with priority given to notions of bodily transcendence. The search for the body in nursing has further shown that while representations of the body in Australian nursing documentation tend to reflect medical dominance, the oral handover provides an indication of the rich and complex ways in which nurses constitute patients as embodied beings through their talk. However it has also been noted that the ephemeral nature of the spoken word tends to reinforce nursing invisibility in the hospital context.

Some issues surrounding nursing invisibility and the body have been explored in relation to the work of writers concerned with embodied and body practices in nursing and critiques offered of both Cartesian metaphysics and medical dominance in nursing. The search has concluded with some speculations about the value of Kristeva's postmodern feminist formulation of the abject body in facilitating deeper understanding of nurses' particular relationship to the body and the practices which sustain this relationship.

348

NOTE

Handover excerpts reported in this chapter are part of the study of the Nursing Handover and Patient Progress Notes funded by the Victorian Nursing Council and the Australian Research Council Small Grants Scheme.

REFERENCES

Ariès P 1974 Western attitudes towards death from the middle ages to the present. Translated by P M Ranum. John Hopkins, Baltimore

Benner P 1988 Nursing as a caring profession. Paper presented at American Academy of Nursing, Missouri

Benner P 1991 The role of experience narrative and community in skilled ethical comportment. Advances in Nursing Science 14(2):1-21

Benner P, Wrubel J 1982 Skilled clinical knowledge: the value of perceptual awareness. Nurse Educator May-June 7:11-17

Benner P, Wrubel J 1988 The primacy of caring: stress and coping in health and illness. Addison-Wesley, Menlo Park

Capra F 1982 The turning point: science, society and the rising culture. Simon & Schuster, New York

Cohen J S 1991 Two portraits of caring: a comparison of the artists, Leininger and Watson. Journal of Advanced Nursing 16:899-909

Creed B 1993 The monstrous-feminine: film, feminism, psychoanalysis. Routledge, London

Elias N 1978 The civilizing process: the history of manners. Translated by E Jephcott. Urizen Books, New York

Ehrenreich B, English D 1973 Complaints and disorders: the sexual politics of sickness. SUNY, New York

Foucault M 1972 The archeology of knowledge and the discourse of language. Harper & Row, New York

Foucault M 1980 Two lectures. In: Gordon C (ed) Power and knowledge: selected interviews and other writings by Michel Foucault 1972-1977. Pantheon, New York

Fraser N, Nicholson L J 1990 Social criticism without philosophy: an encounter between feminism and postmodernism. In: Nicholson L J (ed) Feminism/ postmodernism. Routledge, New York

Garfinkel H 1967 Studies in ethnomethodology. Prentice Hall, Engelwood Cliffs

Illich I 1986 A plea for body history (unpublished), pp 1-10

Inglis K S 1958 Hospital and community: a history of the Royal Melbourne Hospital. Melbourne University Press, Melbourne

Johnson D E 1961 The behavioral system model for nursing. In: Riehl J P, Roy C (eds) Conceptual models for nursing practice, 2nd edn. Appleton-Century-Crofts, New York

Kristeva J 1982 Powers of horror: an essay on objection. Leon S Roudies (transl). Columbia University Press, New York

Lawler J 1991 Behind the screens: nursing, somology and the problem of the body. Churchill Livingstone, Melbourne

Leder D 1984 Medicine and paradigms of embodiment. The Journal of Medicine and Philosophy 9:29-43

Leder D 1990 The absent body. University of Chicago Press, Chicago

Leder D 1992 A tale of two bodies: the cartesian corpse and the lived body, the body in medical thought and practice. Kluwer Academic Publishers, the Netherlands, pp 17-35

Levine M 1971 Holistic nursing. Nursing Clinics of North America 6(2):253-264

McNay L 1991 The Foucauldian body and the exclusion of experience. Hypatia 6(3):125-139

Meleis A I 1985 Theoretical nursing: development and progress. J B Lippincott, Philadelphia

Merchant C 1980 The death of nature. Harper & Row, San Francisco

Merleau-Ponty M 1962 Phenomenology of perception. Routledge & Kegan Paul, London

Parker J 1990 Professional nursing education in the university context. The Meredith Memorial Lecture, La Trobe University

Parker J M, Gardner G 1991 The silence and the silencing of the nurses' voice: a reading of patient progress notes Border Crossing Inter-disciplinary Seminar, English Department, La Trobe University

Parker J M, Wiltshire J 1995 The handover: three modes of nursing practice knowledge. In: Gray G, Pratt R (eds) Scholarship in the discipline of nursing. Churchill Livingstone, Melbourne

Rogers M E 1970 An introduction to the theoretical basis of nursing. F A Davis, Philadelphia

Roy C 1970 Adaptation: a conceptual framework for nursing. Nursing Outlook 18(3):42-45

Sacks D 1986 Clinical tales. Literature & Medicine 5:16-23

Street A 1991 Inside nursing: a critical ethnography of clinical nursing practice. State University of New York Press, New York

Trembath R, Hellier D 1987 All care and responsibility: a history of nursing in Victoria 1850-1934. Florence Nightingale Committee, Australia

Watson J 1979 Nursing: the philosophy and science of caring. Little, Brown, Boston

Watson J 1988a Nursing: human science and human care. a theory of nursing. National League of Nursing, New York

Watson J 1988b New dimensions of human caring theory. Nursing Science Quarterly. University of Colorado Health Sciences Center, Denver

Woodham-Smith C 1951 Florence Nightingale. Constable, London

20

Postmodernism and nursing

COLIN A. HOLMES

The theory of postmodernity must be free of the metaphor of progress that informed all competing theories of modern society. The postmodern condition is a site of constant mobility and change, but no clear direction of development (Bauman 1992).

Introduction

This chapter offers some views on what is meant by 'postmodernism' and briefly reviews some possible consequences for nursing: it can only be a personal view because postmodernism is not a set of principles or a specific doctrine, but rather a kind of attitude or a way of viewing the world which has turned its back on the search for certainty and liberation. As Bauman (1992) suggests, postmodernism is 'a state of mind'. That it should also be the subject of a nursing text would seem to be timely for several reasons. Firstly, nurses need to be aware that postmodernism is an increasingly influential, albeit highly controversial, development taking place in the context of Anglo-European and American social, artistic, and intellectual life. Secondly, some nurses may find in postmodernism's apparently anti-philosophical and anti-theoretical stance a resonance with their own feeling that somehow traditional philosophy has run its course and has little to say which illuminates their practice world. Conversely, it will challenge those with an unshaken faith in the potential of the Western intellectual tradition to enlighten and humanise daily life. Thirdly, nurses need to contribute toward postmodernist perspectives in the nursing literature, and to formulate informed responses. Postmodernism will undoubtedly be encountered as nurses engage with a range of intellectual traditions and with colleagues in other disciplines, and it is important that their participation is informed and proactive. Finally, postmodernism offers creative and stimulating new ways of viewing nursing, which may prove to be useful.

This chapter therefore attempts to introduce postmodernist thought, and then briefly discuss some possible implications for nursing; this is not an easy task and some preliminary cautions are in order. Firstly, postmodernism is strongly opposed to pigeon-holing human experience and human knowledge, and has consequently eschewed definition and delineation as characteristic of world views which are no longer productive and against which it sets itself. Secondly, it draws on, and claims to transcend, a very wide range of intellectual traditions, thereby generating different emphases and interests. As a consequence, thirdly, it has developed as an amorphous and indeterminate body of thought which relishes the uncertainty as to its own nature and direction, assiduously avoids summarisation, and defies definition. I can only give an intimation of what postmodernism is about as I see it, and I have chosen to focus on the Lyotardian version; the significance of this will become clear later in the chapter. In any case, my accounts will doubtless raise the hackles of those, including my colleagues, who see it differently.

The literature of postmodernism is vast and diverse. I have found the texts by Kellner (1988), Sarup (1988) and Rosenau (1992), together with the paper by Boyne and Rattansi (1990), particularly helpful when traversing the subject for the first time. Useful collections of readings include Featherstone (1988) and Turner (1990) on sociological aspects, Kvale (1988) on the implications and insights for psychology, Seidman and Wagner (1992) on postmodernism and social science, and Nicholson (1990) on the relationship to feminism. Docherty (1993) also gathers in one place some of the most important statements of, and about, postmodernism.

Postmodernism: the background

Postmodernist commentary has been mediated through a bewildering variety of academic contexts. Early debates, prefigured in the use of the word 'postmodernism' by a number of authors since 1934, notably the historian Arnold Toynbee (Hassan 1987), appeared in the context of literature and the fine arts, and concerned the status of new forms, particularly fictional (e.g. Howe 1959, Hassan 1971), dramatic (Kirby 1975) and architectural (Jencks 1977). Searing attacks on traditional philosophical discourse appeared, especially from Rorty and Derrida; literary critiques dovetailing with poststructuralism, epitomised in the work of Barthes, De Man, and Kristeva; American cultural postmodernism in the work of Jameson and Said on literature and narrative; and wide-ranging social commentary, predominantly from French social theorists, including Foucault, Lyotard, Bataille, and Baudrillard, each announcing in their own idiosyncratic, sometimes perverse way, 'the postmodern condition'. Whilst it may give the reader who is familiar with these names some orientation to the genealogy of postmodernism, this list is made with a weather eye on Boyne and Rattansi's (1990) warning about the misapprehensions that can arise as a result of lumping together so many writers from such diverse fields under a single rubric. It has to be recognised, for example, that Foucault's position is notoriously ambiguous and his allegiance has been claimed by both the political left and right and by postmodernists and critical theorists, perhaps bearing testimony to his own denial of any allegiances at all (McNay 1992). Nevertheless, the list serves to draw attention to the diversity of postmodernism's origins and to intimate the ubiquity of its influence.

In some respects postmodernism is, as the word suggests, a reaction against, and in some sense posterior to, something called 'modernism'. What, then, is 'modernism'? Boyne and Rattansi (1990) describe modernity as seeking to expose the hidden truths of the world, not as the result of positivist science, but through a continuing process of uncovering and reflexive questioning. In this respect modernism is an agent of its own critique and therefore paradoxically engages with postmodernism. In a well-known but perhaps politically short-sighted defence of modernism, Habermas (1983) described it as a form of consciousness which 'relates itself to the past of antiquity, in order to view itself as the result of a transition from the old to the new'. One of the ways in which it does this is by 'forever inventing the new', in both theory and practice. Thus, modernism constantly invents new '-isms', and new technologies (Ellul 1965). Forever striving after the new, modernity is a *temporally conscientious* attitude, the recent origins of which Habermas ascribes to the French philosopher, Henri Bergson. Interestingly, Bergson, irrationalism, and the problem of time, figure significantly in recent theoretical constructions of nursing, particularly in the work of Martha Rogers, Margaret Newman and Barbara Sarter. As Habermas points out in his paper, modernism, in its celebration of dynamism, betrays a 'longing for an undefiled, immaculate and stable present' (1983). Postmodernism, by contrast, marks the end of the search for absolutes, an aspect presaged by Bell's 'end of ideology' thesis (Bell 1961), and its offshoots (Lipset 1981, Bell 1988). It may be regarded as a 'posthistorical' world view which makes a conscious break with the constraints of the historical process—a break with the tradition of the 'new' in culture, thought, and behaviour. In the eyes of postmodernists, the modernist search is endless and self-defeating, which is why Bell (1976) suggested that modernistic culture is incompatible with the moral basis of a purposive rational conduct of life. He argued that current crises may be traced to a split between culture and society, a split that had been noted many years earlier in the work of Max Weber.

For Weber, reason had become partitioned into three autonomous spheres—science, art and morality. These had developed hand in glove with their related discourses, which correspond to professional groupings characterised by their own distinctive rationality, and under the control of their own 'experts'. A gap subsequently developed between the culture of the experts and that of the larger public, with a consequent impoverishment of the everyday life world. This led to the development, especially in the period after the First World War, to a series of efforts to 'negate' the culture of expertise. Habermas, however, believes that the project of modernity has not yet been fulfilled, and that we should learn from the mistakes of these programs, rather than reject modernity as a lost cause. Many commentators share the view of Kellner (1989), however, that Habermas' response to postmodernism is 'defensive and hostile', and it is not too difficult to identify weaknesses in his arguments, particularly in his depiction of the claims and scope of postmodernism. Although this is not the place to discuss the contest between Habermas and the postmodernists, it is an absorbing exchange which must be a part of any serious exploration of either postmodernism or critical theory.

It also has to be added that whilst postmodernism is claimed by some authors to be posterior to something called modernism, many others regard this 'posteriority' not as a sudden and radical severance with existing traditions of thought but rather as a natural outworking or transcending of that tradition, and therefore an extension of the modernist project. From this perspective it is difficult to see why postmodernism may not be classed as a form of avant-gardism: in other words, as yet another '-ism' seeking to challenge and disrupt what has gone before, much as dadaism, futurism and surrealism did in the early decades of the century. A glib response, which hints at a more sophisticated one, is that, unlike these, postmodernism has no theoretical doctrines, no set of epistemological rules, and no program of political action. It constitutes instead a form of radical eclecticism in which everything is permissible because the universal absolutes which previously served as a bedrock of predictability, and as utterly reliable guides for human behaviour, are no longer treated as incontrovertible. In this respect, postmodernists make a radical break with the past, accepting uncertainty and risk, and glorying in a new found freedom rather than struggling to invent new certainties with which to tie down the thoughts and practices of themselves and others. Post-modernism, then, although it commonly refutes liberatory projects such as Marxism, humanism, and religion, might justifiably be regarded as a quintessentially emancipatory attitude.

The postmodernism of Jean-Francois Lyotard

One philosopher who regards postmodernism as representing a radical break with the past, and a powerful opponent of Habermas' defence of modernity, is Jean-Francois Lyotard. A clear account of Lyotard's main theses is given in Kellner's (1988) overview of postmodernism, and Benjamin (1989) offers an invaluable collection of his most important work. Sarup's (1988) introductory comments on Lyotard focus on areas of especial concern to nurses—science and the nature of knowledge, and the ways in which knowledge is legitimated and marketed. In contrast to Habermas' 'aesthetic' definition of modernism discussed above, Lyotard (1984) provides an 'epistemological' one, using the term 'modern' 'to designate any science that legitimates itself with references to a metadiscourse...making an explicit appeal to some grand narrative, such as the dialectics of the Spirit, the hermeneutics of meaning, the emancipation of the rational or working subject or the creation of wealth'. Lyotard points to the increasing hegemony of language in science and technology, and the transforming effects of technology on knowledge. He believes that, in the light of the impact of computer technology, everything we have hitherto regarded as knowledge must be quantifiable if it is to retain its status as knowledge, and that knowledge is increasingly a marketable consumer product. The old adage that 'knowledge is power' has been given a new potency, and he asks who decides what knowledge is, who shall have access to it, and by what media. The answer he gives is that it will be those individuals and organisations who own and control the technology by which knowledge is produced and reproduced. Those who own the most sophisticated technology will exercise the greatest control. This concern with knowledge and power complements that of Foucault, in that Foucault's views are derived from largely historical investigations, whilst Lyotard's view is based on an analysis of contemporary conditions.

Incommensurable discourses

Lyotard distinguishes between forms of discourse, or 'language games', which centre on the true/false distinction, the just/unjust distinction, and the efficient/inefficient distinction. He describes society as a 'flexible network of language games' (Lyotard 1984, Lyotard & Thébaud 1985), and whilst for the philosopher Emanual Lévinas it is possible for persons to move between games without loss of cognitive integrity, Lyotard holds that they are incommensurable and engaged in interminable conflict. Indeed, he refers to language games as being a form of war. He argues that art, morality, and science have become separated within the network of social language games and that their discourses are incommensurable. It is the contemporary fragmentation and incommensurability of language games that defines the new crisis. Postmodernism admits that contradictions and tensions will always be present, and insists that the continual search for some unifying principle may be called off (Lyotard 1984).

Lyotard and forms of knowledge

Lyotard also distinguishes between scientific and narrative knowledge. According to Sarup (1988), narrative knowledge bestows legitimacy upon social institutions, defining what may be said and done. This 'narrative knowledge' takes the form of stories, myths, legends and so forth, transmitting statements about justice, truth, and beauty, and providing guidance as to the set of rules by which the economic and political cohesion of society is maintained. He argues that, since the Second World War, grand narratives of the speculative kind have lost their credibility in the face of the power of technology. Narrative forms have thus given way to statements which form part of the science game, and for which, in contrast, truth/falsity is the only criterion. Truth is largely consensual among the participants in the game, and without players truth remains *incognito*. The rules of the game are learnt and reproduced by each student, who thereby earns her/his right to fully participate in the game. Those who play the science game reject narrative knowledge, but ironically, according to Lyotard, scientific knowledge cannot be made known without recourse to narrative. Furthermore, the legitimation of institutional science is founded on two myths. Firstly, that science is the means to human freedom, and is thus a basic right of all peoples, and secondly, that all knowledge is amenable to a single discourse because knowledge has a transcendent unity. These myths have been pressed into service whenever the state has sought to justify controversial decisions or to obtain public sanction.

Lyotard subsequently acknowledges that the importance attached to narrative in his earlier work is exaggerated, and their identification with knowledge is an over-simplification (Lyotard 1992). He admits that 'countless other stories (continue) to weave the fabric of everyday life', and that there exists 'a sort of sovereignty of minor narratives which allows them to escape the crisis of delegitimation'. Less optimistically, he goes on to admit that they escape 'only because they never had any legitimating function'.

Knowledge as a commodity

Following Foucault, many postmodernists depict language as the ultimate legitimating principle, subordinating even reason itself to its determinations of what will and will not count as valid knowledge, and shows that knowledge, and ipso facto language, functions as a form of social power, maintaining and extending social controls and legitimating the underlying structures. Power—accessing, producing, controlling and disseminating knowledge—is thus acheived through the mastery and manipulation of language. Since, in contemporary society, this manipulation is a matter of the sophistication of technical resources, such as expensive computer facilities and electronic media, power has effectively become a commodity rooted in an 'epistemological economy' in which knowledge is the common coin. The depiction of knowledge as merchandise is not entirely new, and has obvious affinities with the commodification of culture described by Frankfurtian critical theorists and some French Marxist critiques. The postmodernist analysis goes much further, however, and Sarup (1988) sets the scene nicely: technical devices follow the principle of optimal performance, maximising output and minimising input, and 'Technology is, therefore, a game pertaining not to the true, the just or the beautiful, but to efficiency'. In other words, 'performativity', rather than truth, is the goal of science, and concern has shifted from the value of the *ends* of action to the productivity and efficiency of the *means*. Furthermore, science is 'the game of the rich, in which whoever is wealthiest has the best chance of being right...(and) an equation between wealth, efficiency and truth is established'. This type of critique is to be found in many postmodernist texts.

Postmodernism and truth

Laudan (1978), writing as a philosopher of science, has argued that truth ought to be abandoned as the official touchstone of scientific knowledge, firstly because it was never in fact the criterion by which knowledge was legitimated, and secondly because it is philosophically indefensible. Baudrillard, the *enfant terrible* of postmodernism, insists that just as the secret of gambling is that money does not exist, so the secret of theorisation is that truth does not exist (in, Gane 1993). He appears to delight in exploding intellectual projects which make truth claims, and it is little wonder that he refers to himself as a 'theoretical terrorist'! If we go along with these claims, how shall we decide which theoretical statements should be respected and utilised, and which ones cast aside or held in reserve? Laudan suggests that we should judge theoretical statements according to their power to solve empirical problems, balanced against the extent of metaphysical problems which they raise. As Lyotard (1984) puts it, 'truth doesn't speak, *stricto sensu*; it works', and the first consideration is no longer whether knowledge is true but rather how *useful* is it. This question is increasingly tantamount to asking whether it is marketable, and how much it is worth. If it is not a saleable commodity, one which is consistent with the rules of the game, it may be denied the means of expression. Lyotard describes this as 'terrorism' because the offending players, those who threaten to destabilise accepted political, bureaucratic, academic or disciplinary positions, are silenced by actual or threatened elimination from the language game.

Clearly, developments in postmodern epistemology have largely taken place in the context of studies of language, in particular the development of textual 'deconstruction'. This is associated particularly with Jacques Derrida, although his position in postmodernism has been a matter of debate, with Habermas (1987) and Norris (1989) taking opposing views. Deconstruction is predicated on the view that language is not an empirical representation of reality, but is interpreted within experience, and the value of statements is determined other than by truth-value (Murphy 1988). 'In fact, knowledge is seduced by language, or made to submit to the whims of interlocutors. Methodological rigor, therefore, is insufficient to rescue truth. Instead of adopting Reason, only passionate overture can gain a researcher access to facts' (Murphy 1988).

For Lyotard, the body is the origin of all philosophy (1984), and passion cannot be separated neatly from fact. Thus, Deleuze and Guattari (1977) and Donzelot (1979) claim that diagnosis of certain forms of mental illness, in which the passions may become superordinate to thinking, is founded on a rationalist absolutism which fails to understand the facticity of passionate discourse. Schizophrenia, for example, may be seen as a passionate, post-rational challenge to the status quo, expressed in linguistic forms which lie outside the conventional language games and regarded as 'irrational' or 'meaningless'. To these analyses, Foucault adds the notion that such forms are also 'unproductive' in terms of their value in the linguistic marketplace, and Deleuze and Guattari suggest that individuals whose language games are at odds with those legitimated by society should not be disempowered. The whole point of this analysis ('schizo-analysis') is that language is over-determining in relation to the form and content of thought, and the semantics of absolutism promote an excessive faith in the possibility of absolute knowledge.

Postmodernism and theories

Resistance to theories, as distinct from theorisation, is a basic feature of postmodernism, and its explicit rejection of totalising thought undermines what it sees as dualism's stranglehold on the Anglophone intellectual tradition. Lyotard, like all postmodernists, rejects metanarratives of every stripe—Marxist, Hegelian, Platonic, indeed any 'universal' philosophy. He says that 'master narratives', which purport to offer humankind mastery over nature and over its own destiny, have lost all credibility, and no longer succeed in evoking consensual legitimation. On these grounds, Lyotard, like Foucault, is often regarded by modernists as unequivocally neoconservative, though it must be noted that they both also reject the metanarratives of liberal-democratic politics, and their work has been called to serve the purposes of theorists of the political left (Poulantzas and Giddens for example) as well as the right. For his part, Lyotard rejects all grand theories, systematic philosophies, ideologies, and totalising, holistic discourses. Instead, he champions multiple, small scale narratives, individual creativity, pluralist explanations, competing localised accounts, and the fragmentation of language games, time, the subject and society. For Lyotard, not only are the assumptions about language which are inherent in systematised theories unjustified, more importantly, consensus is a counterproductive goal. Our aim should be to fragment and overthrow the language games of science and other grand discourses rather than homogenise them! Postmodernists are thus generally antiphilosophical in the sense that they deliberately operate in ways that place them at odds with traditional philosophy, which is seen as largely moribund or irrelevant, and they are antitheoretical in the sense of not setting out to understand or comment upon the world in ways that conform to predetermined systematised discourses.

Lyotard is scathing of the various emancipatory enterprises and techniques to which humankind has thus far given allegiance, and offers a brief but brilliant dismissal in a recent collection of letters (Lyotard 1992). The legitimacy of grand theories has been irrevocably undermined, he concludes, by their manifest failures. Despite this, and although Baudrillard suggests that the crowning achievement of theory may be the theorisation of its own dis-appearance (in Gane 1993), some commentators, sometimes referred to as 'neo-modernists' or 'affirmative postmodernists' (Rosenau 1992), continue to attempt a rapprochement of postmodernism with modernist theories. Unwilling to completely renounce enlightenment principles, they therefore see antifoundationalism as without hope. Many have attempted reconciliation with Marxist thought generally (e.g. Hall 1987, 1988, Graham 1988, Keane 1988, Kellner 1989), or with Frankfurtian and Habermasian critical theory (e.g. Norris 1989, Best & Kellner 1991). Other Marxists and postmodernists are uncompromising in their view that the two are quite irreconcilable (Eagleton 1985, Callinicos 1982, 1990a, 1990b). A similar situation applies to feminist thought. The fragmentation of discourse, the championship of pluralism, the recognition of tensions and differences, and the de-centring of personal identity, all suggest a sensitivity to the crucial feminist insight that the personal and the political are inseparable (Boyne & Rattansi 1990). Not surprisingly, therefore, there is a burgeoning literature exploring and utilising postmodernist contributions to specifically feminist ends. Some authors argue for a 'postmodern feminism' (Young 1985, 1986a, 1986b, Jardine 1985, Weedon 1987, Diamond & Quinby 1988, Fraser & Nicholson 1988, Poovey 1988, Rabine 1988), whilst others champion forms of 'feminist postmodernism' (Flax 1986a, 1986b, 1987, Benhabib & Cornell 1987, Nicholson 1989, Felski 1989, Boyne 1990, Hekman 1990, Lather 1990). Both trends are accompanied by an equally committed feminist opposition, often directed at postmodernism's Nietzschean origins and claims that it is an androcentric perspective which is unable to provide an analysis of sexual inequality and injustice (Lorde 1981, Hartsock 1987, Lovibond 1990).

Let us just recapitulate the claims and suggestions being made by postmodernists. As Murphy (1988) says, 'postmodernists deny legitimacy to the metaphysical baggage introduced by sociologists to perpetuate the facade that they are scientists', and indeed, leading postmodernists—Baudrillard (1983), for example—proclaim the wholesale demise of sociology (Smart 1990). Furthermore, because they oppose universal theories and systematic philosophy, and thereby set thinking free from the anchor of absolute principles, postmodernists have been criticised for undermining rationality and language as bases not only for sociology but for any systematic construction of knowledge. Critics insist that social order would thereby be destroyed, and that postmodernism's political radicalism (Ross 1985) amounts to nihilism (Crook 1990, 1991). Murphy (1988), on the other hand, suggests that since they show that 'each language game is sustained by values that must be respected', postmodernists actually do not jettison truth and order, nor do their analyses entail the acceptance of just *any* interpretation of reality. Rather, interpretation must be based on a careful consideration of each language game. It is what actually happens in the game that counts, not theoretical principles, and as noted above, postmodernism seeks to establish new rules, governed by utility, rather than to abolish rules. In the closing pages of *The Postmodern Condition*, Lyotard actually rehabilitates a concept of justice and thereby appears to acknowledge a need for social accountability. This revision of grand narratives, rather than their abandonment, is also suggested by the observation that, in its own discourse postmodernism comes very close to establishing implicit 'metanarratives'. Indeed, some critics would argue that it cannot avoid doing so. Crook (1990, 1991) argues, on the other hand, that postmodernism is nihilistic in its inability to specify possible mechanisms for change, or to provide a rationale for change. Whilst opinions clearly differ, we may say that Lyotard's postmodernism recommends the fragmentation of language games, the rejection of metanarratives, and the dissolution of traditional disciplinary boundaries. It heralds a post-disciplinary intellectual process, not in pursuit of any unitary epistemology or holistic explanation, but in order to maximise creativity and to generate knowledge which is useful in the real, unbounded world.

Postmodernism and nursing

Nursing theory

Some references to postmodernist perspectives have begun to appear in the nursing literature (Holmes 1991, 1993, Lister 1991, Mason & Chandley 1992, Ralph 1993). Increasing dissatisfaction with conventional epistemologies, and the science founded upon them, is leading nurse theorists ever nearer to a postmodernist 'antiphilosophical' position. Indeed, the whole notion of 'nursing theories' is being called into question, and postmodernists would regard them as outmoded and unproductive because of their divorce from the vagaries of the real situation, in which individuals are confronted by phenomena which do not conform to neat and tidy theories. Many nurses will sympathise with this view, and share the belief that grand nursing theories are primarily of historical interest. Meleis (1987), for example, tells readers to 'get off their bandwagons and get on with the development of the business of nursing'. She suggests that we should 'revise' some of the positions current in nursing academia. Firstly, we should 'revise' our 'passion for methodology, for science, and for philosophy', and she calls for a 'passion for substance, for the business of nursing...for the knowledge itself, and not how we get the knowledge'. This amounts to nothing short of the postmodernist renunciation of technique as the basis for establishing knowledge. She also recommends that we abandon the old polarised debates concerning particularism and holism, and pursue a 'need for the future development of other modes more congruent with the emerging shape of ontological beliefs'. Although she goes on to suggest that we adopt a 'gender sensitive knowledge', how we can do this without gender-sensitive methodologies and philosophies is not made clear. Without a passion for methodology or philosophy we are faced with postmodernist anti-rationalism, in which each individual is free to construct her/his own 'truths', and whether we are modernists, affirmative postmodernists or sceptical postmodernists, we must ask if this really will serve to promote the goals of nurses.

The postmodernist analysis clearly enjoins us to reject, overthrow or transform, all forms of nursing theory which constitute or rely on grand theories, including those founded on totalising metaphysical, political or ideological metanarratives. In the case of nursing theories the offending grand theories are not difficult to identify. In some cases one or more form the explicit framework within which the theory is constructed. They include systems theory, positivism, holism, evolutionism, panpsychism, humanism, existentialism, and phenomenology. The implicit metanarratives are less easy to discern and thus considered more dangerous by postmodernists. They include liberal-democratic political theory, Aristotelianism, deontological ethics, Platonic idealism, reductionism, behaviourism, Cartesian dualism, Christian theology, fatalism, determinism, verificationism, falsificationism, utilitarianism, racism, ageism, androcentrism, mysticism, rationalism, economism, scientism, technologism, aestheticism, and classicism, among others. Economies of space preclude any attempt here to attach nurse theorists to particular metanarratives, and the reader may in any case find this an interesting exercise. These metanarratives have been branded by some post-modernists as having a common core with totalitarian, fascistic implications. The Heideggerian concept of care, for example, which appears to be popular among nurses, is based on Platonic idealism and has been linked to nazistic fascism (e.g. Farias 1987, Sheehan 1988, Lavine 1990, Wolin 1990, 1991 Grange 1991, Paskow 1991, Habermas 1992, Hindess 1992, Holmes 1992), although some post-modernists, particularly those who recognise the debt of postmodernist thought to Heidegger, have argued for a separation of his value as a politicial activist from his value as a philosopher (e.g. Derrida 1989, Lyotard 1990).

Having abandoned the notion of nursing 'theories', one postmodernist approach to constructing nursing knowledge would be to exclude metanarratives by dealing directly with the world as we find it. It would champion micro-explanation—small scale accounts aimed at localised understandings—perhaps similar to those initiated by Benner (1984), although resisting her attempts to ground these in phenomenological theories. Ethnomethodology might offer a similar opportunity. It would recommend a flexible multiplism which took no offence at contradictions and discontinuities, and it would expect knowledge construction to benefit from the passionate discourse they create. It would expect theorists to make no special claims to expertise or special understanding, and would value clinicians and patients alike as sources of valuable insights and sensitivities. It would recommend that theoretical statements be judged according to their usefulness rather than to the extent that they correspond to some notion of rationality, truth or falsity. Claims concerning truth would be minimal, and once again Benner comes to mind.

Postmodernist knowledge construction would avoid traditional dich-otomies generated by language's over-production of cognitive certainty, including those between health and illness, science and art, objective and subjective, good and bad, right and wrong, and beautiful and ugly. The dichotomisation of health and illness is already giving way to alternatives which see them not as categories but as 'ways of being', so that, as Margaret Newman (1990) says, one person's illness may be another's wellness. Illness and health are outmoded categories which do not adequately represent the experiences of real people, and unnecessarily constrain the relationships between persons—some labelled 'ill' others labelled 'doctor', 'nurse' and so on. The negative valuation of illness is also being reconsidered—a person's condition is 'right' for them at that time, it is neither inherently 'bad' nor 'good', 'ugly' nor 'beautiful'; these are simply ascriptions which we may or may not make depending on our beliefs and attitudes. Reflecting its emergent utopianism, nursing literature speaks increasingly of the beauty in 'illness' rather than the ugliness, of the 'positive' rather than 'negative' aspects of all life's experiences. In such cases there is an inevitable dialectic between the 'positive', beauty for example, and the implicit 'other', ugliness. Post-modernism would collapse this dialectic so that 'ugliness' and 'beauty', 'good' and 'bad', 'right' and 'wrong', become co-existent. The nurse's role clearly requires a major revisioning if this dialectic, and the commonplace categories, are to be abandoned.

361

Even those who are critical of traditional polarities in nursing theory, nevertheless continue to be bewitched by universalism and the cherished illusion of a 'grand theory'. Packard and Polifroni (1991), for example, arguing for the legitimacy of 'pure science' approaches to nursing knowledge, complain of 'the lack of a central direction for all of nursing science as evidenced by the absence of an all encompassing question', and bemoan the resulting confusion, lack of consensual aims, and inconsistencies in the definition of nursing. Suggesting that other disciplines have a history of a single, clearly defined purpose, they hanker after 'the true essence of nursing science', and refer to 'THE question all scholars in a particular discipline are searching to answer' (original emphasis). Significantly, they conclude that if this question cannot be identified, nurses 'should emphasize the creativity of the craft, call themselves artists and lay science to rest'. Postmodernism would relish this lack of a totalising 'paradigmatic' research objective, and the fluidity with which nursing is able to conceptualise its disciplinary purposes. It would oppose all attempts to tie nursing down to absolute definitions and to the implied universal grand theory (Holmes 1994); it would also, of course, reject the implied dichotomy between nursing as science and nursing as art or craft.

Postmodernism also suggests new foci for nursing scholarship which cut across traditional lines of inquiry. The construction of the subject is a key example, and postmodernism has elaborated a variety of discursive and embodied accounts. Textually generated identities, mediated through cultural practices, contribute to the construction of individual subjectivity and to others as subjects (Shotter & Gergen 1988). These constructions subsume the embodied subject, and bodies have become a renewed area of interest for social theorists (Schilling 1993). They are commonly the focus of nursing care, and their presence is normally a prerequisite for nursing practice. Even in those cases where the recipient of nursing care is not physically present, as in telephone counselling, there is an assumption of embodiment, to the extent that the participants will even construct a notional body of the other based on their experience of the interaction. A particularly interesting postmodernist perspective on the body has emerged from the sociology of medicine, with leading contributions from Featherstone, Hepworth and Turner (1991), and Turner (1984, 1992), who has established a multidisciplinary Centre for the Study of Society and the Body at Deakin University, Geelong, Victoria. Thus far, the only postmodernist nursing perspective on the body appears to have been a performance piece by Holmes and Hickson (1992).

Nursing education

A number of extended texts on postmodern education have appeared (e.g. Aronowitz & Giroux 1991, Giroux 1991, McLaren 1993). Postmodernism would suggest that nurse academics could overcome their xenophobic attitude toward other disciplines and develop a truly post-disciplinary curriculum which nevertheless resists the temptation to simply reproduce, albeit eclectically, the metanarratives of other discourses. This would have direct implications for nurse education, but raises problems concerning the structure of educational institutions, the extent to which such an approach is administratively possible, and the willingness of academics to relinquish their cherished illusions of disciplinary purity. This problem might reasonably be regarded as having been intensified by the transfer of nurse education into university settings, where the protection of those illusions is at its most eloquent and steadfast, where the compartmentalisation of discourses is most rigid, and where playing by the rules of the game is essential to success.

Nursing research

Postmodernism would require nurses to examine and expose the metanarratives which underlie their whole research program (Holmes 1993). This would involve analysis of its explicit and implicit objectives, and the strategies by which it seeks to achieve them, including funding arrangements, the approach to prioritisation, the choice of research issues, preferred methodologies, reporting media and styles, and the structures and processes by which these are maintained. It would involve the examination of the discourse of nursing research, as it occurs not only in research reports but in research texts, in research teaching, and in the use of research by nurses. Work on these issues has begun from a poststructuralist perspective (e.g. Dickson 1990), and it may be reasonable to expect that feminist analyses which have exposed the implicit androcentrism of scientific discourse will now inform the future discourse of nursing research, as well as exposing metanarratives of sexism in existing discourse. Whilst social theorists have long since begun to expose the metanarratives which underlie medical discourse and practice (Foucault 1973, Hazelton 1990), especially psychiatry (Foucault 1967), postmodernist enquiry into the nature of nursing—its discourse, its power structures and processes—has been very limited (Weiss 1985, MacPherson 1987, Chapman 1988), and there is a desperate need for historical and contemporary deconstructive analyses. In a pioneering study, Thompson (1983) used Frankfurtian *ideologiecritik* to expose the scientistic consciousness, the bourgeois ideology and the sexism implicit in nursing. Postmodernist research would seek to extend this work and examine the whole gamut of underlying theoretical assumptions implicit in nursing discourse. Thompson's own critique would itself be liable to deconstruction of course, and its own implicit metanarratives and its susceptibility to totalising theoretical commitments exposed.

Analyses of nursing discourse would alert nurses to the extent and sources of the 'incommensurability' of their discourses, written and spoken, with others—those of 'expert' and 'non-expert' alike. This may, for example, be a useful way of understanding the longstanding antagonism between nursing and medicine, which has often been based on a failure to understand or enter into each other's discourses or language games (Vaughan 1985, Roberts 1986 a-d, McLain 1988). They appear to be located in quite different discursive spaces, characterised by antipathetic metanarratives. Lyotard (1984) suggests that it is useful to provisionally accept, and work within, a variety of language games, but then create novel, disturbing variations, disrupting, fragmenting and destabilising the existing game. If he suggests any rule, it is to 'break the rules'. Thus, postmodernist nursing research would pursue a policy of creative pluralism, as recommended by Feyerabend (1975), rejecting 'paradigms' and any types of research which sacrifice creativity or pursuit of understanding to the demands of a particular ideology, theory, or methodology. Linguistically legitimated dichotomies such as qualitative-quantitative, subjective-objective, and science-art, would cease to command respect in methodology or interpretation. Researchers would not be required to establish the probable truth or falsity of their 'findings', rather the research would be judged according to its relevance and usefulness for practitioners. As Avant asserts, 'In the final analysis, nursing science will be judged by whether or not it can solve "significant disciplinary problems" (DeGroot 1988) or "offer defensible interpretations of the multiple realities of interest to nurses" (Coward 1990)' (Avant 1991). This may be achieved through the process of research as much as through the information it generates, and Avant concludes that '[a] postmodernist approach to science is a most appropriate way to achieve these goals'. I have briefly considered the ramifications of this claim elsewhere (Holmes 1991), and space precludes further discussion here.

Nursing practice

Postmodernism suggests a number of 're-visions' of nursing practice. Firstly, the revaluing of the experience and insights of practitioners and their patients, over and above those of 'armchair' theorists, rehabilitates respect for practice and practitioners, and clinical practice would be returned to centre stage. Secondly, as we have already noted, nurses would be enjoined to consciously expose underlying metanarratives, and commence a program of de-mystification by disrupting and undermining the rules of the game. Thirdly, there would be a rejection of underlying universals, absolutes and dichotomies, and the stereotyped 'games that nurses play' would give way to more creative and fruitful discourse. Fourthly, the nurse's role would also be dramatically changed by abandoning traditional notions of illness and wellness, as noted above, since this would entail revising our notions of treatment, cure and care. Finally, nurses would be encouraged to recognise and accept tensions, discontinuities and differences between their own understandings, and those of colleagues and patients. In nursing, the notion of 'multiple truths', championed by Peggy Chinn among others, could be brought to bear directly on clinical practice, although the existing underlying metanarratives of American liberal-democratic ideology, which characterises these writers, would be unacceptable to postmodernists. We should note that Foucault's analyses also support the postmodernist position against humanistic psychology, to the effect that as knowledge of the nature of persons increases so the notion of the transcendental self or ego, freely choosing and creating, evaporates (Soper 1986, Schwartz 1990). Another strand to this position is the view that the humanist subject is, in any case, a masculinist concept (Weedon 1987, Soper 1990). In nursing, which has generally assumed a humanistic psychology in its conceptualisation of persons, their needs, their problems, and the various techniques to which they are susceptible, a postmodern perspective would entail a major turnabout, and perhaps this is immanent in the work of feminist nurse scholars.

A cautionary comment

Ralph (1994) correctly points out that Lyotard's advice to disrupt teleological thinking mitigates against ending this chapter with a conventional 'conclusion', with its implication of 'possible solutions'. Instead, I will bring it to a close with some brief cautionary remarks. Whilst entertaining a tutored scepticism toward the claims of science and rationalism, we must be careful, not only in practice but in theory, to avoid the pitfalls of unbridled subjectivism and unprincipled irrationalism. Most recently, there has been a huge upsurge of 'spiritualist', 'extra-scientific', 'post-positivist', or 'quasi-rational' thinking in nurse theorising, and the scientists cited by Margaret Newman, for example, assume the reality of 'paranormal' and 'psychic' phenomena (LeShan & Margenau 1982, Young 1976, Jones 1982). Not surprisingly, there is already a tendency for nurses to assume that 'paranormal' phenomena are legitimated by Martha Roger's theory and Newman's notion of 'expanded consciousness'. Barnum (1989), for example, uses the latter term to include 'extrasensory phenomena' such as clairvoyance, 'suprasensory phenomena' such as out-of-body experiences, and phenomena attributed to religious belief such as miracles. Expressing disappointment that Barnum's article did not refer specifically to her theory, Newman (1990) clearly approved of its general thrust. There are many examples of these trends. Sanchez (1989) reports a study which includes an examination of telepathy between mothers and their daughters, suggesting that empathy is 'significantly ($p< .05$) related to telepathy'. The authors seem insensitive to the misgivings that many of their readers will surely have concerning the uncritical acceptance a notion such as 'telepathy'. No effort is made to explicate or substantiate it, nor to place it in the context of a modernist epistemological framework or any wider philosophical perspective. Rogers' theory alone seems to be considered sufficient justification and explanation. Equally, from a postmodern perspective, notions such as 'empathy' and 'telepathy', and their implied cause-effect relationship, reflect unjustified modernist versions of 'faith' and 'hope', and are constructed around an enlightenment framework which is both fraudulent and covert.

Whilst remaining critical of received science and other dominant paradigms, we must be careful not to commit intellectual suicide in the name of postmodernist inquiry. Whilst rejecting the hegemony of positivistic epistemologies, practitioners need to distinguish intuition from guesswork founded on ignorance, and avoid being dragged into, and reproducing, a world of irrational fears and superstitions. In eschewing the academic isolationism of our colleagues in other disciplines, and pursuing a broader range of post-disciplinary conceptual and methodological approaches, we can continue to be sensitive to the actual and potential uses and abuses of nursing theory and the interests which they ultimately serve. We can sympathise with the postmodernist critique of universals and absolutes, and the constraining effects of definition, and still not lose sight of our true purpose as nurses, which is the provision and enhancement of quality nursing care to all those who need it. It is hoped that this paper will have intrigued the reader sufficiently for him or her to explore further in order to form an opinion as to whether postmodernism can be used to the betterment of nursing, or whether it should be treated as a dangerous tendency.

ACKNOWLEDGEMENT

I am grateful to my friend Tony Ralph, of the School of Nursing, University of Tasmania, for his helpful and intriguing comments on this chapter.

REFERENCES

Aronowitz S, Giroux H A 1991 Postmodern education: politics, culture and social criticism. University of Minnesota Press, Minneapolis

Avant K 1991 The theory-research dialectic: a different approach. Nursing Science Quarterly 4(1):2

Barnum B J 1989 Expanded consciousness: nurses' experiences. Nursing Outlook 37(6):260-266

Baudrillard J 1983 In the shadow of the silent majorities. Semiotext(e), New York

Bauman Z 1992 Intimations of postmodernity. Routledge, London

Bell D 1961 The end of ideology: on the exhaustion of political ideas in the fifties. Collier Books, New York

Bell D 1976 The cultural contradictions of capitalism. Basic Books, New York

Bell D 1988 The end of ideology: on the exhaustion of political ideas in the fifties, 2nd revised edn. Collier Books, New York

Benhabib S, Cornell D (eds) 1987 Feminism as critique. Polity Press, Cambridge

Benjamin A (ed) 1989 The Lyotard reader. Blackwell, Oxford

Benner P 1984 From novice to expert: excellence and power in clinical nursing practice. Addison Wesley, Menlo Park, California

Best S, Kellner D 1991 Postmodern theory: critical interrogations. Guilford Press, New York

Boyne R 1990 Foucault and Derrida: the other side of reason. Unwin-Hyman, London

Boyne R, Rattansi A 1990 The theory and politics of postmodernism: by way of an introduction. In: Boyne R, Rattansi A (eds) Postmodernism and society. Macmillan, Basingstoke

Callinicos A 1982 Is there a future for Marxism? Macmillan, London

Callinicos A 1990a Against postmodernism. Polity Press, Oxford

Callinicos A 1990b Reactionary postmodernism? In: Boyne R, Rattansi A (eds) Postmodernism and society. Macmillan, Basingstoke

Chapman G E 1988 Reporting therapeutic discourse in a therapeutic community. Journal of Advanced Nursing 13(2):255-264

Crook S 1990 Radicalism, modernism and postmodernism. In: Boyne R, Rattansi A (eds) Postmodernism and society. Macmillan, Basingstoke

Crook S 1991 Modernist radicalism and its aftermath. Routledge, London

Deleuze G, Guattari F 1977 Anti-Oedipus: capitalism and schizophrenia. Viking Press, New York

Derrida J 1989 Of spirit: Heidegger and the question. University of Chicago Press, Chicago

Diamond I, Quinby L 1988 Introduction. In: Diamond I, Quinby L (eds) Feminism and Foucault: reflections on resistance. Northeastern University Press, Boston

Dickson G L 1990 The metalanguage of menopause research. Image: Journal of Nursing Scholarship 22(3):168-172

Docherty T (ed) 1993 Postmodernism: a reader. Harvester Wheatsheaf, New York

Donzelot J 1979 The policing of families. Pantheon, New York

Eagleton T 1985 Capitalism, modernism and post-modernism. New Left Review 152:60-73

Ellul J 1965 The technological society. Wilkinson J (trans). Jonathan Cape, London

Farias V 1987 Heidegger and nazism. English trans. 1989. Temple University Press, Philadelphia

Featherstone M (ed) 1988 Postmodernism. Sage, London

Featherstone M, Hepworth M, Turner B S (eds) 1991 The body: social process and cultural theory. Sage, London

Felski R 1989 Feminist theory and social change. Theory, Culture & Society 6(2):219-240

Feyerabend P 1975 Against method: outline of an anarchistic theory of knowledge. NLB, London

Flax J 1986a Gender as a social problem: in and for feminism. American Studies, pp 193-213

Flax J 1986b Psychoanalysis as deconstruction and myth: on gender, narcissism and modernity's discontents. In: Shell K (ed) The crisis of modernity: recent theories of culture in the United States and West Germany. Westview Press, Boulder, Colorado

Flax J 1987 Postmodernism and gender relations in feminist theory. Signs 12(4):621-643

Foucault M 1967 Madness and civilization. Tavistock, London

Foucault M 1973 The birth of the clinic. Tavistock, London

Fraser N, Nicholson L 1988 Social criticism without philosophy: an encounter between feminism and postmodernism. Theory, Culture & Society 5(2/3):373-394

Gane M (ed) 1993 Baudrillard live: selected interviews. Routledge, London

Giroux H (ed) 1991 Postmodernism, feminism and cultural politics: redrawing educational boundaries. State University of New York Press, Albany

Graham J 1988 Post-modernism and Marxism. Antipode 20(1):60-66

Grange J 1991 Heidegger as Nazi—a postmodern scandal. Philosophy East & West 41(4):515-527

Habermas J 1983 Modernity—an incomplete project. In: Foster H (ed) Postmodern culture. Pluto Press, London

Habermas J 1987 The philosophical discourse of modernity. Cambridge University Press, Cambridge

Habermas J 1992 Work and weltanschauung: the Heidegger controversy from a German perspective. Foreword to the German edition of Farias V, Heidegger and nazism. Reprinted in English translation by MacCumber J, with author's prefaratory note. In: Dreyfus H, Hall H (eds) Heidegger: a critical reader. Blackwell, Cambridge, Massachusetts

Hall S 1987 Minimal selves. In: Bhabha H (ed) Identity. ICA, London

Hall S 1988 The toad in the garden: Thatcherism among the theorists. In: Nelson C, Grossberg L (eds) Marxism and the interpretation of culture. Macmillan, London

Hartsock N 1987 Re-thinking modernism: minority vs majority theories. Cultural Critique 7:187-206

Hassan I 1971 POSTmodernISM. New Literary History 3(1):5-30

Hassan I 1987 The postmodern turn. Ohio State University Press, Columbus

Hazelton M 1990 Medical discourse on contemporary nurse education: an ideological analysis. Australian & New Zealand Journal of Sociology 26(1):107-125

Hekman S J 1990 Gender and knowledge: elements of a postmodern feminism. Polity, Cambridge

Hindess B 1992 Heidegger and the nazis: cautionary tales of the relations between theory and practice. Thesis Eleven 31:115-130

Holmes C A 1991 Is nursing a postmodernist science? Proceedings of Conference, Science, Reflectivity and Nursing Care: exploring the dialectic. Department of Nursing, La Trobe University, Melbourne

Holmes C A 1992 The politics of phenomenological research in nursing. Proceedings of conference, 1st Nursing Research Conference: Scholarship for Practice. School of Nursing, Deakin University, Geelong

Holmes C A 1993 Postmodernism and the (dis)integration of theory, research and practice. Proceedings of conference, Effective Collaboration: Effective Practice in Nursing—The nexus between theory, practice and research. Charles Sturt University, Wagga Wagga

Holmes C A 1994 Nursing theory and the search for the philosopher's stone. Paper presented at The Discursive Construction of Knowledge: An International Conference. Office of Continuing Education, University of Adelaide, Adelaide

Holmes C A, Hickson P M 1992/3 Nursing, feminism and the postmodern body: a touching case. A performance piece first broadcast in an edited form on ABC Radio's Health Report in 1992, also in extended version at inaugural conference of the Centre for the Social Study of the Body and Society, Deakin University, entitled 'The Outrageous Body'. Deakin University, Geelong. Publication version in Nursing Inquiry 1(1):3-14

Howe I 1959 Mass society and postmodern fiction. Partisan Review 26(Summer): 420-436

Jardine A 1985 Gynesis: configurations of woman and modernity. Cornell University Press, Ithaca, New York

Jencks C 1977 The language of post-modern architecture. Rizzoli, New York

Jones R S 1982 Physics as metaphor. University of Minnesota Press, Minneapolis

Keane J 1988 Democracy and civil society. Verso, London

Kellner D 1988 Postmodernism as social theory: some challenges and problems. Theory, Culture and Society 5(2/3):239-269

Kellner D 1989 Boundaries and borderlines: reflections on Jean Baudrillard and critical theory. Current Perspectives in Social Theory 9:5-22

Kirby M 1975 Special issue of The Drama Review, vol. 19

Kvale S (ed) 1992 Psychology and postmodernism. Sage, London

Lather P 1990 Getting smart: feminist research and pedagogy with/in the postmodern. Routledge, New York

Laudan L 1978 Progress and its problems: toward a theory of scientific growth. University of California Press, Berkeley

Lavine T Z 1990 Thinking like a Nazi: a review essay of Victor Farias' Heidegger and nazism. International Journal of Group Tensions 20(3):279-285.

LeShan L, Margenau H 1982 Einstein's space and Van Gogh's sky: physical reality and beyond. Collier, New York

Lipset S M 1981 Political man, 2nd edn. John Hopkins University Press, Baltimore

Lister P 1991 Approaching models of nursing from a postmodernist perspective. Journal of Advanced Nursing 16:206-212

Lorde A 1981 The master's tools will never dismantle the master's house. In: Moraga C, Anzaldua G (eds) This bridge called my back. Kitchen Table Press, New York

Lovibond S 1990 Feminism and postmodernism. In: Boyne R, Rattansi A (eds) Postmodernism and society. Macmillan, Basingstoke

Lyotard J-F 1984 The postmodern condition: a report on knowledge. Manchester University Press, Manchester

Lyotard J-F 1990 Heidegger and 'the Jews'. Michel A, Roberts M S (trans). University of Minnesota Press, Minneapolis

Lyotard J-F 1992 The postmodern explained to children: correspondence 1982-1985. Power Publications, University of Sydney, Sydney

Lyotard J-F, Thébaud J-L 1985 Just gaming. Trans. Wlad Godzich. University of Minnesota Press, Minneapolis

McLain B R 1988 Collaborative practice: a critical theory perspective. Research in Nursing and Health 11(6):391-398

McLaren P 1993 Multiculturalism and the postmodern critique: towards a pedagogy of resistance and transformation. Cultural Studies 7(1):118-146

McNay L 1992 Foucault and feminism: power, gender and the self. Polity, Cambridge

MacPherson K I 1987 Health care policy, values and nursing. Advances in Nursing Science 9(3):1-11

Mason T, Chandley M 1992 Nursing models in a special hospital: cybernetics, hyperreality and beyond. Journal of Advanced Nursing 17:1350-1354

Meleis A 1987 ReVisions in knowledge development: a passion for substance. Scholarly Inquiry for Nursing Practice 1(1):5-19

Murphy J W 1988 The relevance of postmodernism for social science. Diogenes 143:93-110

Newman M 1990 Letter to editor, and response from Barnum. Nursing Outlook 38(2):58

Nicholson C 1989 Postmodernism, feminism and education: the need for solidarity. Educational Theory 39(3):197-205

Nicholson L J (ed) 1990 Feminism/postmodernism. Routledge, New York

Norris C 1989 Deconstruction, postmodernism and philosophy: Habermas on Derrida. Praxis International 8(4):426-446

Packard S A, Polifroni E C 1991 The dilemma of nursing science: current quandries and lack of direction. Nursing Science Quarterly 4(1):7-13

Paskow A 1991 Heidegger and nazism. Philosophy East and West 41(4):522-527

Poovey M 1988 Feminism and deconstruction. Feminist Studies 14(1):51-65

Rabine L 1988 A feminist politics of non-identity. Feminist Studies 14(1):11-30

Ralph A 1993 Nursing in the void: postmodernity and the Baudrillard scene. Proceedings of Conference, 2nd Nursing Research Conference: Scholarship for Practice. School of Nursing, Deakin University, Geelong

Ralph A 1994 Personal communication

Roberts J D 1986a Games nurses play: merry-go-round and catch...to avoid constructive action on a problem, Part 1. American Journal of Nursing 86(7):848-849

Roberts J D 1986b Games nurses play: pass to a higher authority and trivial pursuit, Part 2. American Journal of Nursing 86(8):945-946

Roberts J D 1986c Games nurses play: monopoly and make a wish...most exasperating coworker, Part 3. American Journal of Nursing 86(9):1041-1042

Roberts J D 1986d Games nurses play: pin the tail on the donkey and war, Part 4. American Journal of Nursing 86(10):1101-1102

Rosenau P M 1992 Post-modernism and the social sciences: insights, inroads, and intrusions. Princeton University Press, Princeton

Ross S D 1985 Foucault's radical politics. Praxis International 5(2):131-144

Sanchez R 1989 Empathy, diversity, and telepathy in mother-daughter dyads: an empirical investigation utilizing Rogers' conceptual framework. Scholarly Inquiry for Nursing Practice 3(1):29-44

Sarup M 1988 An introductory guide to post-structuralism and postmodernism. Harvester Wheatsheaf, New York

Schwartz J 1990 Antihumanism in the humanities. Quadrant November, 46-54

Seidman S, Wagner D G (eds) 1992 Postmodernism and social theory: the debate over general theory. Blackwell, Cambridge, Massachusetts

Sheehan T 1988 Heidegger and the nazis. New York Review of Books XXXV(16 June):38-47

Shilling C 1993 The body and social theory. Sage, London

Shotter J, Gergen K J (eds) 1988 Texts of identity. Sage, London

Smart B 1990 On the disorder of things: sociology, postmodernity and the 'end of the social'. Sociology 24(3):397-416

Soper K 1986 Humanism and antihumanism. Open Court, La Salle, Illinois

Soper K 1990 Feminism, humanism and postmodernism. Radical Philosophy 55:11-17

Thompson J L 1983 Toward a critical nursing process: nursing praxis. Doctoral Thesis. College of Nursing, University of Utah

Turner B S 1984 The body and society. Blackwell, Oxford

Turner B S 1990 Theories of modernity and postmodernity. Sage, London

Turner B S 1992 Regulating bodies: essays in medical sociology. Routledge, London

Vaughan B 1985 Ward games...doctors and nurses. Nursing Practice 1(2):72-75

Weedon C 1987 Feminist practice and poststructuralist theory. Blackwell, Oxford

Weiss S J 1985 The influence of discourse on collaboration among nurses, physicians, and consumers. Research in Nursing and Health 8(1):49-59

Wolin R (ed) 1991 The Heidegger controversy: a critical reader. MIT Press, Cambridge, Massachusetts

Wolin R 1990 The politics of being: the political thought of Martin Heidegger. New York

Young A M 1976 The reflexive universe: evolution of consciousness. Delacorte Press, Robert Briggs Associates, San Francisco

Young I 1985 Mothering: essays on feminist theory. Roman & Allanheld, Totowa, New York

Young I 1986a The ideal of community and the politics of difference. Social Theory and Practice 12:1-26

Young I 1986b Impartiality and the civic public sphere: some implications of feminist critiques of moral and political theory. Praxis International 5:381-401

21

Beyond postmodernism: the case for a feminist hermeneutics

JANICE OWENS

Introduction

As nurses we need 'to develop our faculties rather than avenge our weaknesses with moral and epistemological gestures, to fight for a world rather than conduct process on the existing one' (Brown 1991). Whilst Brown was discussing feminist politics and the direction sought to explain the feminist position, such a statement describes a potential pathway for scholars to not only explain nursing, but to answer the challenge of developing the discipline of nursing, of being proactive and emancipatory, of problematising what we want to be rather than flogging the arguments of who we are. Such a stance demands a politics and vision for possibilities rather than allowing the future to be directed by probabilities derived from the assumptions and arguments of historical and current attachments. This is not to disregard the importance of historical analysis and contemporary critique but emphasises the requirement for nursing to develop post-ontological and non-instrumental modes and criteria for reviewing and judging the scope of the discipline. The goal of a transformative future requires a delicate balance between connectedness and distancing. Thus an argument centred on these themes must search for a way to loosen the chains of metanarratives, stereotypes, categorisations, existing dominations and dogmas. Connor (1989) adds weight to this argument when he calls for 'the dissolution of every kind of totalising narrative which claims to govern the whole complex field of social activity and representation'.

If we don the mantle of 'heterotopia', Foucault's name for this state of non-absoluteness, we simultaneously dispose of its rigidity, static nature and the ability to predict outcomes for all situations. We begin to emphasise the importance of experience, contextual and temporal factors to the development of any knowledge base. We are no longer compelled to assent to any one line of thinking. There is here a danger, a feeling of discomfort and insecurity without the 'truth' as we have known it. Questions, dilemmas and quandaries arise on what to value and then to what degree these structures, processes and knowledge should be valued. Nursing is in a double bind being strongly influenced by several other disciplines; indeed some would argue that the discipline of nursing is non-existent. If, however, the stand is taken that some ideological borrowing is acceptable, if not necessary, then the real issue becomes the protection of our own analytic structures. The deconstruction, re-construction, analysis and synthesis of nursing theory, knowledge and practice is dependent on the use of a nursing perspective. For example, the study of sociology may clarify the structure and nature of society but does not make explicit the place of nursing within these structures, much less the processes of nursing practice. The second strand of the double bind is the placing of value on nursing knowledge, traditionally devalued by other disciplines. Connor (1989) suggests that the overthrow of the absolutes, rather than diminishing questions of value and legitimacy, actually intensifies the struggle to generate and grant legitimacy and value in contemporary practice.

The challenge for nursing scholars and practitioners is to relocate away from secure, one best way approaches (Caputo's 1987 'post-paradigmatic diaspora') to an engagement in a complex heterogeneity of discourses that will allow a re-inscription of nursing. If this challenge is to be met there is an urgent need for an analytical and interpretative framework to facilitate the process. The remainder of this chapter is directed to the discussion of such a framework based on the philosophy and practice of a feminist hermeneutics and placed beyond the current infatuation with postmodernism.

Postmodernism and beyond

'What are we calling post-modernity?...I must say that I have trouble answering this...because I've never clearly understood what was meant...by the word "modernity"' (Foucault cited in Smart 1993). There is an uncertainty and ambiguity surrounding the labelling of the social condition and its processes; is the traditional form of society truly past, is the notion of modernity outdated and irrelevant, is the emergence of postmodernism complete? In addition, uncertainty exists concerning the outcome of modernity or postmodernity. Can either state be thought of as a bounded entity divorced from the other or is it more likely that one is an extension or development of the other? Bauman 1991 (cited in Smart 1993) has considered this possibility: 'Postmodernity is modernity coming of age...looking at itself at a distance rather than from inside, making a full inventory of its gains and losses...Postmodernity is modernity coming to terms with its own impossibility; a self-monitoring modernity, one that consciously discards what it was once unconsciously doing'. While some writers have put dates on the beginning of postmodernism, Harvey (cited in Crook et al 1993) set 1973 as the date, others (Crook et al 1993) have advised caution in the labelling of any social change that infers a 'genuinely new historical configuration'. They suggest that postmodernism as an emerging social form is still indeterminate and problematic: that there is no knowledge of what it is, only that it is not modernity. Out of this intellectual foment and indecision two things are certain, that social change is taking place radically and rapidly and that there is a need to describe and give meaning to both the structures and the processes that have initiated and facilitated these changes.

A further issue that must be considered when discussing social life and its transitions is the place of nursing and nurses within the overall fabric of society. Questioning the identity and situations of nursing, the relevance and inclusiveness of social labels and the usefulness of current social theorising to nursing frameworks, and charting the reactions and responses of nursing to social change are mandatory if nursing is to progress in understanding its epistemological and ontological foundations as well as its political circumstances. For the present discussion, the most important of these questions is the usefulness of current social theorising to nursing frameworks, e.g. does the notion of postmodernism offer concepts and theoretical pathways that illustrate nursing processes or is it diversionary, destructive or merely redundant?

Having stated that uncertainty exists concerning postmodernism it must also be acknowledged that it has been embraced enthusiastically by many scholars. Recognition of the transitional nature of society, and the knowledge that some conceptualisations are past, has resulted in a plethora of 'posts', e.g. theological explorations of Thiering (cited in McGregor 1994) that she labels post-christianity and Brown's 1991 eloquent expose of the experience of 'being after' post-industrialism, post-philosophy, post-structuralism, post-histoire and post-foundationalism. While it is understandable that there is a desire to dispose of the master narratives steeped in exclusions and violations based on oppressiveness, boundaries and absolutes, the postmodern disorganisation and fragmentation may not hold a satisfactory solution. It is easy to be seduced by the postmodern rhetoric—challenging the dominant discourses, avoiding dogmatism, deconstructing polarities and engaging in counter-hegemonic work (Lather 1992).

The very nature of nursing, its traditions, values and image of second class citizenry to medicine, and its largely female work force that has suffered exploitation and domination at the hands of a patriarchal authority has set the scene for the seduction by postmodernist ideology. However, to submit to this force places nursing in a position of being imposed upon, just when a nursing standpoint theory or perspective seems a possibility. Nursing is, as Harding (cited in Lather 1992) described feminism, 'caught in a paradox of needing both a successor regime powerful enough to unseat scientific orthodoxy but with a keen awareness of the limits of any new approach'. This is not to recommend resistance to the new because, as Foucault makes clear, 'resistance is a product of any reaction to power, not an arrogation of it, resistance goes nowhere in particular, has no particular attachments and hails no particular visions' (Brown 1991). What is recommended is a critical, reflective stance that draws together historical and contemporary cultural, political and social influences into a complex interpretative cycle. Such a process, activated by nurses, allows the authentic voice of nurses to be heard and reverses the tendency for nurses to be as others want them to be.

This is an important point, nursing no longer constrained, bounded and cluttered by modernist metanarratives, must take advantage of the postmodern ruptures and lack of definitive alliances to create their own epistemologies and truths. As Brown 1991 warns, the spaces evacuated by the meta-theories and truths do not remain empty, but grow crowded with other technical truths—'instrumentalist discourses dangerously cut loose from regulating values and substantive, accountable aims' (Brown 1991). We are in danger of being subsumed by the hegemony of technical reason or means-end rationality. To allow this to go unchallenged could destroy what is considered at this point to be the very essence of nursing and return it to the reductionistic, task orientation of the past.

With the postmodern tendency to value fragmentation, dissolving boundaries, de-territorialisation, heterogeneity and multiple idioms and representations, Frederic Jameson identifies a further problem, that of disorientation, existential bewilderment and an inability to cognitively map out spaces: 'all profiles have disappeared. This is bewildering, and I use existential bewilderment in this new post-modern space to make a final diagnosis of the loss of our ability to position ourselves within this space and cognitively map it (cited in Brown 1991). With a history favouring others' interpretations of nursing, this viewpoint of postmodernism should sound alarm bells. How easy would it be to develop affiliations and political alignments that, rather than redressing the historical position of nursing, may actually increase its powerlessness. This is a trap of immense danger for a fledgling discipline, positioning without mapping, situating ourselves without a comprehensive analysis of our circumstances and identity. Hartsock (cited in Brown 1991) writes: 'We need to be assured that some systematic knowledge about out world and ourselves is possible...We need to constitute ourselves as subjects as well as objects of history...We need a theory of power that recognizes that our practical daily activity contains an understanding of the world'. Although these statements would seem to have an element of reactionary foundationalism about them, they also reflect a fundamental need to know who we are, where we are located and the meaning to be attributed to our activities and location.

A further contradiction encased in postmodernism concerns the interpretation of its relationship to political action. Postmodernism is said by some to be politically bankrupt (Hekman 1990), that the postmodern critique of modernism offers us no more than the 'weakest of constructive proposals' (Borgmann 1992), that postmodernism leads to a form of conservative reaction aligned to maintaining the status quo and perpetuating existing injustices (Habermas cited in Hekman 1990) and that it further hinders those groups relegated to the periphery of society (Hartsock cited in Hekman 1990). On the other hand, writers such as Brown 1991 suggest that the constitutive elements of politics do not disappear in postmodernity but are starkly featured within it: that issues of human plurality, power and stratification are revealed through its deconstructive projects. To situate nursing in this picture demonstrates a professional group that has been marginalised on the basis of its dominant gender and on its submissive relationship to medicine.

To politically centre nursing will require a distancing from the current epistemological conflagrations, including postmodernism, and an acute awareness of the damaging possibilities of judging all others against our own moralities. In allowing a politics of difference to direct our intellectual searching and theorising we need to be wary that we do not depend on our assumptions and constructed knowledge as a base for one-point comparisons. To take an essentialist approach to nursing would deprive the discipline of the richness afforded by the acknowledgment of diversity, complexity and multiple perspectives and realities. Nursing cannot align itself to a similar conceptualisation to that suggested by Jardine and Young when discussing feminism 'from modernism through to postmodernism to an essentialist gynocentrism' (citedin Hekman 1990). An evolution from modernism through to postmodernism to nurse centrism would merely replace one set of privileged concepts with another and do nothing to overcome the scorned dualisms and hierarchical divisions of power and prestige.

From the preceding discussion, it is clear that the notion, postmodernism, invokes slavish adherence to the ideas spawned by the discourses surrounding it. With equal vehemence there are those who spurn the explanations derived from its ideology. There are still others who remain uncertain of its usefulness in expressing their realities, others in reactionary mode grasp at what has served them well in the past, others ignore the whole chaotic litany. Lyotard (cited in Smart 1993) most succinctly summarises this turbulence by asking:

> Is this the sense in which we are not modern?...is this the continuation of romanticism?...A well executed work of mourning for Being?...the hope of redemption?...Or, is postmodernity the pastime of an old man who scrounges in the garbage heaps of finality looking for leftovers, who brandishes unconsciousness, lapses, limits, confines, goulags, parataxis, non-senses or paradoxes and who turns this into the glory of his novelty, into his promise of change?

Within this turmoil of ideas and explanations who should one follow? There does not seem to be a straight uncluttered pathway. There are twists, turns, obstacles, entanglements, thorns, some enchanting scenery, heady perfumes and vibrant colours and movement. However, one will not find on this path the tranquillity of certain answers.

The pathway of postmodernism does indeed have some attractive features, the deconstruction of constraining metanarratives that encourage domination, stratification and truths based on the socially and politically powerful, the recognition of multiple voices and realities and the public accountability that derives from impersonal debate. There are, however, some barren stretches along the postmodernist pathway exemplified by the inability of postmodernism to take the deconstructive, descriptive processes to a level that could achieve resolutions and transformative action; the tendency to reduce discourse to rhetoric.

Where does all of this leave nursing? Modernism is anathema to nursing and the profession should resist any return to the philosophical and ideological stance advocated by this conceptualisation. Reactionary foundationalism as a response to postmodernism is also untenable despite its posturing as a link to the best of the past. Harkaway (cited in Brown 1991) has identified postmodernism as being 'ubiquitous, liminal and highly toxic in small and fluid doses'. While the discussion has so far been less virulent in its description of postmodernism, it remains an imperative that nursing be cognisant of the dangers of following blindly along this pathway. Hence the argument for beyond postmodernism; 'beyond' indicating in this instance non-alignment. The opportunity is available for nursing to develop its own standpoint epistemology, one that emanates from and explores the discipline of nursing in a contextually appropriate manner, free from whatever social categorisations exist. There is a need for an interpretative process to fill the void, a cycle that allows critical discourse that counters social fragmentations and acknowledges diversity, inclusivity and complexity. Unlike Feher and Heller (cited in Brown 1991) who declared all attempts at hermeneutics to be 'politically subversive', my belief is that a feminist hermeneutics can meet the criteria identified above. To clarify this stance further, the following section will review the hermeneutic tradition, and explain the influence of feminism on the hermeneutic process before proceeding with a description, explanation and application of the feminist hermeneutic model to nursing practice and scholarship.

The hermeneutic tradition

Hermeneutics has been defined as a theory or philosophy of the interpretation of meaning (Bleicher 1980). Thompson (1990) has added to this definition the phrase 'practice of interpretation', an important addition considering that a primary focus of hermeneutics is the explication of theory-practice relationships and contextualised issues. Hiley, Bohman and Shusterman (1991) agree with this emphasis on hermeneutics as practical wisdom. The pragmatic model of interpretation is derived from the Aristotelian 'phronesis', is supported by Gadamer and Rorty (see Mueller-Vollmer 1988 and Skinner 1990) and justified by Hiley et al (1991) with four specific reasons namely:
1 The intentionality of hermeneutics
2 The use of a particular perspective to shape in a large part the interpretation
3 The formative contextuality of the interpretations, and
4 The purposiveness of all interpretative situations.

Hiley et al (1991) further explain that interpretative theory, hermeneutics, 'is founded on practice and itself constitutes a practice', that its motives are characteristic of an applied and practical process. Inde (1971) is less certain, stating that 'hermeneutics is not a well defined field...there is no unified or agreed upon criteria for interpretation'. Dreyfus (1987) epitomises this indefiniteness with his comment 'anyone can define hermeneutics anyway he (sic) pleases'. Hermeneutic philosophy and interpretation has also been cited as an alternative to empiricist and historicist accounts of science (Hekman 1991), as guiding contemporary, methodological paradigms (Lincoln & Guba 1985) and as an interpretative base congruent with feminist theories (Bleier 1984 cited in Thompson 1990). Buker (in Hiley et al 1991) explains that 'the radical hermeneutics that engages feminists not only makes explicit the ways in which feminist theories involve quests for the good and just life (for both men and women) but also benefits from the critical reflections embodied in a variety of social theories'. In a similar way Polkinghorne (cited in Thompson 1990) points out that hermeneutic inquiry is influential in reminding us of the political and ethical standpoints we internalise as cultural agents. In summary, while it is difficult to identify one specific definition for hermeneutics, there are clearly some dimensions that are descriptive of hermeneutics—intepretation, understanding, contextuality and pragmatism, an inquiry process devised to reveal political, social and cultural conditions in a non-positivist approach.

It is not only the definition that is complicated and problematic for scholars and practitioners. The various origins, evaluations and methods involved in doing hermeneutics is equally complex and confusing. The word hermeneutics is said to derive from the name of the wing-footed, messenger god of the Greeks, Hermes, whose task was to deliver the messages of the gods to mortals. In order to achieve this Hermes had to be conversant with the idiom of the gods as well as that of the mortals, he needed to interpret the gods' messages and then articulate their intentions to the mortals. The task for Hermes was complex and is no less so for the contemporary practitioner of hermeneutics. From antiquity, hermeneutics was used for various tasks and in differing ways until the time of the Renaissance and thereafter when it became more specialised and located in the areas of theology, classical philology, jurisprudence and philosophy. Following the Enlightenment period, philosophers began to search for a universal hermeneutics that transcended the confines of individual disciplines. Following Schleiermacher and Dilthey, Heidegger employed a hermeneutics based on a two step downward spiral towards a deep concealed truth, a process that included going back and forth between details and the whole. Heidegger later modified his stance to concentrate on 'specific entities which, during a specific epoch, incarnate for a people and for the interpreters what being means' (Dreyfus 1987). His interpretations revolved around ontological-existential questions of experiencing rather than emphasising epistemological questions of knowing.

Gadamer introduced the fusion of horizons as his metaphor for understanding, identifying horizon as the range of vision that includes everything that can be seen from a particular vantage point (1975, cited in Bleicher 1980). According to Gadamer understanding occurs when the horizon of the scholar intersects or joins with the horizon or context of the object of inquiry. He further explains this notion:

> The historical movement of human life consists in the fact that it is never utterly bound to any one standpoint, and hence can never have a truly closed horizon. The horizon is, rather something into which we move and that moves with us. Horizons change for a person who is moving. Thus the horizon of the past, out of which all human life lives and which exists in the form of tradition, is always in motion (Gadamer 1975 cited in Thompson 1990).

This illustrates some contradictory elements in Gadamer's explanation of the fusion of horizons; the historical and temporal features of life, the presence of limits but also openness, within the fusion the retention of individual identities to form an I-Thou relationship, but the requirement to be able to tolerate relaxing one's own preconceptions in order to be open to another's standpoint. Gadamer does not consider this description to be intellectually lacking but rather explains it as a positive structure of understanding resulting in greater self-understanding, moral awareness and an appreciation of others' viewpoints. For him, understanding is synonymous with wisdom and different to knowledge.

> The truly experienced person, one who has wisdom and not just knowledge, has learned the limitations, the finitude of all expectation. Experience teaches him (or her) not so much a storehouse of facts that will enable (her or) him to solve the same problem better next time, but how to expect the unexpected, to be open to new experience. It teaches him (sic), in short, the poverty of knowledge in comparison with experience (Gadamer 1969 cited in Thompson 1990).

Contemporary hermeneutics cannot be discussed without mentioning critical hermeneutics and Habermas's stance on the implication of what he perceives to be a non-critical interpretation of the human condition by conservative, philosophical hermeneutics. He maintains that ideological structures of half-truths, manipulation and oppression may remain hidden unless scholars are sceptical of taken-for-granted meanings and critically examine cultural and political practices.

From this brief review of the evolution of hermeneutics, the reader may feel empathy with Ricouer's statement that 'there is no general hermeneutics, no universal canon for exegesis, but only disparate and opposed theories concerning the rules of interpretation' (1970).

Knowing the complexity and diversity inherent in the hermeneutical method, it may be helpful to consider the following questions from Hiley et al (1991) as a preface to the remainder of this discussion. Four questions were formulated to direct the approach to and thinking around hermeneutics as interpretation, questions which can be usefully modified and incorporated into nursing discourse and analysis.

First, what is interpretation? It can be asked what emphasis interpretation should take, if any. What is its purpose? For example, should the focus be explanation of a phenomena including issues of parameters, causality and characteristics or understanding that seeks to address both dimensions and context and a depth of knowledge acquisition associated with an event or critical analysis in the form of identification of false consciousness pertaining to social structures, processes and relationships? Should there be a contrast class or should the project of interpretation take a holistic stance that includes meaning, experience, evidence, context, beliefs and traditions, social relations and practices? Such fundamental questions are significant if the mistakes of modernity are not to be repeated with an outcome of a meta-hermeneutics. There is a critical ambiguity to be resolved between the universality of hermeneutic interpretation as a broad process or methodology and the desire to retain a situation, experience specific focus.

Second, what makes an interpretation correct or better than another interpretation? Will the acceptance of one interpretation in preference to another lead us down the path of seeking absolute truths, will our propensity to conceptualise in single, explanatory forms mitigate against the interpretative turn, will the interpretative cycle simply reintroduce older epistemological questions centred around the discovery of truth and validity? The advent of deconstructionist formulae have not prevented 'life explanations' from being in danger; the intellectualisation of meaning is a frail process at risk of corruption unless constant attention is paid to how we develop and articulate our understandings.

Third, is interpretation a relativistic and ethnocentric process in light of its fallible and circular nature particularly in the presence of the notion that the only avenue of appeal is interpretation? It takes considerable effort to make and maintain a paradigm shift that values phenomenologically based knowledge in the face of positivistic domination. If the belief is that hermeneutic interpretation emanates from and subsequently influences practice, particularly practice-in-context, then this third question becomes less problematic. It is only when there is an insistence on dividing theorising from practice, of adhering to a hierarchy of inquiry that places 'pure theory' above that of practical concerns, that the artificiality of such a divide is ignored and questions of relativism and ethnocentrism are raised. Gadamer (cited Hiley et al 1991) claims that 'interpretative understanding is always already application, since the situation that prestructures interpretation always calls for an application, always demands some response from us in the pursuit of the purposes through which we encounter the situation', a statement that supports the futility of decontextualised explanation.

Fourth, if the argument of interpretative practices rejecting universal reason and neutral evidence is pursued, do these practices become nihilistic or the result of power and authority? This places interpretative practice firmly in the social and political arena. Traditionally, hermeneutics has been associated with notions of asocial and apolitical interpretation, an idealistic promise of pure, uncontaminated, distanced knowledge. The political nature, including relations of power, domination and oppression, of all knowledge generation is indisputable. Knowledge manipulation in all disciplines has been at the hand (and minds) of those who hold the balance of power. Critical and imaginative reflection on practice-in-context and by inference theory and knowledge formation results in the recognition of the perspectival character of under-standing and therefore the inevitable influence and intrusion of political and social forces. Nursing is no more or less a part of these processes and forces than any other discipline or social group.

By addressing these questions it is possible to identify the characteristics of hermeneutic interpretation, the problems associated with this process and the possibilities of interpretative practice for nursing. To summarise the characteristics, hermeneutics as interpretation is a practical wisdom which acknowledges the intentional, perspectival, contextual and purposive nature

379

of those who engage in the process. By emphasising practice as the central focus of interpretation the ubiquitous theory-practice gap is minimised, practice is legimated through the explanatory power of hermeneutics while theory originates in and develops from practice. 'Theory-practice gap' arguments become redundant in the face of enlightenment interpretation. Closely related to this proposition is the use of critical reflection in and on practice as both evaluative and change enhancing. If a stepped approach is used, the next stage incorporates the broadening of critical reflection to include imagination and creativity based on critical pluralism (Bohman 1991), the rejection of a univocal language and the exploration of the relationship between object and subject, how we constitute object and subject and what forces influence those constitutions—fraud, domination or participative processes. Inherent in this broader reflection is the explication of the relationship between the interpreter and the subjects or the situations of interpretation. Acknowledgment of the contextual dimensions of reflection/interpretation is the next stage and must closely examine the political, social, moral and value assumptions and possibilities that shape our understandings.

The cyclical, broad nature of hermeneutics has given rise to the notion that the epistemic practices of interpretation may result in a closer alignment to holism than other epistemological constructions. Bohman (1991) wrote at length on this claim stating that interpretation as holism was an enabling, perspectival, reflective-transcendental concept that should be a public offering. He denies that interpretation is a romantic whim or sceptical subjectivity stating that it is a distinct way to establish a claim to knowledge being governed by evidence and normative warrants. The relationship of interpretation to holism will be further discussed later in the chapter.

The greatest criticism of interpretation comes from the empiricist steeped in an ideology that claims objectivism as its central focus and who raises questions concerning the validity of such knowledge. In addition, the multiplicity of types of interpretation and interpretative contexts are seen by some to be problematic. Both questions do not reflect problems of the interpretative process as such, but are the result of evaluating one paradigm from the stance of another. Hermeneutic interpretation is better served by criticisms of rigour and integrity derived from its own standpoint.

Hermeneutic interpretation as it stands, has much to recommend it to the analysis of nursing processes, philosophy and theoretical constructions. One may then question the necessity to further qualify it with the addition of feminist. Will feminist hermeneutic interpretation constitute a more powerful analysis, capable of answering the broad, holistic questions of nursing practice or will it serve to narrow the focus both intellectually and contextually thus damaging what, at this point, appears to be a useful framework? Feminism has an array of ideological themes, some conceptual uncertainties and flaws in reasoning. Although the feminist movement has sought to offer women a perspective that eliminates injustices based on the social constructions of language and gender, there has been a tendency for feminism to result in division and a perpetuation of power differences. Within these inconsistencies it is possible to locate some central and enduring themes, these being the concept of human mutuality, inclusiveness and the acknowledgment of the complexity of human understanding. For these reasons hermeneutic interpretation can benefit from the inclusion of feminist analysis. In particular, nursing has much to gain from a feminist hermeneutic model of analysis and interpretation.

The nursing connection

I began this chapter by stating that nursing needed to protect its own analytic structures, that we need to develop a nursing standpoint from which a knowledge base can be nurtured and from which a nursing identity can be assumed with a measure of certainty. This is not to infer that nursing should be isolationist, (we are of and in the world), but that we should map, affirm and value that which is uniquely nursing. To further explicate both these ideas and the feminist hermeneutic framework each of the four dimensions of the framework—historical, critical, reflective and interpretative—will be considered separately before integrating these entities to a method suitable for use in the analysis of nursing. There is also an explanation needed for the use of nursing without the usual appendages of scholarship, research or practice. An interpretive model, by definition, is one that must consider the derivation of meaning and the giving of meaning; it cannot consider research without practice, practice without scholarship, scholarship without research. It must in the interest of logic make all the connections explicit if meaning is to truly represent the phenomena. The historical dimension is the beginning process where one is required to view not only the current structures, symbols and circumstances that influence nursing but also must review past explanations, constraints, reproductions and actions that will allow understanding of the present to occur. Without this step one runs the risk of being trapped in a 'theoretical cul-de-sac' (Anderson 1989). It is so much easier to answer the question of today in the most facile way than to explore the origins of behaviour, to debate the possibilities and conceptions of false consciousness and the place of human agency and to penetrate the constraints of social structures that have led to the current condition. An interpretive model that is ahistorical, apolitical and does not attempt to map a position must raise serious questions as to its ability to be an adequate explanatory vehicle. Ricoeur (cited in Inde 1986) adds credence to this stance by stating there is a requirement for both clarity and depth in philosophical thought, a search for distinctions and bonds; that clarity without depth is empty, depth without rational clarity 'effuse romanticism'. One cannot fully know the distinctions or the bonds without an historical excursion.

The critical dimension of the feminist hermeneutic framework centres on the unravelling of the 'taken-for-granted', the routine, the habitual. It attempts to deconstruct the dominant discourses concerning the phenomenon of study while concurrently negotiating a democratic space to reconstruct the phenomena unfettered by hegemonic relationships. Such a project requires courage and commitment to the process. The question changes from what is nursing? to the investigative, why is nursing? Epistemologies, ontologies and language are all unveiled—what is nursing knowledge, why has it developed the way it has, what does being a nurse mean, how does the language of nursing construct nursing reality? Critical theorists believe that this type of questioning leads to not just enlightenment but also to empowerment and emancipation. Critical thinking is a complex of processes including reflexivity, historical cognition, and a search for meaning. This may result in understanding; it may also result in emancipation; but one should not be tempted to assume that this is always the case. Nursing is at an infantile stage in addressing the challenge of critical review. Small segments have been diligently researched but the synthesis is incomplete. As Sontag (1992) has warned, simplistic and reductive analyses diminish understanding, complexity is equated with clarity, and obfuscation with over-simplification. Complexity is a notion worthy of much more attention and thought; how to transfer this knowing to others, how to analyse the complex without loss, and, in teaching nursing tasks, how to ascertain competence in doing while maintaining the integrity of the whole.

The third dimension of the feminist hermeneutic framework is that of reflexivity. Again there has been a tendency to over-simplify a complex process in much of the nursing literature. Reflection combines analysis, judgement, synthesis and theorising through a dialectical process that includes cognisance of:

- personal constructs
- personal ideological and theoretical biases
- others constructs
- the here and now situation
- the historical and structural forces that informed the social construction of the now situation.

This process allows a micro-social level of analysis as well as exploring the location of self within social systems. This systematised and integrating form of reflection parallels the notion of holism. It rejects the reproduction of social constructions and relationships in favour of a representational theorising.

Interpretation, the fourth dimension of feminist hermeneutics, is the central focus, the outcome of historical, critical, reflective thinking, the conferring of meaning. The discussion earlier in the chapter explained much about this process, however it must be reiterated that interpretative integrity is easily corrupted, particularly at the whim of the intellectual power brokers.

I have previously alluded to the relationship between interpretation, reflection and holism. The unexplored concept of holism has been embraced by nursing; unexplored because of the indeterminate and vague explanations given for such a complex notion. Nurses, in general, have grasped at holism to supposedly guide their practice with little thought for the implications. Holism has been variously described as delusional (Adorno cited in Owen & Holmes 1993), cultural hegemony (Feher 1985), rhetorical flourish (Owen & Holmes 1993) and a conservative philosophy which works within the status quo (Bruni 1989 cited in Owen & Holmes 1993). It has also been suggested that holism should not be thought of as a single concept but referred to as holisms. The common understanding of holism is based on the belief of the unification of interrelated and interdependent parts to form a whole leading to an expectation in nursing that all dimensions of a client be integrated so that care is considered for a 'whole being'. A laudable sentiment, opposing reductionistic practices, but in reality an unattainable myth. Our understanding of ourselves is limited, our potential to fully understand another is impossible. The point of this discussion is that reflection and interpretation can bring us a little closer to this desirable state if they remain contextually grounded.

Conclusion

I have proposed that there are some attractive and useful ideas in the postmodern rhetoric, but that it cannot fulfil the needs of a nursing analytic model; that it has some serious flaws that indicate nursing should move beyond this current immersion. Instead, I have proposed a feminist hermeneutic framework that seeks to utilise the feminist ideologies of inclusivity, justice, freedom from oppressive dominations and open discourse. Hermeneutics in this instance has centred on interpretation. Together, the framework involves the processes of historical, critical, reflective and interpretative analysis and synthesis. Nursing has a unique identity but is vulnerable to those who would mould and dominate it. In this context nursing has many imperatives to deal with, however, it is my belief that nursing discourse, analysis and synthesis must take a high priority. A feminist hermeneutic process can help this to happen. Kappeler (cited Lather 1992) stated:

> I do not really wish to conclude and sum up, rounding off the argument so as to dump it in a nutshell on the reader. A lot more could be said about any of the topics I have touched upon...I have meant to ask the questions, to break the frame...The point is not a set of answers, but making possible a different practice.

It is a fitting conclusion, a challenge to inspire action.

REFERENCES

Anderson G L 1989 Critical ethnography in education: origins, current status, and new directions. Review of Educational Research 59(3):249-270

Bleicher J 1980 Contemporary hermeneutics: hermeneutics as method, philosophy and critique. Routledge & Kegan Paul, London

Bohman J F 1991 Holism without scepticism: contextualism and the limits of interpretation. In: Hiley D R, Bohman J F, Shusterman R (eds) The interpretive turn: philosophy, science, culture. Cornell University Press, New York

Borgmann A 1992 Crossing the postmodern divide. The University of Chicago Press, Chicago

Brown W 1991 Feminist hesitations, postmodern exposure. Differences: A Journal of Feminist Cultural Studies 3(1):63-84

Caputo J 1987 Radical hermeneutics: repetition, deconstruction and the hermeneutic project. University of Indiana Press, Bloomington

Connor S 1989 Postmodernist culture: an introduction to theories of the contemporary. Blackwell, Oxford

Crook S, Pakulski J, Waters M 1992 Postmodernization change in advanced society. Sage Publications, London

Dreyfus H L 1987 Beyond hermeneutics: interpretation in late Heidegger and recent Foucault. In: Gibbons M T (ed) Interpreting politics. Basic Blackwell, Oxford

Dreyfus, H L 1991 Heidegger's hermeneutic realism. In: Hiley D R, Bohman J F, Shusterman R (eds) The interpretive turn: philosophy, science, culture. Cornwell University Press, New York

Feher F 1985 Grandeur and decline of a holistic philosophy. Theory and society 14(6):883-878

Hekman S J 1990 Gender and knowledge: elements of a postmodern feminism. Polity Press, Cambridge

Hiley D R, Bohman J F, Shusterman R 1991 The interpretative turn: philosophy, science, culture. Cornell University Press, New York

Inde D 1971 Hermeneutic phenomenology: the philosophy of Paul Ricoeur. Northwestern University Press, Evanston

Lather P 1992 Critical frames in educational research: feminist and post-structural perspectives. Qualitative Issues in Educational Research 31(2):87-99

Lincoln Y S, Guba E G 1985 Naturalistic inquiry. Sage Publications, Newbury Park

McGregor A 1994 Thiering strikes again. The Australian Magazine 22 Jan:28-31

Mueller-Vollmer B (ed) 1988 The hermeneutics reader. Continuum Publishing Company, New York

Owen M J, Holmes C A 1993 Holism in the discourse of nursing. Journal of Advanced Nursing 18:1688-1695

Ricouer P 1970 Freud and philosophy: an essay on interpretation. Yale University Press, New Haven

Skinner Q (ed) 1990 The return of grand theory in the human sciences. Cambridge University Press, Cambridge

Smart B 1993 Post modernity. Routledge, London

Sontag S 1992 A Susan Sontag reader. Penguin Books, London

Thompson J 1990 Hermeneutic inquiry. In: Moody L E (ed) Advancing nursing science through research, vol. 2. Sage, Newbury Park

22

Nursing: a rhythm of human awakening

ELIZABETH DAVIES, SANDRA LYNCH

Introduction

In Bryce Courtenay's *The Power of One* Professor Von Vollensteen teaches the six year old Peekay:

> Everything fits...Nothing is unexplained. Nature is a chain reaction. One thing follows the other, every thing is dependent on something else. The smallest is as important as the largest...always in life an idea starts small, it is only a sapling idea, but the vines will come and they will try to choke your idea so it cannot grow and it will die and you will never know you had a big idea...the vines are people who are afraid of originality, of new things...always listen to yourself...It is better to be wrong than simply follow convention. If you are wrong...you have learned something and you will grow stronger...If you are right you have taken another step towards a fulfilling life (1992).

What does Von Vollensteen's insight tell us about 'being in the world'? These words speak explicitly of the importance of intuition, of believing in yourself and learning by your mistakes, but they imply more. Von Vollensteen suggests that to reach one's full potential, to become the possible human, one will be faced with the prospect of conflict which will require negotiation with others before a new state of being is achieved. In order for nursing to reach a new state of being as a discipline the same difficulties will be faced. The 'possible future of nursing' and its relationship to the 'possible human' will be explored in this chapter by a heuristic pathway using the notion of transformation.

Nursing research and scholarship construct the meaning of nursing. Currently such work is contributing to the reconceptualisation of a number of critical concepts, namely, caring, the nature of humankind and the education of nurses.

This process of reconceptualisation, apart from having obvious implications for the future of nursing and its scholarship, has ramifications for society.

Houston advises that 'the Rhythm that is coming brings the search for the possible human in ways that it has never been sought before' (1982). Nursing has the potential to be a 'rhythm of human awakening' that will assist with the recovery of the future by acting as a midwife to a fresh vision of reality, to the birth of a new mode of consciousness that will bring forth new ways of knowing, doing and being. Nursing's search for meaning has the potential to make an endowment to the reconstruction of a caring society by augmenting a new life-offering world view.

Use of the word 'recovery' implies that the future can no longer be assumed but must be achieved (Slaughter 1988). In light of such an assumption it becomes imperative that we 'enrich our understanding and ability to act now in the present...To begin to move out of our unconscious immersion in a limited here and now to a wider extended present' (Slaughter 1988). The intention 'here and now', is to extend our understanding of nursing in light of its reconceptualisation by nurse scholars.

The transformative cycle

In order to gain an understanding of the reconceptualisation process that is occurring in nursing and to assess the consequences of such a process, it is helpful to 'operationalise the notion of an extended present by looking at recurring stages that arise again and again in many contexts' (Slaughter 1988). In order to gain such insight Slaughter offers the transformative or T-cycle (see Fig. 22.1) as a device for illustrating continuity and change. The T-cycle uses a dynamic approach which can be divided into four main stages.

The initial stage, 'breakdown of meaning' makes reference to 'understandings, concepts, values and agreements which once served to support social interaction but which now, for one reason or another, have become problematic' (Slaughter 1988). In other words, what once was taken for granted, what constituted 'common sense' seems to dissipate.

The introduction of new ideas that challenge those that already exist are part of the process of 'reconceptualisation', the second stage of the T-cycle. The consequences of such challenges are many Slaughter argues, and '...it is characteristic of new ideas that they almost invariably challenge existing structures...and the interests embedded within them. Hence very many...fail to make any impact [and]...all new ideas...if they represent a significant departure from existing social perception or social practice encounter disinterest or resistance'.

If ideas are pursued with passion, then the third stage of the T-cycle namely 'conflict and negotiations' is inevitable. Not all conflicts will lead to negotiation and sometimes the two can occur simultaneously. Conflict is inevitable when an established structure (and the interests supported by it) 'perceives a threat to its continued existence and mobilises resources to defend itself and repel the threat' (Slaughter 1988). For a conflict to reach the negotiation stage the conflicting interests must be prepared to listen to each other, which implies some degree of equivalence between the opposing groups. As a result of the negotiation process, conflicts can be resolved and new resolutions can emerge.

The fourth and last stage involves 'selective legitimation' of those proposals that have been the focus of negotiation, although not all such proposals, not even the 'best' proposals, will be implemented. Furthermore, notes Slaughter: 'The public realm is itself one of the mainstays of the old order which has suffered under the onslaught of modernism. So it may well be that the process of selective legitimation directly serves particular interests and validates meaning which work against the majority' (1988).

The recovery of the future involves change. Interactions with other human beings are integral to nursing. By the nature of such interactions nurses understand change, because these interactions embrace not only the present but the past and the future, and clearly reflect the transient nature of the here and now. Each authentic human experience brings about change, even transmutation (Slaughter 1988). Birch (1993) suggests that such change is in fact creative transformation, through which each discovers a special sense of reality that makes us subject, not object, and gives us '...a new feeling of possession and participation in the world'.

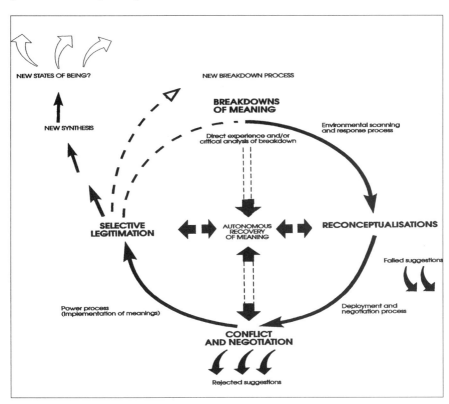

Fig. 22.1 The transformative cycle. Reproduced with permission from Slaughter (1988)

Shifting paradigms

Evidence of transformation or change is manifested in the currently accepted frameworks for nursing knowledge, practice and research. Such 'frameworks of thought' (Ferguson 1980) often form patterns that emerge from the knowledge of a discipline. Thomas Kuhn (1962) in his seminal discourse *The Structure of Scientific Revolutions,* named these patterns 'paradigms'. A scientific paradigm according to Kuhn, is that framework shared by a scientific community, within which science is pursued as it seeks to define problems and solutions and includes concepts, values and techniques (Capra et al 1992). The term has been widely adopted across diverse disciplines, and the term 'world view' is not uncommonly used as a synonym (Fawcett 1993).

Kuhn, says Ferguson (1980) 'by naming a sharply recognisable phenomenon', and describing paradigm shifts in science, has given us considerable insight into how change or transformation occurs in the development of knowledge in any discipline, and the nature of the resistance that is inherent when old ways of thinking are replaced by new ways of addressing the old problems of a discipline. The frameworks and theories of nursing are 'works in process' (Smith 1992a) and are therefore evolving. Embedded in nursing knowledge are paradigmatic perspectives about the nature of human beings, the nature of human interaction with the universe and the nature of health, amongst other variables (Parse 1992a).

Kuhn's definition has been extended to include the notion of society also having a paradigm. Capra (Capra et al 1992) defines a social paradigm as 'a constellation of concepts, values, perceptions, and practices shared by a community that forms a particular vision of reality that is based on the way the community organises itself'. Caring has been described 'as a new paradigm for nursing' (Gaut 1993). Capra's definition of a social paradigm could be applied to the caring paradigm in the context of nursing.

According to Slaughter (1989) the world view of industrial society based on the legacy of Newton and Descartes places value on 'certainty, predictability, control and instrumental rationality'. Capra has said that 'we are in a situation in society where the social paradigm has reached its limits...severe problems can no longer be solved in the old paradigm' (Capra et al 1992). Houston summarises society's dilemma succinctly:

> The 'single vision and Newton's sleep' dominating Western consciousness since the eighteenth century has brought with it the ideal of mind modelled on mechanism, resulting in turn in the materialisation of values, the standardisation of society through industrialisation, and the inability to consider anything other than cause-and-effect relationships as underlying events. In the interest of an extraordinarily narrow notion of 'progress', culture is disintegrating, computers are replacing consciousness, and the erosion of human reality is being enacted and mirrored on the stage of nature in the erosion of the planetary ecosystem (1982).

Slaughter (1989) endorses this conclusion stating that society has experienced erosion of many core values and beliefs with a resultant loss of meaning and associated fragmentation and breakdown of societal norms.

It is in the light of these shifting paradigms that nursing is attempting to recreate its meanings. In a recent analysis of four stated sets of world views from the nursing literature, Fawcett (1993) identified the paradigm shifts in nursing and named the emergent paradigm 'The simultaneous action worldview'. This paradigm, which is a synthesis of the work of Parse, Rogers and Newman, offers the following perspective:

- Unitary human beings are identified by patterns
- Human beings are in mutual rhythmical interchange with their environments
- Human beings change continuously, evolving as self-organised fields
- Change is unidirectional and unpredictable as human beings move through stages of organisation and disorganisation to more complex organisation
- Phenomena of interest are personal becoming and pattern recognition.

As the profession struggles to regain its meanings and to reconceptualise its domain and its practice it must, of necessity, also reconceptualise its body of knowledge. A critical aspect of this reconceptualisation involves an examination of the ways in which that knowledge is transmitted. This examination is vital because of the very real danger that exists in attempting to transmit knowledge in ways which are incongruent with the nature of that knowledge. Another critical reason for such an examination is vested in the obvious contention that any state of knowing lasts for a very short space of time. Just as nursing itself is destined to be continually reconceptualised, so too is the 'scholarly socialisation of its members' (Meleis 1991). Just as nursing absorbs nurses and humans into a web of interaction, so too education absorbs faculty and students. It is within the educative arena that the modelling for future caring encounters begins and the value of lifelong learning is inculcated. It is within this arena also that the process of becoming nurse through nurse becoming is begun.

Recreating meaning in nursing

If we accept that beliefs about caring, humankind, and the education of nurses underpin nursing, then the current challenge is to recognise the breakdowns of meaning that have occurred and to recapture the meaning of these concepts and their interrelationships through reconceptualisation within nursing's emergent world view.

Caring

Mayeroff's (1971) discourse *On Caring* accents the interdependence of caring and being 'in place' in the world. Grounded in the old paradigm, the nature of reality for Western society does not imply stability, because it is not centred in caring and there is no sense of belonging for much of human kind; 'He is nowhere'.

Nursing represents a contradictory metaphor in that Western society, while refusing to value caring (Colliere 1986, Reverby 1987) demands that the nursing profession does so. It demands not only that nurses care, but that they do so within health systems which, because of rigid policies and protocols, are unable to value individuality or cultural differences (Reverby 1987).

Nursing's predicament has been exacerbated by the notion argued by Colliere that:

> The development of an ideology of care based upon dedication to the poor and salvation of the soul took the place of a fundamental knowledge of body care practices. This paved the way during the nineteenth century for the increased value of cure and consideration of care as menial work, worthless, requiring no ability, no knowledge, and therefore socially and economically unrecognised (1986).

The reality of nursing as a discipline is 'practice', which absorbs nurses into a web of interaction with human beings within a context of health and illness. Nursing practice has been likened to a tapestry that is woven of 'taken-for-granted ways of being in the world as nurses' (Arndt 1992). As the nature of nursing has been exposed by nurse scholars the meaning of the brilliant colour and the intricate texture of the tapestry of nursing practice has been illuminated.

From the collective of nursing knowledge, caring has emerged for many as the concept that connects nurses to the health and illness matters of other human beings. The use of the participle 'caring', with the 'ing' ending, makes explicit a dynamic process orientation (Parse 1992a) and, by the nature of this vitality, caring has the capacity to be the warp of the tapestry of practice. Such a notion makes caring 'everydayness' (Arndt 1992), as caring practices are bound in the lived experience of being a nurse, and suggests that caring may be the essence of nursing and therefore a reflection of nurses' being, doing and knowing.

Currently any attempt to analyse the nursing literature on caring is bound to give rise to considerable bewilderment. Such confusion arises, in essence, from the immense diversity in definitions and conceptualisations of caring. Scholarship has done little to expose the intimate nature of caring and has simply identified its elusiveness as a concept (Morse et al 1990).

There is a further complication in that 'the human lives at multidimensional realms of the universe all at once, freely choosing ways of becoming as meaning is given in situations. The possibles are the cherished hopes and dreams that a person is incarnating with his or her life' (Parse 1992a). Thus each person will make meaning of the concept of caring within the spectrum of their own reality and such a construct further magnifies the pluri-dimensional complexity of caring.

While calls for 'theoretical preciseness, clarity and parsimony, especially when describing such complex concepts as care and caring' (Morse et al 1991) are well meaning, they belie the notion that what may be critical is not the production of a unifying definition, but the process of reconceptualising caring; 'You shall know the truth and the truth shall make you you' (Brunner cited in Ferguson 1980).

In order to reveal some of the dimensions of the caring phenomenon, some ontological, anthropological and ontical perspectives of caring are presented in Figures 22.2, 22.3 and 22.4. These perspectives are taken from a recent systematic analysis of major theoretical works related to nursing, carried out by Boykin and Schoenhofer (1990). The framework for this analysis utilised five categories of questions proposed by Roach (1987 cited in Boykin and Schoenhofer 1990). The three categories identified in Figures 22.2, 22.3, and 22.4 allowed the extant theory to be analysed and integrated. Two other categories which will not be discussed further were epistemological and pedagogical dimensions which allow the substantive knowledge about caring in nursing to be organised for the purpose of teaching and learning (Boykin & Schoenhofer 1990).

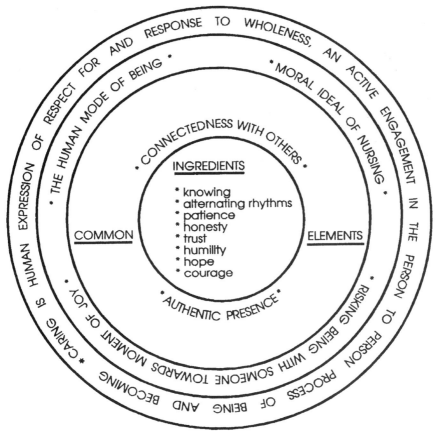

Fig. 22.2 The revelation of an ontological analysis of extant theory about caring in nursing. Source: Boykin and Schoenhofer (1990)

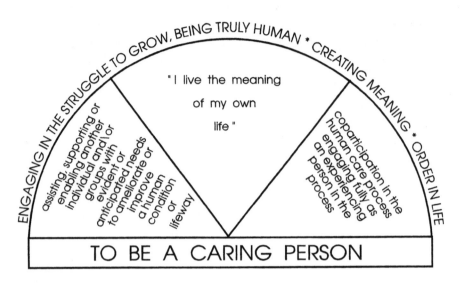

Fig. 22.3 The revelation of an anthropological analysis of extant theory about caring in nursing. Source: Boykin and Schoenhofer (1990)

Given that Roach views caring as an intrinsic human expression, the ontological questions of the analysis focus on the 'being' of caring, and Figure 22.2 presents this perspective. Figure 22.3 represents the dimensions of caring revealed by questions of an anthropological nature which asked, 'what does it mean to be a caring person?' (Boykin & Schoenhofer 1990). Some overlap with the ontological dimensions are manifest. The ontological nature of caring relates to the function and ethic of caring. Their interrelationship becomes obvious when one asks, 'what is a nurse doing when he or she is caring?' and 'what obligations are entailed in caring?' (Boykin & Schoenhofer 1990). The dimensions revealed by these questions are outlined in Figure 22.4.

Critical analysis of the philosophic claims of caring theory in nursing reveals something of the values and beliefs of nursing. Such values and beliefs guide the development of nursing knowledge (Fawcett 1993), and offer a scheme for understanding and explaining the reality of nursing.

The concept of creative transformation can extend even further the relationship of care to the practice of nursing, beyond the pervasive view. Parse states that nursing practice '...is a subject-to-subject interrelationship, a true loving presence with the other to enhance the quality of life' (1987 cited in Parse 1992a). Caring should not be the exclusive domain of nurses, humanity needs to regain the attributes of caring. Rogers notes that 'every one needs to care; the nature of caring in a given field depends entirely on the body of scientific knowledge specific to the field. Caring is simply a way of using knowledge' (1992). The reconceptualisation of caring by nurse scholars gives nurses the opportunity to use the knowledge they gain to enhance practice.

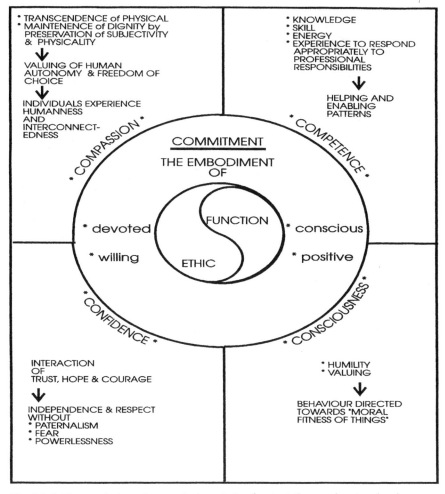

Fig. 22.4 The revelation of an ontical analysis of extant theory about caring in nursing. Source: Boykin and Schoenhofer (1990)

Houston contends that '...breakdown is always the signal for breakthrough. After the harvest during winter's parentheses of life, the sere and decaying stalks of the previous year's vegetation collapse to supply nutrients for the spring breakthrough of the reseeded earth' (1982). So too with the re-conceptualisation of caring. By identifying the 'everydayness' of caring practices and creating powerful images of caring, the image becomes 'selectively empowered' and behaviour possibilities are generated as the concept explodes into a realised future (Boulding cited in Slaughter 1988) not just for nursing but as a rhythm of awakening for society.

The nature of humankind

A recent analysis of four nursing frameworks serves as a vehicle to explore some of the meanings that are held in relation to human beings, and their ways of being in the world. Mitchell and Cody (1992) analysed the works of Paterson and Zderad (humanistic nursing), Newman (model of expanding consciousness), Watson (human science and human care) and Parse (theory of human becoming). They identified inconsistencies in the frameworks of the first three and suggested that Parse's 'theory of human becoming' could eliminate these inconsistencies.

Unarguably there is a common nursing value that focuses on the wholeness of human beings. However, analysis of recently emerging theories reveals that conceptualisations of the person do not always support this notion of wholeness. Instead they may focus on discrete parts (Paterson & Zderad); physiological, psychological and emotional processes (Newman); and body, mind, spirit and soul (Watson). These approaches could be seen to be inconsistent with the concepts of totality and connectedness that feature in the emergent nursing paradigm.

Similarly, the paradigm position that human beings are intentional and inherently free willed is not always incorporated. Paterson and Zderad contend that the nurse should monitor choices made by people to determine if they are responsible ones. Newman believes that people lose freedom which can only be regained by reaching a state of expanded consciousness which is facilitated by the nurse. While Watson describes humans as self-determining and free to choose, she also sees nurses making decisions about interventions and correcting conditions to increase harmony for the person. These conceptualisations suggest that the nurse determines what is best, right, and appropriate. Once again, this is an inconsistency that is not able to be reconciled with the ideal of self-determination.

The meaning of people's 'being in the world' proposed by these theorists is also critiqued. It is concluded that they hold an 'essentially dichotomous view' which separates the person's experience of the world from the world as it actually is. Mitchell and Cody (1992) propose that the work of Parse overcomes inconsistencies in the areas of the nature of human beings, self-determination and being in the world. They suggest that Parse provides new meanings through reconceptualisation. Parse's theory is based on Rogers' (1970) science of unitary human beings. The Rogerian approach is combined with existential phenomenology to present a human science perspective. Such a perspective does provide a real alternative to nurses wishing to practise beyond the natural science-based biomedical modality.

The wholeness of the person, intentionality and free will and the nature of reality are harmonised and inextricably interconnected by Parse's focus on a 'unitary human being's experience of living and creating health'. At all times human beings are referred to as living unities, and there is no attempt to reduce them to parts in order to understand them. Free choice is another tenet in the theory of human becoming. Humans are seen to freely choose meaning in situations and to bear responsibility for those choices. The place of the nurse in the area of intentionality and free will is one of co-participation as the person chooses his or her own way. The nurse does not judge or stereotype the person but is a presence with the person as meaning is created.

394

In relation to the nature of reality, there is no subject-object dichotomy. Instead the person actually co-creates reality through a process of co-constitution with the environment.

Similarly, the concept of health can be shown to have lost some of its meaning. The current, commonly held meaning of health as physical, mental, social and spiritual well being, achieved when body, mind and spirit are in equilibrium, is rooted in the totality paradigm. An examination of the values underlying this approach reveals a separation of body, mind and spirit. As a result, the goal of nursing, which is to promote health, prevent illness and restore health, is achieved through interactions which focus on the bio-psycho-socio-spiritual facets of the person. This is essentially carried out in a context where curing remains the dominant and ultimate objective. As an alternative to this way of understanding health there is an emerging meaning which emphasises the maintenance and restoration of health through caring and healing (Parse 1992a 1992b, Quinn 1992, Rogers 1992, Newman 1989, Watson 1988a, 1988b).

Watson (1988b) suggests that nurses need to undergo a 'radical transformation' in relation to their concept of health. She sees the future as one where nurses have developed a new consciousness of human caring and healing as a result of their challenge to the medical ideology that currently dominates health and healing. This will enable them to develop many new options. Watson forecasts that nurses will be in a position to achieve 'new human possibilities that accommodate transcendence and other metaphysical concepts in relation to health and illness' (1988b). As the changing relationships between cure and care come into focus, nurses will work with people by 'restoring and preserving the human center', not only in the one being cared for but also in the one caring.

Newman (1989) sees that the concern of the nurse has to do with the 'wholeness of life'. The way that nurses will work with people towards health will be through attuning them to a 'higher consciousness'. Nurses will assist people to identify their patterns of interaction with the environment, to isolate areas where blocks to energy flow exist and to search for new possibilities. Disease is presented as an opportunity for people to recognise the pattern of their existence. Dealing with disease enables people to experience the patterns of their lives more fully and is part of the 'ongoing process of expanding consciousness'.

For Rogers (1992) health is a value which enhances humanness in the striving for human betterment. Rogers stresses that in our study of human health we must be part of a 'new worldview compatible with the most progressive knowledge available'. Her own science of unitary human beings proposes that we are in a process of accelerated evolution and that there is a speeding up of human field rhythms co-ordinating with higher frequency environmental patterns. This is likely to be manifested in new norms and wider ranges of individual differences in phenomena such as blood pressure, waking patterns and child behaviour. Ageing is seen, not as a process of decline and running down, but as increasing diversity and complexity. Ideas such as these will, indeed, lead to serious reconceptualisation of the notion of health.

Healing as harmony in the human-environment relationship is a concept of health proposed by Quinn (1992). Re-patterning enables people's consciousness to expand and empowers them to move towards health. This process of healing occurs when there is 'right relationship at, between and among all the levels of human being' (Quinn 1992). Even though no one person can heal another (that must come from within) nurses are able to remove barriers to healing. They are seen as 'midwives' to the process of healing as they create environments that can support healing.

In her theory of human becoming, Parse (1981) describes health as a 'process of becoming, a cocreated process of living value priorities'. Health is manifested in the daily living of rhythmic patterns. The healthy person is able to move on in life in the way that they choose for themselves. It is their very own process of becoming. They participate with the universe in the co-creation of health. They 'live their health incarnating personal values which are each individual's unique connection with the universe' (Parse 1992a).

The reconceptualisations that are emerging in the ways nurses know humankind are coming into sharper focus. Humans are being viewed as intentional beings striving for harmony with their environment and healing within themselves.

Education

Education is about 'the learner within, waiting to be free' (Ferguson 1980); it is about a process that is liberating, enlightening and exciting. Like Michelangelo, educators strive to free the shape from the stone which encloses it so that it can emerge in all its uniqueness and beauty. Already there have been many reforms. Those of particular relevance for nursing have focused on the development of independence in learners, curriculum as a means of social change and the importance of practice as a curriculum focus.

The desire to develop independence in learners has lead to a criticism of curriculum as a means of conveying technical, non-context specific knowledge in professional education (Schön 1983 1987, Bevis 1988, Benner 1984, Benner & Wrubel 1989). Such an approach is seen to place emphasis on issues and to use processes which have very little relevance to day-to-day professional practice. As a result students have little opportunity to deal with a diversity of situations that are complex and context specific. In addition, this approach is unlikely to enable students to develop autonomy, independence and a sense of inquiry.

Instead, curriculum as a means to achieve freedom through dialogue has been proposed. Richardson (1988) suggests that it is time for democratisation of the faculty/student relationship so that they can become partners in the learning process. Similar ideas are expressed by Watson (1988a), Moccia (1988) and Diekelmann (1988) who suggest respectively a shift, a reclamation and a reconciliation in the relationship between faculty and students. A more egalitarian, less hierarchical relationship, based on the sharing of power, is suggested by Hedin and Donovan (1989) as an emancipatory measure for students who could then become members of the collective working towards educational goals. De-emphasising evaluation, power and grading is proposed by Bevis and Krulik (1991) in support of achieving a balance of power. Nelms (1991) shares a vision of faculty and students working in a dialogical relationship in what is termed the educational journey, while Tanner (1990) envisages 'a transaction among students, faculty and the people who are participants in health care'.

Perceptions of faculty as brokers of knowledge are also undergoing change. The notion of faculty as expert learners is supported by Watson (1988a), Hedin and Donovan (1989) and Bevis and Krulik (1991). Faculty as facilitators of learning is a role favoured by Richardson (1988) who sees learning as an unfinished process in which faculty and students interact through dialogue. Along similar lines, Nelms suggests that it is 'time to remove the boundaries between who does the learning and who does the teaching. Students should be helped to accept that they can discover the answers and that they must be responsible for their own learning' (1991).

Student expectations in relation to faculty and knowledge also provide some insights. In the general sense Belenky et al (1986) found that women as learners 'wished to be treated as containers of knowledge rather than empty receptacles'. The kind of teacher they wanted was the 'midwife teacher' who could 'assist the students in giving birth to their own ideas, in making their own knowledge explicit and elaborating it'. Studies specific to expectations of nursing students found that the students expected faculty to be knowledgeable and willing to share knowledge and experiences (Brown 1981, Windsor 1987, Howie 1988).

How faculty implement their role, their doing, in relation to their interactions with students has also received attention. At the practical level, it is suggested that faculty should encourage inquiry and problem solving (Richardson 1988, Bevis & Krulik 1991); promote active learning through attending to processes and allowing for diversity (Hedin & Donovan 1989); engage in critical dialogue with students (Bevis & Krulik 1991, Hedin & Donovan 1989); and establish a balance between challenge and support (Valiga 1988).

Another reform movement has focused on curriculum as a vehicle for social change rather than as a system for 'reproducing an obsolete past' (Slaughter 1989). This view is supported by Habermas (1971) who resists the over extension of technical processes into areas where other factors such as power and ideology should be considered. This idea of social responsibility is most evident in his contention that education be directed towards emancipation and liberation through the critique of mystification, domination and repression. In analysing the major thrusts of the curriculum revolution in nursing, Tanner (1990) designates social responsibility as the primary theme. Such a position could be interpreted as evidence of the place of education in preparing individuals to engage in 'the process of cultural reconstruction and renewal' (Slaughter 1989). Similarly, Gough (1989) suggests that it is time to take an eco-political approach to curriculum (grounded in Aristotelian philosophy) to allow for a '...re-emergence of a deeper continuity in our culture'.

Munhall (1988) emphasises the ethic of care in curriculum and proposes that curricula need to protest unsafe and inhuman patient conditions as well as those factors which demean the status of nurses. She envisages this will occur through higher professional self-esteem leading to social consciousness and, ultimately, to action. Moccia (1990) clearly designates the need for curriculum in nursing education to transform existing power relationships from dominance to liberation. Tanner (1990) also pleads for egalitarian, co-operative communities with the abilities to critique and transform the health care system.

It is also evident, in emergent ideas relevant to alternative pedagogies, that practice should become a major focus for curriculum (Schon 1983 1987, Benner 1984, Bevis 1988). From a nursing perspective this idea is encapsulated by Deikelmann (1988) who stresses that 'caring as an ontological state is fundamental to the curriculum'. Speedy (1989) identifies context specifically as one of particular relevance to nursing and urges nurses to perceive the people they deal with 'from their viewpoints within their particular contexts'. The development of creative, context-responsive practitioners is seen by Bevis & Clayton (1988) to be the major objective of programs of nurse education. Bevis (1988) contends that practice as a source of learning is critical for neophytes to discover the character, uniqueness, values, aesthetics and general philosophy of their profession.

Maclean (1989) suggests that curriculum should allow learners the opportunity to develop frameworks grounded in experience. Gough (1989) sees a future wherein education, built on understandings of reality, nature and human nature will provide the impetus for learners to 'search their environments' to learn. Doll (1989) expounds that learners need exposure to systems that feed on the flow of matter and energy from the environment. This triggers a state of non-balance within the learner who must re-organise concepts to regain balance. In this fashion growth and development occur.

Practice is also an invaluable source of meaning and understandings derived from practice can lead learners to the acceptance of multiple realities, and to the realisation of their own potential (Maclean 1989). Similarly, Slaughter (1989) stresses the importance of meaning which, he suggests, '...is derived from an active process of involvement and participation'. Benner and Wrubel (1989) have declared that it is time for theory development to focus not on the 'imagined ideal' but on 'actual expert nursing as it is practised day to day'.

But are these reforms sufficient to move education from the narrow, oppressive, content focused, rigid, compartmentalised endeavour that it has become? Ferguson suggests that what we have been doing in education has been founded on 'mending' rather than 'metamorphosis': '...we have been trying to attach wings to a caterpillar. Our interventions in the learning process to date have been almost that crude. It is high time we freed ourselves of attachment to old forms and eased the flight of the unfettered human mind' (1980). She is of the opinion that we have surrendered to custom and authority and lost our way and our meaning in an increasingly technological and depersonalised world. She believes that we have deteriorated to the extent that we are 'swimming in knowledge we have not claimed'. As we struggle for a 'second chance at meaning', we may be able to reconcile mind and heart, fuse intellect and emotion and achieve 'simultaneous and equal co-operation of logical and intuitive thinking' (Ferguson 1980).

It is Ferguson's contention that, as a society, we aspire towards reclamation of knowledge and meaning through the personal transformation of individuals. While this process of transformation is open to all, as yet very few have experienced it. Perhaps the raison d'etre of education is to make it possible for people to begin their own personal transformation so that each one may achieve full potential. The origin of the word 'educate' is from the Latin, 'ex', out of, and 'ducere', to lead; to lead out of. It may be that what we really need to do as educators is to lead into, i.e. into the self, so that, through the inner journey, the self can achieve transformation.

Butler (1992) also argues for this inner transformation, this process of personal becoming as the means to the fulfilment of human potential. He is critical of entrenched educative practices in professional education and refers to the 'common illusion...that knowledge can produce change'. Rather than basing educational experiences on the premise that thought leads to action, Butler suggests that a reversal is required. As educators of professionals for the future we need to appreciate that meaning is derived from within the person through an active process of involvement and participation—a situation where there can be a two-way relationship between action and thought.

Munhall (1993) takes a similar approach in the contention that 'unknowing' is 'critical to the evolution and development of knowledge'. By taking possession of what they do not know about clients, situations and contexts, and by being prepared to engage in authentic encounters with them, nurses open themselves to an understanding of the client's perspective and subjectivity. This understanding is able to emerge as the nurse engages in a process of de-centring which leads to being 'authentically present for the patient'.

It is Butler's (1992) belief that professional practice is grounded in a person's world view and their personal practical knowledge. Their practice, therefore, conforms to an 'inner agenda' emanating from the personal, from values, beliefs, assumptions. Even though there is a lack of trust in the knowledge gained by personal experience, such knowledge Butler contends, is a form of rationality. This is supported by the utility of personal knowledge in comprehending the social world, by its constructivist mode of operation and by positioning truth in the present and immediate context. This view is supported by Smith (1992b) who asks nurses to consider the question 'Is all knowing personal knowing?' She suggests that self knowledge makes knowing others in significant ways a possibility.

If the purpose of professional education is to change individuals from lay persons to knowledgable, competent practitioners, how can this be achieved? Butler (1992) proposes that it can happen by inviting each individual to engage in a process of self-exploration and self-discovery. It is not possible to impose or facilitate change, it must come from within as a result of the self interacting with the external environment. This is outlined in the model of human action illustrated in Figure 22.5. This model provides the basis for a 'reflective dialogue' that can enhance the self and enrich professional practice. Public knowledge represents givens such as theories, formal knowledge, policies and mores. Professional practice refers to the choices regarding what is to be done in particular situations. The world view represents the values and rules that govern the actions of the person at that particular point in time. Personal practical knowledge is all that the person has come to know and understand through their being in the world.

The application of this model can be operationalised through a process of action learning. This process situates the teacher in relationship with learners as they 'collect data on the outcomes of the actions and... understand, interpret and evaluate the data within the requirements of the context' (Butler 1992). Consequently, 'the choice of what to do in a particular situation is the beginning rather than the end of thinking, justification, learning and reflection' (Butler 1992). The teaching role becomes one of 'helping development' as the practitioners of the future become ready to continue as 'creators of our practice'.

Slaughter (1989) situates these ideas of personal transformation in the broader context. He suggests that 'fractures and dislocations in our ways of understanding' can result from the 'stale conventionalisation' of educational processes. He urges educators to make shifts in curriculum theory and practice which will provide opportunities for learners to derive meaning from active involvement and participation. This, he envisages, will enable them to move beyond the 'cultural editing' that is present in Western societies so that they can see wider patterns, broaden spans of time and space and reach higher levels of awareness. To assist learners to develop in these ways educators can provide access 'through clarity of insight, through deepened perceptions, creativity and certain forms of spiritual practice' (Slaughter 1989). It is in this way that we can 'refine the instrument of knowing' and set our beginners on a 'journey which leads up and out of the abyss towards new stages of personal and cultural development' (Slaughter 1989). The reconceptualisations that are emerging in relation to education do seem to be pointing towards a metamorphosis. The strong theme of personal transformation casts education as 'a discipline in transcendence, body to mind to soul' (Wilber 1983 cited in Slaughter 1989).

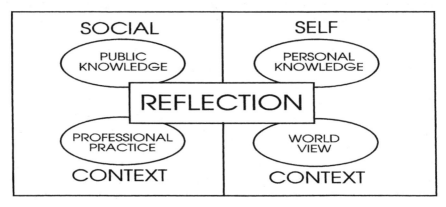

Fig. 22.5 The components of the model of human action. Reproduced with permission from Butler (1992)

Creative transformation for the future

The recreation of meanings in nursing that have been explored are beginning to impact on our way of 'being in the world'. Nursing is undergoing a cultural reconstruction. This in turn exerts influence on the domain and nature of nursing practice and the development of the discipline through enquiry and the preparation of neophytes for nursing practice. In short, nursing itself is undergoing transformation. This, Ferguson (1980) explains, is a process comprising entry, exploration, integration and conspiracy.

The entry point can usually only be identified in retrospect and is often associated with some event or circumstance that 'shakes up the old understanding of the world' (Ferguson 1980). It gives a hint of a more meaningful dimension imbued with brightness, diversity, richness and complexity way beyond previous experiences and imaginings. It provides a glimpse of possibilities free of repression, hesitation, isolation and fear of the self. In short, it opens up to other ways of knowing.

To be able to progress to the next stage, exploration, a deliberate decision to go on must be made. That decision means being prepared to let go, to let inner knowledge come forward. In this process the quest is the transformation, the 'letting' is the intentional release of 'psychic spasm' that must be quiet before change can occur. Through exploration it is possible to discover that there are systems to bring about the other ways of knowing.

The third stage, integration, marks an end to the dissonance between the old and the new and results in the emergence of a new self—a self which finds itself emerged into an old culture—a self which may need to reinterpret old values, relationships and aspirations. At this stage there is experimentation with ideas, testing and refining, sharpening and expanding thinking through reflection. There is the discovery that, in addition to other ways of knowing, there are other ways of being in the world.

The final stage, conspiracy, leads to the discovery of 'other sources of power, and ways to use it for fulfilment and in service to others' (Ferguson 1980). The discovery that the mind can heal and transform is realised. Transformation has occurred. Among the treasures discovered through the transformative process is the body-mind connection, a sense of vocation and responsibility for giving back and freedom.

It is inevitable that such a transformation will lead to conflict. It represents a direct challenge to established and legitimised ways of knowing, systems to bring about that knowing, ways of being in the world and sources of power. However, Ferguson (1980) reminds us that 'dissolution and pain are necessary stages in renewal'. It brings with it a freedom that implies release from the tyranny of culture and habit, restoration of autonomy, and the space to communicate, to change and to create. If these are our aspirations for the nurses of the future, we must seriously begin to search for ways to achieve them. It is suggested that the search begins within and that it is integral to the transformative journey of each one of us. It is in this way that, collectively, we will ensure the survival and flourishing of our discipline.

REFERENCES

Arndt M 1992 Caring as everydayness. Journal of Holistic Nursing 10(4):285-293

Belenky M, Clinchy B, Goldberger N, Tarule J 1986 Women's ways of knowing. Basic Books, New York

Benner P 1984 From novice to expert: excellence and power in clinical nursing practice. Addison-Wesley, Menlo Park

Benner P, Wrubel J 1989 The primacy of caring: stress and coping in health and illness. Addison-Wesley, Menlo Park

Bevis E 1988 New directions for a new age. In: Curriculum revolution: mandate for change. National League for Nursing, New York

Bevis E, Clayton G 1988 Needed: a new curriculum development design. Nurse Education 24(7):301-303

Bevis E, Krulik T 1991 Nationwide faculty development: a model for a shift from diploma to baccalaureate education. Journal of Advanced Nursing 3 (16):362-370

Birch C 1993 Regaining compassion for humanity and nature. NSW University Press, Kensington

Boykin A, Schoenhofer S 1990 Caring in nursing. Nursing Science Quarterly 3(4):149-155

Brown S 1981 Faculty and student perceptions of effective clinical teachers. Journal of Nursing Education 20(9):4-15

Butler J 1992 From action to thought: the fulfilment of human potential. Paper presented at the Fifth International Thinking Conference, Townsville

Capra F, Steindl-Rast D, Matus T 1992 Belonging to the universe. Penguin, London

Colliere M 1986 Invisible care and invisible women as health care-providers. International Journal of Nursing Studies 23(2):95-112

Courtenay B 1992 The power of one. Mandarin, Melbourne

Diekelmann N 1988 Curriculum revolution: a theoretical and philosophical mandate for change. In: Curriculum revolution: mandate for change. National League for Nursing, New York

Doll W 1989 Foundations for a post-modern curriculum. Journal of Curriculum Studies 21(3):243-253

Fawcett J 1993 From a plethora of paradigms to parsimony in world views. Nursing Science Quarterly 6(2):56-58

Ferguson M 1980 The Aquarian conspiracy: personal and social transformation in the 1980s. Tarcher, Los Angeles

Gaut D 1993 A vision of wholeness for nursing. Journal of Holistic Nursing 11(2):164-171

Gough N 1989 From epistemology to ecopolitics: renewing a paradigm for curriculum. Journal of Curriculum Studies 21(3):225-241

Habermas J 1971 Towards a rational society. Heinemann, London

Hedin B, Donovan J 1989 A feminist perspective on nurse education. Nurse Education 14(4):8-13

Howie J 1988 The effective clinical teacher: a role model. Australian Journal of Advanced Nursing 5(2):23-26

Houston J 1982 The possible human. Tarcher, Los Angeles

Kuhn T 1962 The structure of scientific revolution. University of Chicago Press, Chicago

Maclean H 1989 Linking person-centred teaching to qualitative research training. In: Boud D, Griffin V (eds) Appreciating adults learning: from the learners' perspective. Kogan Page, London

Mayeroff M 1971 On caring. Harper Row, New York

Meleis A 1991 Theoretical nursing: development and progress, 2nd edn. Lippincott, New York

Mitchell G, Cody W 1992 Nursing knowledge and human science: ontological and epistemological considerations. Nursing Science Quarterly 5(2):54-61

Moccia P 1988 Curriculum revolution: an agenda for change. In: Curriculum revolution: mandate for change. National League for Nursing, New York

Moccia P 1990 No sire, it's a revolution. Journal of Nursing Education 29(7):307-311

Morse J, Solberg S, Neander W, Bottorff J, Johnson J 1990 Concepts of caring and caring as a concept. Advanced Nursing Science 13(1):1-14

Morse J, Bottorff J, Neander W, Solberg S 1991 Comparative analysis of conceptualizations and theories of caring. Image: Journal of Nursing Scholarship 23(2):119-126

Munhall P 1988 Curriculum revolution: a social mandate for change. In: Curriculum revolution: mandate for change. National League for Nursing, New York

Munhall P 1993 'Unknowing':toward another pattern of knowing in nursing. Nursing Outlook 41(3):125-128

Nelms T 1991 Has the curriculum revolution revolutionised the definition of curriculum. Journal of Nursing Education 30(1):5-8

Newman M 1989 The spirit of nursing. Holistic Nursing Practice 3(3):1-6

Parse R 1981 Man-living-health: a theory of nursing. Wiley, New York

Parse R 1992a Human becoming: Parse's theory of nursing. Nursing Science Quarterly 5(1):35-42

Parse R 1992b Nursing knowledge for the 21st century: an international commitment. Nursing Science Quarterly 5(1):8-12

Quinn J 1992 Holding sacred space: the nurse as healing environment. Holistic Nursing Practice 6(4):26-36

Reverby S 1987 A caring dilemma: womanhood and nursing in historical perspective. Nursing Research 36(1):5-11

Richardson M 1988 Innovating androgogy in a basic nursing course: an evaluation of the independent study contract with basic nursing students. Nurse Education Today 8(6):315-324

Rogers M 1970 An introduction to the theoretical basis for nursing. Davis, Philadelphia

Rogers M 1992 Nursing science and the space age. Nursing Science Quarterly 5(1):27-34

Schon D 1983 The reflective practitioner: how professionals think in action. Basic Books, New York

Schon D 1987 Educating the reflective practitioner. Josey Bass, San Francisco

Slaughter R 1988 Recovering the future. Monash University Press, Melbourne

Slaughter R 1989 Cultural reconstruction in the post-modern world. Journal of Curriculum Studies 21(3):255-270

Smith M 1992a The distinctiveness of nursing knowledge. Nursing Science Quarterly 5(4):148-149

Smith M 1992b Is all knowing personal knowing. Nursing Science Quarterly 5(1):2-3

Speedy S 1989 Theory practice debate: setting the scene. Australian Journal of Advanced Nursing 6(3):12-20

Tanner C 1990 Caring as a value in nurse education. Nursing Outlook 38(2):70-72

Valiga T 1988 Curriculum outcomes and cognitive development: new perspectives for nursing education. In: Curriculum revolution: mandate for change. National League for Nursing, New York

Watson J 1988a Human caring as a moral context for nursing education. Journal of Nursing and Health Care 9(8):150-154

Watson J 1988b New dimensions of human caring theory. Nursing Science Quarterly 1(4):175-181

Windsor A 1987 Nursing students perceptions of clinical experience. Journal of Nursing Education 26(3):150-154

Index